D0172344

# The
# *Wellness Project*™

## A Rocket Scientist's
## Blueprint for Health

Designed by Nature
Researched by a Rocket Scientist

## Roy Mankovitz, BS, JD, CNC

With a Foreword by
Dr. David Brownstein, MD

Montecito Wellness LLC
Santa Barbara

## Notices

The information contained in this book is based upon the research and personal experience of the author. It is not intended as a substitute for consulting with your physician or other healthcare providers. If you choose to follow any of the ideas in this book, you might want to consider first consulting with your doctor about the appropriateness of these suggestions for your particular situation. Nature, not the author, is responsible for any positive (or adverse) effects or consequences resulting from the use of the suggestions or procedures discussed in this book.

Portions of the material presented in this book are the subject of US and foreign issued patents and pending patent applications. No license is granted to the purchaser or reader of this book or to any other individual or entity to commercially or otherwise exploit or offer to others any of these inventions, some of which are listed in Appendix A of this book. The following are trademarks of the author or publisher, or used under license: The Wellness Project™, The Wellness Diet™, Hypothesis for Health™, A Rocket Scientist's Blueprint for Health™, The Dirt Diet™, Officizer™, CellFrame™, Clayodine™, HealthBra™, ABC Food Test™, The Dirt Detox Protocol™, The Mercury-Yeast Spectrum Disorder™, and Whispers of Wisdom®.

Copyright © 2008 Roy J. Mankovitz

All rights reserved. No part of this publication may be reproduced, stored in a retrieval system, or transmitted in any form or by any means including electronic, mechanical, photocopying, recording, or otherwise, without the prior written permission of the publisher.

Published by:

Montecito Wellness LLC
1482 East Valley Road, Suite 808
Santa Barbara, CA 93108

info@montecitowellness.com
www.montecitowellness.com

ISBN: 978-0-9801584-5-8

## Dedication

To my mother Sarah for giving me life, to my wife Kathleen, my children Jill, Alan, Miriam, and Andrea, my grandchildren Alexa and Jordyn, and my sister Toby for their patience and support, and to my father Benjamin and my uncle Solomon, both of whom had their lives cut short as a result of medical errors.

## Acknowledgements

In the field of medicine, I wish to acknowledge Dr. Orion Truss, Dr. John Trowbridge, Dr. Broda Barnes, Dr. William Jefferies, Dr. Laszlo Belenyessy, Dr. Hans Gruenn and his wife Annika, Dr. Deitrich Klinghardt, Dr. Michael Gershon, Dr. Guy Abraham, Dr. David Brownstein, Dr. Jorge Flechas, Dr. Paul Dantzig, Dr. Mildred Seelig, Dr. C. Norman Shealy, and Dr. Lawrence Wilson for their courage in pursuing alternative approaches to research and healing. In the field of dentistry, I wish to acknowledge Dr. Weston A. Price, Dr. George Meinig, Dr. Hal Huggins, Dr. David Villarreal, and Leo Cashman for their courage in pursuing alternative approaches to treatment. In the field of anthropology, I wish to acknowledge Vilhjalmur Stefansson, Jared Diamond, and Cindy Engel for their pioneering studies, which opened many windows into our past. In the field of cellular biology, I wish to acknowledge Dr. Leslie Wilson and Dr. George Ayoub of the University of California at Santa Barbara for their research skills and support. In the field of emotional detoxification, I would like to acknowledge Bert Hellinger, JoAnna Chartrand, and Dyrian Benz for their work in healing the psyche. Last but not least, I wish to acknowledge the support of John Posa, Esq., and Dr. Julie Staple, Esq.

# Contents

# Foreword

By Dr. David Brownstein, MD

Once in a while, you read a book that strikes you as a needed addition to your library. The Wellness Project by Roy Mankovitz is one such book. This book should be required reading by all who are interested in safe and effective natural therapies.

Modern medicine is a mess. In the United States, we spend over 16% of our gross national product on health care. We spend more than any other country on the face of the earth. Do we have better health care because of this? No. The United States ranks near the bottom in almost every health indicator as compared to other Western countries. Why would that be?

Conventional medicine has been corrupted by Big Pharma. For every diagnosis, there is a drug that can be prescribed to treat that diagnosis. Unfortunately, nearly all commonly prescribed drugs do not treat the underlying cause of the illness. The drugs merely treat the symptoms of the illness. The long-term use of most drug therapies is detrimental to the patient.

We cannot go on spending the amount of money we are spending on health care. We cannot afford it and we are not getting value for our money as it is currently spent. There needs to be another way.

Roy Mankovitz is offering a different approach. He describes his own illness, how he searched for help in the conventional medical model and was not satisfied with the answers or the medical care he was receiving. Roy took things into his own hands, formed his own hypothesis, and experimented on himself to find the answers that would help his condition.

He found that he was suffering from a yeast problem known as Candida. He found out that he had many food allergies and was suffering from heavy metal toxicity. He also had an adverse effect to a childhood vaccination, DPT. Roy embarked on a program to clean up his diet and take the right supplements necessary to supply his body with the nutrients needed to heal his system. Finally, Roy discovered the power of detoxification. This book describes his thought processes and how he implemented a holistic plan to heal himself.

But this book is not only about Roy's health condition. He provides the reader with a wealth of knowledge about a wide variety of holistic principals. He describes how the conventional model is failing those with chronic illness. In particular, he writes in great detail about diet.

There is no question that the standard American diet is making us ill. It lacks basic nutrients and contains a host of toxic chemicals that cause illness. I spend every day in my office trying to educate my patients on the importance of eating a healthy diet. Roy makes it clear that we have to eat a diet that properly supports out body. Eating a diet that our ancient ancestors ate, free of chemicals, provides our body with the proper nutrients that it needs to optimally function. Roy recommends a diet that contains (free-range) animal protein, non-bitter fruit, mineral rich water, and soil. It was fascinating to read about ancient man's diet and how Roy adapted this diet to our present time. I learned a lot from this section.

A significant part of the book deals with detoxification. My clinical experience has clearly shown that living in a polluted society has consequences. The consequences of these toxicities include a poorly functioning immune system and the onset of illness. Roy devotes a great deal of his book to describing the various toxic items we are exposed to and what they are doing in the body.

Roy describes, in detail, various methods of helping the body detoxify from these toxic chemicals. I have used many of these methods successfully in my practice. I also learned a lot of new information that I cannot wait to implement in my practice. This section could have been a new book in its own right.

I cannot recommend The Wellness Project highly enough. It is an enlightening book that offers hope to all of us and especially offers hope to those suffering from chronic illness. Implementing the holistic treatment plan as outlined by Roy Mankovitz is bound to improve your health. This book is a must-read for all who are interested in achieving their optimal health.

David Brownstein, M.D.            www.drbrownstein.com


Author of:

*Iodine: Why You Need It, Why You Can't Live Without It, 3rd Edition*

*Overcoming Thyroid Disorders, 2nd Edition*

*Drugs that Don't' Work and Natural Therapies that Do*

*The Miracle of Natural Hormones, 3rd Edition*

*Salt: Your Way to Health*

*Overcoming Arthritis*

*The Guide to Healthy Eating*

*The Guide to a Gluten-Free Diet*

# Section One - The Hypothesis for Health

*Common sense is not so common* - Voltaire

It does not take a rocket scientist to realize that something is very wrong with the health of our present population, and that the medical community has not been able to reverse what seems to be a relentless trend downward with respect to the prevention or cure of dozens of chronic illnesses. The goal of this book is to present a program which is designed to reverse that trend, but in a very unusual way. Over the last twenty years, I have voraciously read everything I could get my hands on that had to do with health, including most of the texts used in medical schools. I applied the skills I developed in the fields of rocket science, engineering, and even law, to try to arrive at an understanding of the problems in the health field that prevent a reversal of the trend toward illness. It became clear to me that the medical community is primarily devoted to the treatment of symptoms, not the prevention of illness. In a pragmatic sense, illness prevention is bad for business. My years of self-experimentation and research produced the program that is presented in this book, and I have been following it for several decades with great success. My reason for now publishing it is in the hope that likeminded others might also profit from trying all or parts of the program to evaluate its impact on their health.

More specifically, this book was written for those who are concerned about illness and are interested in a program (designed by Nature in this instance) to enable the body to restore health. It may also appeal to those who are intellectually curious about a health program (The Wellness Project) written by someone with a background in rocket science. They may wish to learn about it in the event illness becomes a concern to them in the future. Then there are those readers who like to self-experiment (which include me). They may find the information in this book of interest from the perspective of illness prevention.

Most popular books on health are directed to a particular illness such as diabetes, arthritis, cancer, etc. One of the unusual aspects of The Wellness Project is that it is not illness, diagnosis, or symptom specific - a result of my hypothesis for the causes of illness. This hypothesis was arrived at by observing patterns found in Nature and making some sense of them, and here is the result. Virtually all illnesses result from some failure of the body's defenses (which I will refer to as *the defense system*). This failure can arise as an inability to cope with a pathogen or toxin that entered the body, as in the case of an infectious disease or poisoning from ingesting a toxic substance. This failure can also arise as an inability to cope with some biological abnormality that arises within us, such as cancerous cells forming tumors, or foreign deposits in our arteries. Last, but not least, this defense system failure can arise as an inability to distinguish friend from foe, whereby the defense system mistakenly attacks what appear to be healthy parts of the body, resulting in autoimmune diseases such as MS, rheumatoid arthritis, lupus, and the like. I discuss the defense system and autoimmunity in more detail below.

The common denominator in all of these instances is some issue dealing with the body's defenses. Rather than viewing the problem as a defense system defect or disorder, I view it as an overburden of toxins in the body that either interferes with the defense system's ability to fully perform, or leads to a malfunction in its performance. I define a toxin, sometimes referred to as a poison, as any substance, natural or human-made, that is capable of activating the defense system and producing a deleterious effect on the body of a particular individual. The immune system is a part of the defense system and is traditionally thought of in terms of special cells in the blood and lymph fluid, such as T cells, which deal with infectious pathogens. In addition to the immune system, my definition of the defense system encompasses the bacteria in our intestines, the acid in our stomach, all of the detoxification properties of our liver and other organs, and undoubtedly, other portions of our body we have yet to identify that defend us against a host of pathogenic and toxic substances.

A corollary to my hypothesis is that if the defense system can be relieved of this toxin overburden, it is then available to restore and maintain health, regardless of the illness. Some might take exception to the above statement when it comes to autoimmune diseases, where a traditional approach to treatment is to suppress the immune system to alleviate symptoms, on the basis that the immune system has become defective and is attacking healthy tissue. I have an alternate theory with respect to autoimmune conditions, based on my research in the field of detoxification. The theory is that the immune system is not defective and is simply doing its job of attacking cells that, while they might appear to be healthy, are not. I will spend some time defining the word *healthy* below, but suffice to say that what the medical community defines as healthy is only so to the extent cellular defects can, or cannot, be measured. Put another way, I believe that the cells that are attacked in an autoimmune condition are not healthy, but are in fact infiltrated by toxins and hence deemed "foreign" by the immune system. In the detoxification sections below, in support of my theory I will discuss examples of how some detoxification strategies have resulted in autoimmune illness remission.

In this book, Nature is used as a template to unburden the defense system from having to deal (often on a daily basis) with a lifetime of toxins. In its unburdened state, the defense system is then fully available to respond in a proper manner to existing illnesses, and to ward off future ones. Of course, the extent to which health can be restored in an individual is controlled by many factors, including any permanent damage that may have occurred in the past affecting the defense or other systems.

My analyses have also shown that it is the defense system, not drugs, chemotherapy, radiation, or a supplement that ultimately cures the person. While medical intervention may assist the defense system in coping with the problem, the actual restoration of health results from the defense system restoring equilibrium. We know this fact from persons who have a compromised defense system, as in the case of AIDS, where no amount of medical intervention appears to be able to stop the ravages of illness.

The term *Project,* as used in this book, refers to a set of plans describing how to operate and maintain a complex chemical factory – the human body. The overall plan includes a diet plan to put the good stuff in our body, a detoxification program to get a lifetime of bad stuff out of our body, and suggested changes in lifestyle to enhance our health. In every instance, in keeping with the hypothesis, the goal is to minimize the intake of toxins, and to maximize the elimination of any toxins already in our body. This is a good place to point out that foods are a potential source of toxins, especially ones put there by nature to discourage their being eaten. This will be covered in great depth in the diet section below.

As my research progressed, my toxin hypothesis for health evolved, based simply on observing nature. For example, here is a critically important point when it comes to our health: living things thrive when their environment is in alignment with their evolution. I will define all of these terms in detail below, but simple examples will suffice for now. Herbivores (animals evolved to eat plants) do very poorly if placed in an environment that forces them to eat meat. Fresh water fish do very poorly in salt water. Tropical plants do very poorly in cold climates. Humans do very poorly if they eat foods that their heritage did not evolve them to eat. In each case, Nature designed a particular species to thrive in a particular environment, and this synergy between evolution and environment took place over a very long period of time (sometimes millions of years). Put another way, and in keeping with my central theme, an environment that is not right for a living thing is actually toxic to it. Hence, an important factor in minimizing illness is to bring one's environment and evolution into alignment, which forms a major premise of The Wellness Project. While this may sound complicated, it really is not, as long as we pay attention to Nature and follow her cues. In fact, it can be quite a lot of fun to learn, among other things, what we were originally designed to eat, as we take a multi-million year stroll back towards the origins of our species to find the answers. The side box entitled Hypothesis for Health is a recap of what we have covered so far.

## The Hypothesis for Health™

1) Illness results from a failure or malfunction of the body's defense system.

2) The body's defense system may fail or malfunction as a result of an overburden of toxins in the body (including those from food).

3) The body may be overburdened by toxins as a result of a misalignment between the body's evolutionary history and its present environment.

# Chapter 1 – A Search for Answers

## Human Evolution and Environment

In this section, we are going to concentrate on the evolution/environment portion of the hypothesis. From what we know of evolution, whether in the plant or animal kingdom, there is a constant tension between an evolving species and its environment, which is usually also evolving. Those species that, from an evolutionary perspective, most closely align with their present environment end up as the survivors, and through reproduction, spawn more survivors. The *others* die out. Random mutations along the way introduce new "test cases," and if they fit the environment even better, they go on to success. Otherwise, they too die out. Thus, we have the survivors and the *others*. Put another way, a measure of a person's health and chances of survival is the degree to which their heritage is in alignment with their present environment.

From my research, I have concluded that most of the current health crises are explainable by the above evolutionary summary. Our species has been naturally and quite successfully evolving for about 2.5 million years (say 100,000 generations). However, because of recent human technological "advances" (in hindsight, mostly blunders over the last 400 generations) we have altered our environment at a pace that, for many of us, far exceeds our ability to adapt to it. That is the case for many of us except for a lucky few who would not be reading this book or even going near a book section on health. These are the *winners* in our environment, individuals that seemingly can eat anything, smoke, drink, get little sleep, never exercise, work in a toxic environment, and live a perfectly healthy symptom-free life into triple digit years. They have acquired, probably by random chance, the evolutionary makeup that fits our modern environment, at least for the moment. How do you know if you are one of the winners in our present day Western society? You have no aches or pains, lots of energy, a cheery disposition, no illnesses, radiant skin, no weight problems, take no medications, eat whatever you want, and can't understand why others don't share your good fortune.

An important point to consider is that winners can only remain so in the environment to which their ancestors, and hence they, have adapted. Put them into a new environment or change their environment quickly, and they are no longer winners. If you would like to see what winners looked like in each of several different indigenous environments around the world in studies done about 75 years ago, you can go to the website of the Price-Pottenger Nutrition Foundation (I am a member of their Advisory Board) [1]. You can also thumb through the book *Nutrition and Physical Degeneration* by Weston Price [2], where you will see pictures of the *others* in each of these environments who foolishly changed their ancestral diets to mimic the one we eat today.

This is certainly a lesson for many of us, the *others* that die out, or would do so except for the "miracles of medicine," which keep us going at least long enough to reproduce progeny who for the most part inherit our "otherness" and who also need the miracles of medicine to survive.

The tension between evolutionary heritage and environment for all living things is a conflict that, barring a catastrophic incident such as volcanic eruptions or asteroid bombardment, plays out very slowly over millions of years. By the term "evolutionary heritage," I include not only genetic variations and mutations that have occurred over the millennia, but also non-genetic changes that have evolved in our body that we have yet to discover or define, and about which we can only speculate, as I will take the liberty of doing later in the book.

By the term "environment," I include everything external to our body, inclusive of everything put into or on our body. Of course, there are the traditional environmental factors such as the air we breathe and the water and food we ingest. My definition also includes the vaccinations and other drugs we have been injected with and have taken orally, our dental work, other things we put in our mouths (including toothpaste, chewing gum, and mouthwash), and on our skin (including soap, cosmetics and sunscreens), and our emotional interactions with everyone and everything around us.

Because of its uniqueness, the several pounds of bacteria that reside in our gut require special mention. In my frame of reference, these microflora, which can have a great impact on our health, are unique because they bridge the gap between evolutionary heritage and environment, sharing a part of each. This subject is discussed more thoroughly under the category of probiotics (friendly bacteria) throughout the book.

From an environment point of view, what we have today is quite different from what our ancestors experienced. A good part of our environment, from the food we eat to the toxins we have spawned, is becoming more and more of an artificial human creation and it continues to evolve at a frantic pace. There is the constant addition of genetically modified foods and food processing techniques to create products that never existed in nature, and innumerable newly created chemical toxins being added to the environment. There is big money in these ventures, and they are unlikely to stop any time soon. So, the heritage/environment tension is in fact increasing and, at this rate, even the offspring of the *winners* will have a tough time keeping up. There are some optimists out there who, at least on a statistical basis, see an acceleration of human adaptive evolution driven in part by the large size of our population [3]. However, from my perspective, what I see happening is that each generation is getting sicker sooner. Enter the geneticists.

If we are not willing to change our environment, how about changing our genetic heritage to align with the present environment? The genome-tweaking industry is off and running with stem cell research and other approaches to doing exactly that. As a bystander and usually optimistic technologist (and an *other*), who is carefully watching this game of cat and mouse between human heritage and environment play out, I have reached a conclusion. While it is theoretically possible that the geneticists will in the distant future be able to catch up to the environment shifters, I don't particularly like the odds or the timetable, of which there is none. Enter The Wellness Project.

I have no aspirations toward changing my genetic heritage during my lifetime, so if I want to align with my environment, it is not rocket science to conclude that I must change my environment. The key word here is *my*, since I also have no aspirations toward changing the greater environment, other than participating in the various causes attempting to do so.

This book is all about how, over the last twenty years, I have used my training in science, engineering, and even law, coupled with common sense, to find out how to go back in time to discover the environment to which I was most likely attuned. I have taken this environment, in which my ancestors were likely to have been winners, and sought to recreate it to the practical extent possible in today's world. As a corollary to this basic premise, I have found that when our heritage and environment are in alignment, our defense system is able to perform at its peak, because none of the health issues that result from misalignment burden it. I think you will find the results of my research quite interesting, if not downright startling. One reason for writing this book is to bring this information to the public, because what I learned during this journey is that this same wellness plan has every likelihood of working for all the other *others,* all of us who are trying to survive in an incompatible environment!

## A Rocket Scientist's Search for Answers

*Be careful about reading health books. You may die of a misprint!-*
Mark Twain

In this section, I am going to describe the steps I took in my journey from the hypothesis for health to the Wellness Project. I am a technologist at heart and have a continuing fascination and curiosity about how things work. Perhaps because I have a science and engineering background, not having operating instructions for my body has been a particularly frustrating experience. Here is an example. One of the simplest of questions I had been trying to get answered over the last twenty-five years from the healthcare community was "What should I eat to prevent illness and keep myself healthy"? After all, knowing what to eat can't be as difficult as rocket science! Since foods can be a source of toxins, and we usually eat three times per day, eating the wrong foods could add up to a very large load on the defense system. So, I needed the right answers, and I made it my first goal to find out what foods would be in alignment with my evolutionary history, and hence would prove lowest in potential toxins.

I consulted with many nutritionists, and each gave me a different answer. Out of frustration, I read every book I could find on nutrition, and studied for and passed a test to become certified as a nutritional consultant. However, neither the books on health nor the certification brought me any closer to finding my answers. In fact, I was somewhat alarmed to realize that the "science of nutrition" lacked the rigors of my field that enabled rockets to get off the launch pad, and DVD players to work. Did you know that there is no agreed upon definition for the words *fruit, vegetable, nut, seed,* or *bean* – or even the term *Vitamin E*; that we do not know the complete composition of any food or how these various food elements interact with each other in the body; that we have not identified the majority of friendly bacteria in our gut that are critical to digestion and keep us alive; or that we only recently discovered that our gut has its own nervous system that can act independently of our brain; or that the gut produces more serotonin than our brain and can have a major impact on our emotions [4]? Keep this in mind the next time you have a "gut feeling" about something.

It took me twenty years of independent research to find the right answers, and now that I am a nutritionist, I feel comfortable answering the question for others and myself. It is an answer unlike any given to me by those who are supposed to have the answers, is one I had never seen in print before, and it forms the backbone of the diet section of the Wellness Project. Guess what? There is one particular diet that all humans originally evolved to eat, just as other species of mammals have a diet that has uniquely evolved to keep them healthy.

Please note carefully that the previous sentence does not state that there is *only* one diet for each individual that must be followed to produce health. In fact, there may be many diets each person can adopt that will yield an illness-free life. My point is that among these various dietary choices, there appears to be one in particular (the Wellness Diet) that is safe for every person to eat, based on our common human heritage. This is a very subtle but important point. Here is a simple analogy. All modern gasoline engine powered cars can run smoothly and safely on 91-octane fuel. Some can also run smoothly and safely on 89-octane fuel, or perhaps some form of biogas. If you were given such a car with no operating instructions, the safe thing to do would be to fill it with 91-octane fuel, rather than risk using the wrong stuff. As you read this book, you will see the importance of this simple analogy as it relates to the entire field of nutrition and dietary choices.

In fact, this book is filled with answers to incredibly simple questions regarding health for which the healthcare community has never been trained to answer. Why do we need toilet paper when our human ancestors for the previous 99,990 generations (about 2.5 million years), and every other mammal in Nature (including our pets) can do without it? Why do we need to brush, floss, or use mouthwash when our ancestors for all but the last 400 generations (10,000 years) had perfectly straight, cavity-free teeth (including wisdom teeth) without the need for any dental care (chewing on bones is not the correct answer)? The answers to these and other simple questions (and their health implications), are found in this book.

I refer to our ancestors often because that is where I finally found the answers I was looking for. I am not referring to the "ancient" Greeks or Romans or Egyptians, or Eastern medicine such as Ayurveda, or Biblical times or Aztecs or Mayans. I found my answers before any of these (or written language, or farms, or villages, or towns, or empires) were in existence. Humans have been roaming the Earth for about 2.5 million years, and all of the above took place within the last 5000 to 10000 years, so none of what we normally think of as ancient is really ancient at all.

As you will see, to get the answers I needed, I went back in time before fire was used for cooking, estimated to be somewhere between 20,000 and 150,000 years ago (800 to 6000 generations ago), defined as the Paleolithic era (I will abbreviate it as Paleo in the book). But isn't it true that our ancestors way back then lived short lives because of illness, and also had high infant mortality? No, that is not true. Incredibly, our Paleo Ancestors of that time (from skeletal evidence) were on average taller than we are today, had bone strength higher than ours, and had virtually perfect teeth, all strong indicators of robust health. Paleontologists believe that our early ancestors would have lived long healthy lives except for three things: starvation, predators, and accidents, none of which has anything to do with illness [2, 5-7]. Take away your supermarket; put yourself in a wild animal park; and suffer an arm or leg fracture; and you too would be challenged to reach a nice, ripe old age. If there was a high infant mortality back then (we have no evidence that there was), the odds of us being here today would be quite slim.

From my research in anthropology and Paleopathology, it actually appears that our species reached its pinnacle of health somewhere around 10,000 years ago (400 generations). Something happened in the last 400 generations to reverse this course and take us backward and downward. These "somethings" are covered in some detail in this book. Further, I have spent a great deal of time researching, understanding, and recreating in today's world the environment of our ancestors at that time. (No, it does not require eating raw meat or walking around in a loincloth.) I actually use some high tech tricks right out of a rocket scientist's toolbox to recreate that past environment in a way that is fun and simple to do.

Out of my studies came the framework for the Wellness Project. The concept is to use Nature as the template for bringing our current lifestyle into alignment with our evolutionary heritage at that time in the past when we were so healthy. The premise is that if we perform such an alignment, our body will return to and stay at a pinnacle of health with an unburdened defense system. Unfortunately, the "height" of the health pinnacle for each of us is not readily predictable, because it is affected by many personal variables including certain genetic defects, as well as permanent damage to and removal of important body parts, discussed in more detail below.

The word "detox" will be used extensively in this book. The word itself has many meanings, such as spending time in a rehab center for drug and alcohol abuse. In this book, it has a much broader meaning, which is to either remove or render harmless foreign elements and compounds that have collected in our bodies over a lifetime. They range from parasites (usually collected from restaurant meals), to mercury (from dental work, fish, and vaccinations), to a host of other chemicals (from drinking out of plastic bottles, sitting on furniture made with toxic fire retardants, and a host of other activities). We will even deal with drugs and alcohol, but not in the ways you would expect. The drugs include prescriptions widely dispensed to very young children (antibiotics), and the alcohol issues result from a fungal overgrowth (Candida), having nothing to do with drinking alcoholic beverages, but producing similar symptoms. These toxins tend to set a limit as to how high our pinnacle of health can reach, so it behooves us to deal with them now.

The Wellness Project has been in the making for over 20 years, and I am finally bringing my findings to the public in this book, based largely on experimentation coupled with years of research. Therefore, unlike other books on diet and health, it not filled with stories of how well John C. or Mary L. improved their life, or enjoyed the recipes (none are needed) such as a soy burger made with fifteen herbs. A reader might well wonder then if this book is premature for lack of such real-life testimonials. For any of the modern health programs in print, that would be true, but in the case of the Wellness Project, it is based on the largest health "study" ever conducted in the history of our species. It extended over a period of about 2.4 million years (about 96,000 generations), involved millions of our ancestors, and flies in the face of virtually every health program written to date.

My hypothesis for health is not based on dispensing drugs or supplements to be taken for a lifetime. It is not a weight loss program; it is not an exercise program; it is neither symptom nor diagnosis based. In a nutshell, it is designed to restore a human body as closely as possible to the condition intended by Nature, to the extent our current knowledge allows. In an engineering sense, it is designed to restore the body to its "factory default," or baseline state in as many areas as possible, based on the rationale that such a state yields optimum health. It uses very simple principles, including common sense and humility, along with approaches used in my fields of endeavor to produce a program designed to yield positive results.

While the medical community has made great strides, with great successes, in the fields of surgery and repair of the human body, their record of accomplishment in preventing or treating chronic illnesses has not been as successful. They cannot make definitive statements about the "cause" of any major illness, and not surprisingly, have not come up with "cures" for them. I have put quotes around the words *cause* and *cure* because as you will see, it is very important to define these terms. Without a consensus on these and many other definitions, it is hopeless even to begin to discuss health. Disappointed with my lack of answers, I launched into a mission of self-education, reading as much as I could, venturing into what some would consider the unrelated fields of anthropology, zoology, and Paleopathology, and applying to myself what I learned.

I'm an engineer, an inventor, and an attorney with a specialty in intellectual property (IP) rights, such as patents, trademarks, copyrights, and trade secrets. My initial motivation for pursuing a legal career as a second vocation was to learn how to protect my own legal rights as an inventor, which eventually led me down the road of successful entrepreneurship. Strangely, as my odyssey in health research moved forward, I recalled one of the important (and sometimes controversial) principles of our legal system, known as *stare decisis*, meaning roughly to stand by prior decisions. As I conducted my research, this principal took on a new and very important meaning. As Supreme Court Justice Thurgood Marshall explained to the court in 1986, stare decisis is the "means by which we ensure that the law will not merely change erratically, but will develop in a principled and intelligible fashion." While it does not mean that new decisions cannot replace old, it does mean that one should always go back in time and research what took place in the past before proposing something new. Lawyers spend a great deal of time doing just that, known as "Shepardizing a Case" (Shepards ® is a citation service that indexes prior decisions and rules). This exercise is quite fascinating, because you can see the very earliest of decisions and how they subsequently may have been agreed with, modified, or overturned. Well, as you will see below, I ended up doing something quite similar to that in the field of health – finding out what went before that worked, and what subsequently changed it.

During my engineering career, I worked with many smart folks at the Jet Propulsion Laboratory, a NASA facility operated by the California Institute of Technology, designing unmanned spacecraft control systems. Previously, I worked at Rocketdyne designing space-engine control systems for lunar landing missions. I also worked at Teledyne creating and producing patented technology in the field of electronics used today in military and commercial applications worldwide. I am a named inventor in more than 60 U.S. patents and hundreds of corresponding foreign patents (please see Appendix A). I have additional patent applications pending in the U.S. Patent and Trademark Office, some of which are in the field of health, and I will tell you more about a few of them later in the book. I come to the health field with an engineer's and inventor's perspective, and since the body is really a complex chemical factory, these skills work very effectively to help me devise methods to try to understand it. Here are some of the analogies I used.

If I was presented with a complex device (my body) that did not have accompanying operating instructions, and I wanted to find out how it was designed to work, I would have several alternatives. A first approach very familiar to engineers is called "reverse engineering," where we endeavor to take the device apart, ideally without damaging it, so that we can compare its inner workings with our prior knowledge in order to try and figure it out. A second approach that we are all familiar with from our consumer electronics experiences is to just start pushing buttons somewhat randomly and see what happens. (Sometimes we do this even though we were given operating instructions!) This approach is commonly called a "trial and error" approach. A third approach is to contact the manufacturer and communicate directly with the person or team that designed the device. I don't know of a name for this approach so I will make one up: I will call it the "common sense" approach, and as you will see, it forms the backbone of my hypothesis for health. So, let's look at each of these approaches as they apply to the human effort to understand how we are designed to work. The presumption is that if we had this understanding, we would be well along the road to maintaining ourselves in a state of health.

Considering the first approach of reverse engineering, it is believed that somewhere about 300 BCE, Herophilus, referred to as the Father of Anatomy, began dissecting cadavers and documenting what he saw. These crude endeavors continued over the next 1000 years or so to provide us with an anatomical road map that allows skilled surgeons to put us back together when our parts are damaged. Unfortunately, this technique has yet to produce any useful results in finding the causes of the major chronic illnesses that plague us today. Please refer to the side box for important definitions of terms such as "illness," "cause," and "cure." You might find these definitions less than fascinating reading, but they will play a very large role in finding our way in the Wellness Project without getting lost, as has happened to others so many times in the past.

Now, let's explore the second, or button-pushing approach to finding out how our body is designed to work. I will hereafter refer to this as the "trial and error" (T&E) approach, which is actually a form of experiment. As we will see, this approach is the mainstay of the healthcare industry in its efforts to treat illness, from the development of new drugs or supplements to creating treatment protocols.

# Definitions of: Illness, Health, Cause, Prevention and Cure

Let's first try to put a definition around the term **chronic illness**, which is sometimes defined as a condition that persists for 3 months or more. First, we need to define **illness**, but that is not easy because there is no widely accepted definition for this term. How does it compare to disease, syndrome, disorder, medical condition, dysfunction, and so on. I got a headache (is that an illness?) trying to find a definition with which I was comfortable, so let's try this: **illness is an abnormal condition of the body or mind that causes discomfort**. Illness can cause discomfort relatively immediately, or it may take decades for the discomfort to appear, and it can manifest as anything from a rash to death. If you press me for a definition of *abnormal*, I would say any condition of the body not intended by Nature, which is itself defined later in the text. I will use the words *illness* and *disease* somewhat interchangeably in this book. We can now define **health** as **freedom from illness**.

Please note that the term "health" is very different from the term "healthy." **Healthy** implies a comparison to something that is either not healthy or not as healthy, which, as you will see, leads to mass confusion in the health field. The reason for the confusion is that the item to which it is being compared is rarely defined! Here is an example of what I call a junk-science statement: "Olive oil is healthy." Compared to what? Corn oil? Safflower oil? Hydrogenated oil? What turns out to be the case with most of these undefined statements is that the item being declared as healthy may be simply less unhealthy than the alternative. Yes, olive oil is less unhealthy than the other oils listed above, but as you will see it is not a particularly good source of any essential fatty acid, and totally unnecessary in the Wellness Diet. A major reason for creating the Wellness Diet is to establish a baseline standard for comparison to any other diet, so that responsible, intelligent, and scientifically defendable research can be conducted in the field of nutrition with everyone on the same page.

Most of us know of the chronic illness biggies: cancer, heart disease, diabetes, arthritis. Then there are the ones whose names are abbreviated with letters, such as MS, ALS, IBS, UC, SLE, GERD, COPD, etc., followed by those named after the folks that "discovered" them:   Crohn's, Parkinson's, Cushing's, Addison's, Hashimoto's, Paget's, Meniere's, Raynaud's, etc.   Not all chronic illnesses are life threatening, but they can have a major impact on quality of life, such as psoriasis and acne. Writing this list reminds me of a conversation I had with a friend who is a dermatologist. He told me that at least 80% of skin ailments have no known cause, but virtually 100% of them have names. His take on this was that patients believe "If we name it we tame it."

Now that we have some handle on chronic illness, it is time to define the terms "cause," "prevention" and "cure." As you will see, these are critically important in any discussion regarding illness, since they really are a measure of progress towards health. Having studied philosophy, logic, and the scientific method, I feel comfortable stating that the term "**cause**" has no universal definition In fact, attempts to define the term date from Aristotle, and have yet to produce consensus. For purposes of this book, I will offer a definition as related to illness, but first we must acknowledge that the cause of an illness may actually require two or more events to occur, so it is more accurate to talk about the causes of an illness.

Causes can be separated into *necessary* and *sufficient,* and as you will see, this distinction will be very important as we analyze the (usually incorrect) conclusions that have been drawn in many major medical research studies. Here is an example: dermatologists (and perhaps everyone else in the world except a few others and me) believe that at some cumulative level of ultraviolet (UV) light, well within the range of the amount of sun exposure virtually all of us would experience during our lives, skin cancer will occur. If that statement was taken at face value, such that UV light is considered *sufficient* to cause skin cancer, then everyone exposed to the sun would eventually have skin cancer, which is not the case. There are plenty of folks who get enormous doses of UV during their lives with no signs of skin cancer, so at best UV light could be a *necessary*, but not *sufficient* cause. In other words, another cause is missing (from my personal experiments, it is a weakened defense system primarily due to toxins), and given the combination of the two (or even more) causes, skin cancer is likely. I give this example to show the subtleness and complicated nature of causation in the medical field, and yet you hear every day about the efforts to find the "cause of cancer", which may turn out to be a combination of many different events occurring over some yet to be determined time period. So, my definition is this: **the causes of an illness are all of the events that are individually necessary and, in combination, prove sufficient to result in that illness, including all of the causes of each of those events**.

To be the cause of an illness, an event must contribute to the resulting illness. It is an axiom of science that mere correlation does not prove causation. Correlation is when there is a statistical relationship between two or more events, perhaps because they tend to occur together. An example is high cholesterol levels and heart disease. This is actually a poor example because in fact the statistical relationship is very weak. Studies have shown that more than half the people with heart disease have low cholesterol levels. Nevertheless, the medical community has used whatever correlations they can find to jump to the conclusion that there is a causal relationship between the two. I discuss this further in the next section.

Let's go back to the skin cancer example. If the combination of necessary elements sufficient to cause the cancer is a certain cumulative dose of UV *and* a compromised defense system, we then look at the causes of each of these. The UV part is easy – too much tanning, an outdoor job in the tropics, etc. The other part is not easy – what caused the compromised defense system (interestingly, UV itself can temporarily reduce defense system effectiveness). The medical community (including Western, Eastern, and Alternative) does not fully know how the defense system works, so a satisfactory answer to this part is not likely to be forthcoming (other than guesses) in the near future. The present protocol from the medical community to avoid skin cancer is to avoid UV light, which sells a lot of sunscreen. Is that a strategy of "prevention" or is it a strategy to provide billions of dollars of revenue to sunscreen manufacturers?

Let's define prevention. In the medical field, three levels of prevention have been defined. <u>Primary</u> prevention avoids the development of a disease. <u>Secondary</u> prevention activities are aimed at early disease detection, thereby increasing opportunities for interventions to prevent progression of the disease and emergence of symptoms. <u>Tertiary</u> prevention reduces the negative impact of an already established disease by restoring function and reducing disease-related complications. In this book, my definition of **prevention** will be: **the avoidance of the development of an illness in a manner that does not compromise the overall health and well-being of the person.** In general, to prevent an illness, one must eliminate at least one of the necessary events causing that illness, including at least one of the necessary causes of that event.

We can use colonoscopies as an example, since it is offered by the medical community as a means of preventing colon cancer. The objective is to use this procedure as a diagnostic tool to detect polyps and remove them, hopefully before they become cancerous. Under the above medical definitions, this is secondary prevention. Under my definition, this is not really prevention because it does not address the burning question that should be on every patient's mind when told they have polyps: "What caused the polyps?" Many gastro docs will give an answer like: "Its genetics", or "It's aging". I have come to understand these statements as a code for "We don't really know." It is my personal belief, from my research, that polyps are caused by an improper diet and lack of detoxification, both of which form the mainstay of my hypothesis for health. Please understand that I am not discouraging the use of colonoscopies (they have saved many lives), I am merely pointing out that if you do not address the ultimate causes of the problem, there is a very high likelihood that either the same or a different problem will return.

Now let's turn to **cure**, which implies that you already have a condition or symptoms of a condition that you want to reverse. **One definition of cure that I like is the following: to restore the person to good health in a manner that does not compromise the overall wellbeing of that person.** Let's go back to the skin cancer example. Does avoiding ultraviolet (UV) light, as found in sunlight, restore the person to good health? Absolutely not, and in fact, as a result of vitamin D deficiency (UVB light impinging on the skin converts cholesterol to vitamin D), it will likely lead to very debilitating chronic illnesses including systemic cancers of all sorts, osteoporosis, and possibly MS [8]. Further, if topically applied sunscreens are used to block UV light, they will likely also contribute to illness (including skin cancer), since virtually all of them are toxic, as more fully described in the Lifestyle section of this book (along with a description of an exciting university research project I am funding on this subject). So, here is an example of a condition possibly caused by a combination of events (UV light and a compromised defense system) in which the cessation of either one can potentially relieve the condition. However, picking the right event to cease is critical – ceasing UV exposure can lead to major illness, while repairing a compromised defense system theoretically will lead to an immense improvement in all phases of health. As we shall see, if we give the body what Nature intended and remove from it what Nature did not intend, for the most part, the human body cures itself. The best we can do is to give it a hand.

I love electronic gadgets, and am an avid button-pusher, which has gotten me into no end of trouble. In many cases, I either have to resort to reading the instructions (drat!) or, as a final resort, calling the manufacturer to get the answer as to how to restore the gadget to its proper operating condition. Some manufacturers, bless their heart, provide a button on their widget that can be used as a factory reset – if only we humans had such a feature! Personally, my button-pushing behavior can be characterized as somewhat motivated by a sense of arrogance- I don't need anyone to tell me how this thing works, I can figure it out myself!

From a study of the theory of evolution and of the history of our present human species, it is apparent that Nature makes great use of T&E experiments in evolving species. It seems to work like this: random mutations and genetic and probably other variations occur all the time in every species and these can be viewed as the *trials*, while poor reproductive fitness is regarded as the *error*. Thus after long periods of time, well-adapted evolutionary patterns accumulate simply by virtue of their being able to reproduce, while less well-adapted patterns die out. Now "die out" can be a euphemism for many different behaviors, from a failure to reproduce to debilitating birth defects to chronic illness, but the end result is the cessation of that line of evolutionary patterns. So in a T&E experiment run by Nature, a failure is clearly demarcated and is not perpetuated indefinitely.

At about ten to twelve thousand years ago (about 400 generations ago), we gained sufficient intelligence and had developed enough tools to begin some very serious T&E "button pushing" ourselves with respect to virtually all aspects of our lives. Not only that, the scope of these T&E experiments was substantially increased because of the development of societies that were grouped into towns and villages, so that one experiment could effect very large numbers of people. As you will see, humans have conducted experiments that have not only fooled with Nature, but have reversed many of the biological gains made in our health up to that time.

For the human evolutionary period older than 400 generations ago, (a period of about 2.49 million years, or 99,600 generations), it is believed by many in the field of anthropology that our ancestors, living primarily in tropical Africa, led a nomadic life consisting of hunting and gathering. I will refer to this period as the Ancient or Paleo Era (see the side box entitled Defining Ancient for further clarification), and the more recent period following the Paleo Era as the Neolithic era.

The T&E experiments during the Paleo era would have included Nature fiddling with mutations and other variations, the results of which may have taken a very long time to surface (perhaps several hundred thousand years); and some simple experiments devised by humans, such as sampling new sources of food.

The T&E system works very well for humans when the E follows soon after the T, so that a cause and effect relationship can be established. Push the wrong button and the screen goes blank. Eat the wrong food and you soon get sick. In these experiments one quickly learns (and hopefully teaches others) to avoid that behavior. Animals do that all the time with eating and other behavior and, in ways we do not understand, pass a lot of that information on to their offspring. A problem with humans running T&E experiments on themselves is our relatively short lifespan (perhaps 120 years maximum) compared to our 2.5 million year evolutionary heritage. Eating something and getting sick an hour later is a no-brainer, but how about eating something that does not show its damage for a decade, or for three generations, or for 400 generations?

---

## Defining Ancient

The word Ancient has many meanings in the field of health. In this book, the term refers to a prehistoric era distinguished by the development of stone tools. It covers the greatest portion of humanity's time on Earth, extending from about 2.5 million years ago, with the introduction of stone tools to the introduction of fire for cooking, estimated at around 100,000 years ago. **THE TERM "ANCIENT" <u>DOES NOT</u> REFER TO THE FOLLOWING, ALL OF WHICH ARE RELATIVELY <u>MODERN</u>:**

| | |
|---|---|
| Biblical Times | Any Empire or Dynasty |
| Roman Times | Greek Times |
| Egyptian Times | Large city or town |
| Ayurveda/Eastern Medicine | Farms |
| Yoga | Ranches |
| Tai Chi | Growing of crops |
| Domestication of animals | Harvesting |
| Mayans/Incas | Polynesians |
| American Indians | Inuits |
| Eating Dairy | Eating Grains |

---

The problem is compounded by the fact that the human body is not a static device like most human made things, but is alive and constantly evolving, renewing, healing, and adapting to its environment. This is coupled with the fact that we humans continue to run multiple T&E experiments in parallel, in many cases not even realizing these are experiments. (Those of us who like to run experiments know that this behavior is disastrous, leading to chaos and conclusions that are wrong.) All of this is going on during the interval between starting the Trial and recognizing the Error, so that when the Error is finally recognized (if at all), it may be impossible to link it to the correct cause (or combination of causes). Sound like a nightmare? It is, and unfortunately it also could be said to characterize our progress in health (or lack thereof) over the last 400 generations. In the following chapters, I will touch upon examples of what I (and some others) regard as faulty T&E experiments carried out by our fellow humans (many times in good faith), some as far back as 10,000 years ago, that are now manifesting as chronic illnesses.

Let's go on to the third approach (common sense) to finding out how we were designed to work. As you may recall, this approach was to contact the manufacturer of the widget in hopes of communicating with the designer/engineer or team thereof to get the real scoop on how the widget works and how to keep it working that way for as long as possible. Well, "who" or "what" designed us? While I am certainly aware of the faith-based answers to this question, in this book, I refer to our designer as Nature. While I would like to have a side box defining what I mean by the term Nature, I am at a loss for words. The best I can come up with is this: Nature is that which has caused everything in our universe (and probably others) to evolve and exist. Because of our human conceptual limitations, it is much easier to give Nature human attributes in our attempt at definition. So, when I make statements such as Nature does this or that, or Nature intended ...., it is really a combination of ignorance and arrogance on my part. I cannot ultimately "know" what Nature was or is "doing" or "intending", and it is arrogant of me to think that I do know. However, this is the best I can do, so please bear with me.

So, what happens since Nature has not provided us with written operating instructions? Well, in the animal kingdom, a great deal of knowledge is passed from generation to generation regarding what to eat and how to self heal [9]. Since we are also part of the animal kingdom, I presume such information was also passed along in the human chain, but somehow got lost along the way. A large portion of this book is devoted to efforts to reconstruct this lost knowledge to the greatest extent possible, and then to apply what we have learned to our modern lifestyle – this is the essence of The Wellness Project. The goal is to do as good a job as possible to align our environment to our heritage, with the expectation that by doing so we are capitalizing on the successful result of 99,600 generations of Nature's Trial and Error experiments. If one believes the Darwinian model of evolution, then, but for our own interference in Nature's experiments, we now should be at a very high pinnacle of health, having had 100,000 replication cycles to discard untold numbers of failed evolutionary experiments in favor of the ones that produce optimum wellbeing.

I am certainly not alone in believing that a "return to Nature" would be a healthy thing to do as compared with where most of us are now. In furtherance of this goal, several studies have been conducted in the field of anthropology to try to deduce what our Paleo Ancestors ate [10], and yet others have studied modern hunter-gatherer societies to try to determine their lifestyle and its effects on health [2]. Still others have investigated the effects of domestication on the health of our pets [11], from which we can deduce some interesting information about our own diets. A more thorough discussion of these works can be found in Section Two.

Before we move on to the next chapter, I suspect that some readers may continue to take exception to the premise that our Ancient ancestors were healthy or that they should be viewed as a model for us. Why, isn't it true that they rarely lived past 30 or so, certainly not long enough to have gotten the chronic diseases like cancer, atherosclerosis, and diabetes generally associated with aging? Weren't their lives nasty, brutish, and short? Or how about this argument: Nature has no use for us after our reproductive years are over. Although we will address these issues in more depth in later chapters, this is a good place for a sanity check.

Let's try to find some common sense answers to these questions: First, the way evolution works, at least in the animal kingdom, (barring human interference) is that with few exceptions species evolve over time to become stronger, not weaker, and experts such as UCLA environmental historian and Pulitzer Prize winning author Jared Diamond discount statements to the contrary.  As mentioned earlier, these experts argue that our early ancestors would have lived long healthy lives except for three things: starvation, predators, and accidents (none of which has anything to do with illness).

As I also mentioned earlier, our Paleo Ancestors of about 400 generations ago were on average taller than we are today, had bone strength higher than ours, and had virtually perfect teeth, all indicators of robust health.  As we shall see in the following chapters, something happened in the last 400 generations to reverse this course and take us backward and downward.  Oh, regarding the ditty that Nature has no use for us after reproductive years, it is somewhat well established that Nature has endowed our cells with about a 120-year life, and that male humans have reproductive capacity their entire lives.  So, if this idea made any sense, males would far outlive females (they do not), who (for reasons we do not understand) run out of eggs way before 120.

It has puzzled me as to why it is so well entrenched in our culture that our ancestors led short lives filled with illness and high infant mortality.  Where did these stories come from?  Well it finally occurred to me that they were referring to a different group of our ancestors, and this is the reason I went to the trouble of defining the term Ancient with a capital A.  There is no question that the so-called ancient civilizations, such as the Egyptians, Greeks and Romans and their successors did indeed live short lives prone to illness and high infant mortality, and that is what these stories are referring to.  Because we expect, rightly so, that each generation would be healthier than the previous, which is the way Nature works when undisturbed, it is counterintuitive to think that our ancestors living before these civilizations could possibly have been healthier than later generations, but that is the case.  It is why I finally abandoned research into the so-called "ancient" medical wisdom of the Greeks and Romans and the Far East Dynasties, none of which are truly Ancient.  Why should I dwell on this body of knowledge when the generations before them were much healthier?  In my opinion, the Ancient time period is where the real health pearls of wisdom lie and, sure enough, that is what I found.

My research is based on what could be considered the largest "clinical trial" in the history of the human species, having been conducted and refined over a period of about 2.49 million years, and involving millions of our ancestors.  Until recently, (about 10,000 years ago) the results of these trials, from a health point of view, were a great success, which is why our species exists today.  It allowed our ancestors over most of the last two-and-a-half million years to survive in a quite healthy fashion.  This survival over eons has much to offer contemporary man who has strayed far from Nature's blueprint and who, despite the marvels of modern sanitation, medicine, and technology, wallows in chronic illness.

The ideas contained on these pages reflect my experience, an attempt to reconnect with Nature's fundamentals for the sake of my health.  I invite you to consider the ideas as possible tools for your own health.

## How To Use This Book

In the chapter that follows, I document what I call Faulty Human Trials – a list of Trial & Error experiments concocted by humans over the last 400 generations and foisted on virtually all of civilization.  These experiments are ongoing today, and in my humble opinion, either singly or in combination, are the causes of virtually all chronic illnesses because of their potential to produce toxins in the body.  I complete the chapter by disclosing how some of these experiments adversely affected my own life and how, by "opting out" of the experiments and going back in time to a prior point, I have been able to restore and maintain my health.

Section Two (Diet), Section Three (Detoxification), and Section Four (Lifestyle) set forth the entire Wellness Project.  They can act as a guide for readers should they want to follow the same route, and they are intended to nudge one into greater sync with Nature.

Regard this book as a blueprint for better health, and not a cookbook with recipes.  I will lay out my theories of how our heritage developed when we allowed Nature to be in charge.  These suggestions can have a powerful effect, and they helped me achieve relief from many annoying symptoms, giving me the ability to rise to a higher level of health.  The sincere intention of my hypothesis is illness prevention, and for those already ill, the reversal of the condition.  The approach is really a "one-size-fits-all" set of ideas based on alignment with Nature.  They are designed to benefit the body regardless of specific symptoms or illnesses, such as cancer or diabetes or Parkinson's or acne.  They are about proper (non toxic) foods that can be assimilated, periodically detoxifying the body to eliminate accumulated toxins, and shifting our lifestyle to one that is more closely aligned with our natural heritage, while still maintaining most of the comforts of today that we enjoy.

# Chapter 2 - Fooling (With) Mother Nature

*It's not nice to fool Mother Nature! -*
1970s Margarine Commercial

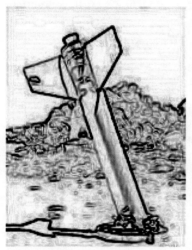

I like the concept of "Mother Nature." Somehow, I find it comforting to think of our designer in feminine terms – soft, comforting, and nurturing. Of course, She does exhibit some behavior that seems out of character – earthquakes, hurricanes, drought, a tiger taking down an antelope and tearing it to pieces. My point is that there are some things we like about Nature and others we do not and would like to change or at least control. We have an inkling about how She works (our so-called Laws of Nature), but for the most part we are quite clueless.

I would like to keep my writing style in this book as gender-neutral as possible, trying to avoid terms like Paleo Man and Mother Nature, so here is a shot at it. I will sometimes refer to our Paleo Ancestor as "PA," and to Mother Nature as "MA," with the caveat that we owe our existence to the fact that PA paid a great deal of attention to MA!

As a techno-geek, I have had an inflated sense that I understand how things work. I get a great deal of satisfaction in inventing and making things that perform, but these are not living things. My research into health has really humbled me. I have read many of the same texts used in medical schools, and it has opened my eyes as to how truly little we know about the world of *living things*. As I write this, I am looking out at an olive tree, realizing that we don't even fully understand the composition of a single leaf, or why it is different from a pear tree leaf. I now know that there is no way in my lifetime that I will be able to understand the workings of nature in sufficient detail to reproduce a living thing from scratch, or even to modify the way my body works in ways that Nature did not intend, without the possibility of causing harm. So, my best bet is to try to find out what Nature did intend for me, and to stick to it as closely as possible. The real beauty of this approach is that I do not have to understand *why* we evolved to eat certain foods or follow a particular lifestyle, or even to understand how the body works – it is enough just to know the plan. This is an enormous relief and allows me to concentrate on preparing the blueprint for wellness, which is really Nature's blueprint, not mine. My task is to figure it out as best as possible and document it.

The reason I have spent the last few paragraphs dwelling on Nature is in preparation for a discussion of what I consider to be some major experiments directly affecting our health. These are in the form of Trial & Error experiments conducted by humans over the last 10,000 years (and still going on today) that undoubtedly had and continue to have a major negative impact on the health of a significant portion of the population by directly or indirectly raising the body's toxin burden. One can look at these experiments as attempts to fool or change Mother Nature in ways that are supposed to provide a benefit to our species that Nature has not provided. In my opinion, we may fool *with* Nature (that is, we have the *ability* to launch these experiments), but to think that in our lifetime, or even over a hundred generations, we can actually cause Nature to modify her plan for us, evolved over 2.5 million years, is somewhat unrealistic. To remind myself of my relationship with Nature, I periodically go to the beach and walk out into the ocean, positioning myself squarely in front of a large breaking wave – very humbling.

## Ten Thousand Years of Human Experiments

Referring to Table 1, I have listed what I consider to be some of the major experiments conducted by humans over the last 400 or so generations, which have the potential of adversely affecting our health and are moving some of us (the *others*) down the road to illness. However, for many of the *winners* in our society, some of the items on this list would not be viewed as a problem at all, because they have little or no negative health impact on their health. For the rest of us, these Trial & Error experiments have proved faulty because their intended outcome, while initially designed to improve our lives, is causing or contributing to illness in our body by increasing its toxic load. In many instances, we have yet to recognize that fact, or if we do recognize it, to take the necessary action to stop it. One reason for our lack of recognition is the long interval between the start of the trial and the manifestation of the error, so that we have lost track of the cause/effect relationship. As part of this problem, we have also lost the reference point or baseline that we started with, leaving us with meaningless comparisons to arbitrary reference points. Another reason is our lack of knowledge of how the body works, leaving us clueless as to how a cause could possibly result in a particular effect. As part of this problem, researchers have confused necessary causes with sufficient causes for various conditions, and confused correlation with causation, leading to incorrect conclusions capable of doing harm. The protocols for treating skin cancer and cholesterol are only two examples of these errors.

I have limited the list (which if it included all of the ecological insults to us and our environment, would have gone on for pages) to those items that are somewhat under our control as individuals and that can be either changed or at least dealt with personally through reasonable effort, and which affect large segments of society. In Section 2 of this book I will discuss each in detail, touching on the motivation for the experiment, the impact it has had on humans, and at least one way to "opt out" of it. In a way, this is an attempt to return to Nature's evolutionary experiment, picking up where we left off before we meddled with the plan.

As I mentioned before, all of these are ongoing experiments, so one must assume that somebody considers them worthwhile. These "somebodies" are very powerful entities indeed, including virtually the entire Western and Eastern health and dental communities (including a substantial portion of the alternative health industry), as well as food, cosmetic and chemical industries (and governments and universities) worldwide. They certainly do not consider the items on my list as faulty, since in many cases they form the backbone of their businesses or are major contributors to their income. There really is no money in discrediting the items on this list. To the contrary, there is enormous money at stake to perpetuate these experiments. How can toilet paper be a faulty experiment in health? (See Chapter 15 for the answer.)

| Table 1 |
|---|
| Ten Thousand Years of Fooling With Mother Nature |
| **A Partial List of Potentially Faulty Human Trials** |

| | |
|---|---|
| Eating Grains | Fluoridation |
| Eating Dairy/Pasteurization | Amalgam Fillings |
| Eating Concentrated Sugars | Root Canals |
| Feeding Unnatural Food to our Food | Heavy Metals in the Environment |
| The Germ Theory | Halogens in the Environment |
| The Cholesterol Theory | Toilet Paper |
| Eating Plants Protected by Nature | Antiperspirants |
| Artificial Sweeteners | The Skin Cancer Theory |
| Infant Formulas | The Osteoporosis Theory |
| Ingesting Ice | Tight Clothing |
| Chlorinated Water | Plastic Food Containers |

# What is an Experiment?

I will admit that in my chosen fields of rocket science and electronics, controlled experiments are much easier to conduct and explain than in the life sciences. One reason is the ease with which we can define a starting point or baseline for a human-made object before we begin the experiment, making it much easier to establish a control and a cause/effect relationship, all of which are important if we expect the conclusions drawn from the experiment to have any validity. Why am I dwelling on experiments? Well, if my goal is to opt out of the dozens of experiments listed in Table 1, I should back up this decision with as much reason, analysis, and common sense as possible. Further, the collective wisdom of modern medicine comes from research experiments that have been documented in various journals, so it behooves us to take a careful look. In the following paragraphs, I will take the reader on a short journey into the world of experiments (I also refer to them as trials) in the life sciences from my "launch pad" perspective. Experiments usually begin with a hypothesis, simply defined as "an educated guess" – a suggested solution based on some knowledge or experience. Another way to define hypothesis is as a proposal suggesting a possible correlation between multiple phenomena. A hypothesis can gain enough strength from successful experiments to eventually graduate to a theory, and then to a law.

For purposes of this book, I am going to define "Experiment" (spelled with a capital E) as a method of research devised by humans and based on a hypothesis that includes an inference of cause and effect. Two groups of subjects neither of which have been nor are undergoing any other human devised experiment, are treated exactly alike in all ways except one, the independent variable. Differences in the behavior of the Experimental and Control group, which cannot be accounted for by experimental error, are then attributed to the effect of the experimental treatment. To me, the underlined phrase is critical to a meaningful definition when it comes to experimentation on living things. This condition of the subject (s) prior to the experiment is what I have called the "Baseline."

Given my definition for Experiment, there also can be a corollary definition for what I will call subsequent experimentation, where one or more human-devised, fully documented experiments have already been conducted on a subject. In this event, any reports on these experiments must fully disclose all previous human experiments to which that subject has been exposed. In my opinion, failure to do so can, produce virtually meaningless results.

A threshold problem I see in the life sciences fields is that there is no consensus as to the "baseline" of the living thing on which they intend to conduct an experiment, whether it is a rat, mouse, guinea pig, monkey, or human. Why do we care about a baseline? Well, here is an example that will hopefully illustrate my point and show the complexity and detail that I believe is necessary to produce meaningful results in the field of medical and health research.

Let's say I want to conduct an experiment on rats to see the effect of a calorie restricted diet (CRD) on their health and longevity. Normally, in the world of animal studies as it exists today, researchers simply contact one of many organizations that supply caged lab rats and purchase a bunch, or they may have their own breeding facilities. These rats come in many varieties, each bred to produce certain traits deemed useful in different experiments. The odds that bred lab rats have been subjected to prior human devised experiments are 100%, based on the fact that selective breeding *is* a human devised experiment. So, you get these rats and, following convention, put them into cages in your lab, begin feeding them rat chow that you bought from a distributor or directly from the manufacturer (usually one of the mega-agricultural companies), and divide them into control and experimental groups in preparation for the experiment. Because of the environment in which these rats were bred and raised, I can name at least three additional human-devised experiments that have simultaneously been running even before you have started your experiment. The rats have been removed from (or never were in) their natural environment, whereby 1) they have been separated from physical contact with the earth; 2) they have been exposed only to artificial lighting, not sunlight; and 3) they have been fed an unnatural diet.

The above example is not hypothetical – this experiment has been and is continuing to be conducted by many research institutions. Some time ago, I had a conversation with an executive of a foundation that has poured millions of dollars into studies of this kind in an effort to advance their mission of "anti-aging" research, hopefully, to be applied to humans. He was proud of the fact that the research had shown that a calorie-restricted diet increased the longevity of the experimental group versus the control group of rats. I told him that from my analysis of the research, what their millions had really proved was that when you feed rats food that contains ingredients that rats are not evolutionarily adapted to eat (rat chow), you are slowly poisoning them. Thus, if you restrict the intake of such poison, they will live longer than those fed larger doses. This is not rocket science; it is common sense and can easily have been predicted without spending a nickel. As you will see from the hypothesis in this book, the same is true for humans. The answer is not calorie restriction – it is to switch to foods that we (and the foods we eat) are evolutionarily adapted to eat. Think about it - does starvation seem synonymous with increased health in the evolutionary scheme of things? The only time I have seen animals voluntarily fast is when they have eaten a toxic substance or are otherwise ill. Analyzing the experiment more closely, we can see that the coexisting experiment of feeding the subjects rat chow has a major impact on the conclusions to be drawn from the current experiment of food reduction.

Let's look at rat chow. One of the most popular lab rat chows contains ground corn, soybean meal, beet pulp, and a variety of other processed foods as well as artificial preservatives and synthetic vitamins. The ratio of macro to micronutrients is fixed by the chow formula. Questions immediately come to mind as to whether the corn or soybeans come from genetically modified (GMO) crops, and whether the ingredients were tested for toxins such as pesticides (after all, a rat is considered a pest!). Certified rat chows are available that are tested for some toxins, as are irradiated chows, designed to be bacteria free. I tried to get answers to some of these questions by researching the CRD studies and the various rat chows used in each, but I could not get definitive answers to these basic questions. If the study is designed to evaluate the effects of restricting the quantity of food given to rats, isn't the food itself a (or maybe *the*) critical variable? Shouldn't it be analyzed to the ultimate extent possible, tracing each ingredient back to its ultimate source? Where were the corn/soybeans grown? What fertilizers and pesticides were used? What was the source of the seed stock? Of course the biggest question of all is which of these ingredients, if any, would be considered natural food for a rat in its native environment?

In aerospace and many military programs, traceability is mandatory. Materials can be traced by lot number back to the mine, if necessary. After suggesting to this fellow that millions may have been wasted to determine that rat chow is lousy cuisine for rats, I offered to discuss a different set of experiments that might prove to be much more interesting, but by then I was talking to the wall. I undoubtedly completely lost him when I also suggested that the very concept of "anti-aging" is fooling with Nature and quite unnecessary. After all, our cellular clocks have a lifetime of 120 years. The trick is not to stop aging, but to age while remaining completely healthy until the clock runs out. To me, anti-aging is another word for death.

Well, you might ask, what was my suggestion for these other experiments? Keep in mind my definition of Experiment (not subsequent experiment), meaning that I want "clean" rats that have not been (or been minimally) tampered with by humans. So, my baseline for rats to be used in this experiment are ones that has lived their whole life out in the wild in an environment shielded from human activity, and who have descended from many similar generations. While I do not know their history out in Nature, at least I do know that humans have not grossly tampered with them. I presume that for far less than the millions already spent, a reasonable sum would be all that is necessary to find these pristine creatures.

I would divide a bunch of these rats into three groups. The first two groups would be put through the same experiment described above – in the cage, one group gets all the rat chow they want, the other group is restricted. The third group is actually left outside in a natural environment that would be fenced off to eliminate predators and to confine the rats, but large enough so as to give them their natural foraging space. This environment would ideally be the one in which they were raised, so that they have full access to all of their clean natural food sources, which they can mix and match to their heart's content. As you will see later in this book, the foraging space should also include products of nature that a rat would use for self-medication, perhaps including certain normally toxic plants, as well as medicinal dirt such as clay. Rodent experts would be consulted to ensure the environment was as naturally correct as possible.

Now, the objective would be to see which group wins the longevity contest. While I am betting on the outside group, I honestly don't know the answer and could be rudely disappointed (not the first time), thus restoring my humility (like standing in front of a wave). Actually, I really would like to see what happens, because the outcome has a strong bearing on the theory that "Mother Nature knows best." If one wanted to take the experiment to another level, a forth group could be added, which would be another, but separated, outside group that had only limited access to their natural food sources, to see the effect of calorie restriction on this naturally raised and fed group. One of my goals in writing this book is to interest others to join with me to fund experiments such as these in an effort to learn more about what Mother Nature had in mind for us.

Some experiments in this direction have been taking place recently with respect to comparing the anti-aging effects of CRDs with non-calorie restricted diets containing various nutritional supplements. In particular, diets supplemented with resveratrol, a chemical naturally found in some plants, particularly in berries such as grapes and blueberries, have compared favorably with CRDs in animal longevity studies. As I write this book, the results of a study were released where the effects on longevity markers in mice fed a CRD were compared to a group on a regular diet supplemented by small amounts or resveratrol. The researchers found that resveratrol, in doses easily achievable in human diets, produced anti-aging results that mimicked, and in some instances surpassed, those achieved for the CRD group [12]. To me, this is clear evidence that eating the right foods can easily achieve all of the anti-aging effects of calorie restriction.

A final point I want to make here again relates to the definition of *healthy*. What the authors of the calorie restricted diet studies are claiming is that these diets are healthy, begging the question "healthy as compared to what?' If the answer is: when compared to eating rat chow or the Standard American Diet (SAD) diet, then I agree. However, the Wellness Diet was established to act as the ultimate reference point for future diet studies, because it is the lowest in natural toxins of all of the conventional diets, and has 99,000 generations of human trials behind it. By the way, an important component of the Wellness Diet is fruit, so it is naturally loaded with resveratrol!

## My Personal Experiences with Faulty Trials

As a prelude to a discussion of The Wellness Project that developed from my heritage/environment hypothesis, I think it may be of interest to the reader if I outline my personal experiences with some of the potentially faulty technology I listed in Table 1. At the time I was a "participant" in these trials, I had no idea they *were* trials, nor did I know that the symptoms I was manifesting were in fact the Error phase of these T&E experiments. How nice it would be if we all had built-in red lights that would illuminate with an error message when we are eating or doing something detrimental to our health. However, as you will see, Nature does provide us with clues; we just need to be cognizant of them. As I write this chronology, I will periodically inject hindsight wisdom that I acquired only decades later and after a great deal of research.

Starting with the first five years since my birth in the 1940s in New York City, I, like every other child in those days, was on the receiving end of multiple vaccinations. Included in those injections was thimerosal, a mercury compound used to protect vaccines against microbes. Today, thimerosal is still used in vaccines (the flu shot contains it) but has become the focus of rising controversy. Some experts say it has contributed to the sharp rise in autism. Mercury is widely considered the second most potent neurotoxin in nature, behind plutonium. It is extremely harmful to the body, and injecting it into humans is truly insane.

I was bottle fed with pasteurized cow's milk, and then weaned to the Standard American Diet (I will refer to this throughout the book as the SAD diet), consisting of grains, dairy, meat, chicken, eggs, some fish, vegetables, and fruit. Foods were sugared to taste. Crisco® (hydrogenated corn oil) and margarine were in wide use. Well, I did quite poorly, becoming a very fussy eater and failing to gain weight. In hindsight – through exhaustive testing and my own trial-and-error experiments over the years, I have discovered that I am gluten intolerant (= no grains); I am lactose, casein and whey intolerant (= no dairy); and egg albumin intolerant (= no egg whites). My well-meaning parents kept trying to push these foods on me and in an effort to please, I ate what I could.

One of the vaccinations I received, including a booster at about 6 years old, was the so-called DPT shot to protect against diphtheria, pertussis, and tetanus. In my case, it did just the opposite and I came down with diphtheria, a bacterial disease that can be life threatening. It is uncommon to develop an infection that is precisely the infection you are being vaccinated against, unless the vaccine is faulty in some way, but I will never know the ultimate cause. I was one of a handful of diphtheria cases in New York at the time, where the incidence was primarily among immigrants who had contracted it before arriving in the United States and to which I had no exposure, so I was an oddity. To keep me alive, one of the doctors plied me with a new medicine called penicillin. They were trying it out somewhat experimentally, using massive doses, and I ended up as a "successful case history." At that time doctors made house calls, and I remember the doctor sticking his finger down my throat to break the membrane that had grown across it, making it very hard to breathe or swallow, a hallmark of diphtheria. The doctor's intervention kept me alive while the penicillin was working. I obviously survived.

I should probably be grateful for the antibiotics, but at most, the gratitude is qualified. If it were not for the vaccination, the odds are very strong that I would not have contracted diphtheria in the first place. The vaccinations introduced mercury into an obviously sensitive body. We are just starting to learn of the devastating effects mercury has on the defense system as well as the nervous system, making it doubly unreasonable to administer a vaccine designed to strengthen the defense system, along with an element that weakens it. I am not arguing that vaccines *per se* are bad, but I am arguing that the way they have been and continue to be implemented is fraught with errors. I can tell you that the "fixes" used in today's vaccines to eliminate thimerosal also border on the dangerous – how do you feel about you or your young children being injected with aluminum (also a neurotoxin), or MSG (a neurotoxic flavoring agent), or formaldehyde (a carcinogen) [13]? Well, the massive doses of penicillin injected into me to control the infection also destroyed the natural beneficial bacterial flora in my intestines that make up a major part of my defense system and perform many other essential functions. I did not know any of this as a child, of course, and neither did the medical community. I did not figure it out until years later.

After the diphtheria episode, strange symptoms started to pop up. For starters, I developed hay fever and allergies to just about everything, along with chronic sore throats and earaches. The doctors decided to remove my tonsils and adenoids because, in their opinion, they were unnecessary and the cause of my problems. Here is a classic example of making the wrong decisions when you don't know how the organism works. Physicians routinely used to remove tonsils and adenoids in those days. Some in the medical community now know that tonsils and adenoids function as part of the immune system, and therefore removal is not as automatic. Tonsils and adenoids are anything but unnecessary. They are all part of the lymph system, the body's garbage collection system, about which doctors know little. I remember going to the UCLA medical school bookstore years later, asking for books devoted to the lymph system, and they couldn't find any! Knowledge, of course, evolves and just as the tonsils and adenoids have been found to have specific roles in the design of the body, so too has the appendix been finally connected with functionality. Researchers at Duke University recently announced that the generally considered superfluous appendix actually supports and protects friendly bacteria in the body [14]. Nature always has its reasons, even if we don't know what they are.

Additional symptoms that cropped up in my teens were odd skin rashes, and an immense craving for foods containing grains, like rye bread and pretzels, which caused excessive weight gain. As far as the rest of my diet was concerned, I was not much different from other kids my age. I ate candy, packaged foods, white bread, bologna, and other processed meats, and guzzled my share of sugared soft drinks. Well, that took its toll on my teeth, leading to the usual cavities and "silver" fillings.

It was not until decades later that I began to find answers to the symptom puzzle. About this time, I stumbled across a series of books that led me out of the wilderness of conventional medicine and towards a promised land of healing. Two of the most important books were by Drs. Orion Truss and William Crook [15] [16]. They believed that a yeast organism called Candida, which normally lives in the human intestine, could multiply under conditions of weakened immunity and secrete quantities of toxins that disrupt normal metabolism, causing or worsening a vast range of health problems. The "yeast syndrome," as it was referred to by yet a third author, John Trowbridge [17], could include localized infections, but also widespread problems; for instance in the digestive tract and skin. I was still suffering from skin problems, food cravings, and allergies. Were these problems related to yeast?

I contacted a dermatology professor referenced in several of the books on yeast overgrowth, and he recommended an anti-fungal medication, which my dermatologist knew nothing about. I tried the UCLA dermatology clinic, but the doctors there knew nothing as well. It turns out that most conventional doctors still do not accept the idea that yeast overgrowth has systemic repercussions. I finally found a holistic MD who agreed to write a prescription for Nizoral®, one of the early azole families of systemic antifungals. Bingo! The rashes, the cravings, and the allergies all disappeared within two weeks. I quickly adopted what is now called the "anti-Candida" diet, essentially free of grains, dairy, and sugars. As you will see, in some respects this diet resembles our Ancient diet, and has been found to restore health in a number of different conditions. I have followed various versions of this diet for more than 20 years.

With the benefit of hindsight and research, it is now obvious that antibiotics destroy beneficial bacteria in the gut that normally control yeast overgrowth, leading to numerous skin problems, even including dandruff (now believed caused by *malassezia*, a genus of fungi), gut problems, and a symptom list that runs for several pages. While we normally refer to *Candida albicans* as the major culprit, there are millions of fungal and related yeast species in Nature, mostly unidentified, some of which have been shown to be quite beneficial to our health. The bottom line is that antibiotic use disturbs the natural flora in our gut in ways that are mostly unpredictable. Very recent studies have further implicated mercury in the gut disturbance equation, and I will discuss this in the next section.

Well, I felt great by following the anti-Candida diet. As part of that diet, I ate fish every day, sometimes twice a day. It's a very healthy food, right? My favorite was tuna, backed up by swordfish, sea bass, and mahi-mahi. Also during this time, I became enamored with alternative health, having read the classic book *Life Extension* by Durk Pearson and Sandy Shaw [18]. I self-experimented with gobs of supplements and was full of energy. I had no idea at the time that these supplements, touted by the alternative health community as great stuff, were in fact feeding the bad guys still in my gut as the result of the mercury in the fish I was eating, all of which was setting me up for more health problems down the road. Periodic visits to the dentist produced the usual metal fillings and crown replacements as the old ones from my childhood wore out.

It took 20 years until another set of odd health symptoms began to appear. Strange skin rashes, one around an ankle, another around the chest area, occasional fatigue, muscle cramps, twitching/zapping sensations, cold hands, dry eyes, chronic nasal congestion, a heel spur, occasional headaches, changes in bowel function, heartburn, frequent urination, hypoglycemia (low blood sugar), and hypotension (low blood pressure). Individually, these symptoms would be merely annoying, but collectively they were a real pain. During this time, I was deeply involved in building a high tech company and taking it public and did not have a lot of time to research these issues.

When I did have time, I consulted with many doctors for this dizzying array of symptoms and got as many different diagnoses. I underwent dozens of tests over a five-year period and saw multiple dermatologists, endocrinologists, gastrointestinal specialists, cardiologists, internists and self-proclaimed alternative health gurus. I was pretty fed up with the repeated failure to get an explanation for my symptoms. For me, conventional medicine—despite all its so-called "breakthroughs" and razzle-dazzle technology—was turning out to be a big bust again as it had been many years before. Fortunately, my company became a Wall Street hit and soon after, I opted to take a brief retirement. After a few years lolling on the beaches of Hawaii to recharge, I decided to jump into the field of health with both feet to attempt not only to figure out my issues, but also to try to finally get some answers as to why the world was in a health crisis. Why was "adult diabetes" appearing in children? Why was autism now an epidemic? Why, after 50 years and billions of dollars were we nowhere in solving the cancer riddle or the heart disease riddle? What was going on with all of these chronic degenerative diseases starting to plague my friends?

I read everything I could find in the fields of Western and Eastern medicine to try to understand their approaches to chronic illness. I explored many of the conventional and exotic areas of alternative health, from chiropractic, muscle testing, osteopathy, homeopathy, naturopathies, energy medicine and "healing machines" of all sorts, every diet program you could think of from vegan to Atkins, meditation and mind-body work from Reich to Rolf. I investigated the claims of the "gurus" in each field that "they had the answer"; and along the way collected various board certifications in nutrition and alternative health. I self-experimented with many modalities and tried hundreds of supplement regimens. The bottom line was I found that all of this stuff lacked the scientific rigor of my profession; the human body was way too complicated to be understood sufficiently to run experiments on large groups of people as was being done; and none of it was likely to get off the launch pad in my lifetime (or that of my grandchildren at the rate they were going).

When I finally grasped the gravity of my conclusions, it deeply saddened me because it was obvious that I could not entrust my health (other than for physical repairs from accidents or injuries) to the health community. I had to take charge and figure it out for myself to the best of my ability, and this was the perfect time in my life to do so. As I got older, I realized that my most important asset was my health, and as any student of business will tell you, it makes sense to devote a substantial portion of your resources to protecting such an asset. As one sage said, "If I don't have a healthy body, where will I live?"

It was at about this point in time that I concluded there was no way I was going to understand how the body worked – it was way too complicated and made rocket science look like child's play. So, I embarked on the road to consulting with our designer, Nature, which provided me with the answers I was looking for. I took steps to align myself with what I perceived was Nature's plan, and sure enough my symptoms slowly resolved. Along the way, I refined my diet to align more closely with what our Paleo Ancestors were likely to have eaten, based on a combination of research, common sense, and educated guesses. I felt good and had quite a bit of symptom relief with this natural diet, but some symptoms persisted, leading me to the suspicion that while the correct diet was a necessary element for health, it was not sufficient. Something was missing, and additional research into the field of animal behavior produced what would turn out to be the answer. Remarkably, animals have been observed to spend a great deal of energy throughout their lifetime performing tasks that we now know (or should know) are designed to cleanse their bodies of toxic organisms and other substances. I say "should know" because even in the field of animal behavior there is controversy as to whether animals possess the ability to self-medicate (known as zoopharmacognosy).

For a sanity check, I went back to the engineering drawing board and took another look at how I would attempt to define the operation of a chemical factory (me). The critical parameters are (1) the input (what are the starting materials –i.e. diet), (2) the output (what is the factory designed to produce when it is working correctly – i.e. a healthy, happy person), and (3) waste management and maintenance (primarily involving the removal of unwanted waste products that interfere with the desired chemical reactions). The missing link for my health study was the removal of unwanted products that interfere with the desired healthy chemical reactions. Others and I refer to this as detoxification (detox for short) and it is dealt with at length in Part Three.

Once I figured that out, I decided to test myself for toxic metals. I was stunned to learn from a hair toxic mineral test that I was 1300 percent over the normal limit for mercury! How could this have happened? I concluded that it probably was partially a result of my habit of eating fish every day for over 20 years. There are now numerous studies that show the large fish I was eating are highly contaminated with mercury, so I stopped eating fish until I could figure out what to do next. Because the half-life of mercury in the body can be as long as 50 years, undoubtedly the thimerosal in the vaccinations I'd had as a kid, and the mercury in the "silver" fillings in my mouth also contributed to this toxic burden. My mercury revelation opened the door to the world of detoxification and I plunged in with great enthusiasm, studying everything I could find, attending lectures, consulting with specialists in the field and, of course, self-experimenting, sometimes with very unexpected results.

In some respects, human detoxification using natural means is a very old phenomenon that has been largely forgotten or ignored, and I have found that studying the habits of animals may be the best way to reconstruct this lost knowledge. Detoxification using artificial means is a relatively new field and is becoming increasingly necessary to help our bodies cope with the toxin types and doses that Nature never intended for our bodies, primarily caused by faulty human experiments. I remain very active in researching this field, and new breakthroughs continue to occur. This is another area where outside research funds are sorely needed, since the usual funding sources either ignore the toxification problem or dismiss it.

As I put myself though various detoxification programs over time, stubborn symptoms began to fall away. Not overnight, but slowly and steadily, and the more I detoxified the healthier I felt. As I saw the problems gradually ebbing, I had confidence in staying the course. As you will see in the section on detox, staying the course can be a challenge because detoxing can initially worsen existing symptoms and/or produce new symptoms. Further, detoxing can be an agonizingly slow process (weeks, months, years) depending upon the toxin, the level and duration of toxicity, and how well the body's natural detox pathways have been operating.

Among many other things, the odd rashes I had disappeared, the same ones that no doctor could figure out. Interestingly, one rash that had been diagnosed as Grover's Disease (a.k.a. transient acantholytic dermatosis, cause and treatment unknown) was recently linked to mercury toxicity by dermatologist Paul Dantzig at my alma mater, Columbia University. Dr. Danzig's pioneering work has also uncovered a link between mercury toxicity and certain forms of psoriasis, discussed more fully in the mercury detox section below [19].

As a recap of my health history (and likely that of plenty of other people), I was duly vaccinated as a child with all of the mercury-containing vaccines developed and approved by the medical community; I was treated with antibiotics, still the drug of choice in the medical community for bacterial infections (which in my case happened to be caused by one of the vaccines), and it wiped out my intestinal flora, causing fungal overgrowth; I had my tonsils and adenoids removed as the approved treatment for sore throats (which were caused by the fungal overgrowth), thus removing an important part of my immune system; I ate FDA food-pyramid approved foods, including lots of fish, the poster child of healthy foods, which turned out to be loaded with mercury (and other toxic chemicals); I had mercury amalgam fillings placed three inches from my brain as the approved practice of the dental community, and which were required as a result of my eating the FDA (Food and Drug Administration) approved foods. Along the way, I started taking all sorts of supplements recommended by the alternative health community, which ended up feeding the disturbed flora in my gut, leading to more health issues.

What's wrong with this picture? Everything. The sad part of all of this is that it took so long for me to realize that I could no longer play by other people's rules when it came to my health, and that I had to become my own doctor. The good news is that it resulted in The Wellness Project, so lets get on to it.

# Chapter 3 - An Overview of the Project

*Life in all its Fullness is Mother Nature Obeyed*

– Weston A. Price

The discussion that follows could be thought of as a roadmap that can be followed by individuals to reach or remain at a pinnacle of health. As mentioned earlier, the hypothesis behind the program states that by increasing our personal alignment with our heritage as evolved in Nature, we increase our chances of leading a life devoid of illness as a result of reducing the toxic burden on our body. Although I sometimes call this "my hypothesis," I am certainly not the first to propose it with respect to diet, and there are many studies available on the subject of Paleo diets [20]. However, the personal path I took to arrive at this hypothesis and the conclusions drawn from it are very different.

What I have found in the literature on the subject of how our Paleo Ancestors may have conducted their lives is almost exclusively directed toward diet, and even then, there is disagreement. The studies I am familiar with either use modern hunter-gatherer societies as their models, or limit their studies to the late Paleo Era, after PA had learned to cook. These models yield vastly different results than the one in this book, which takes into account the approximately 2.4 million years of our heritage that seems to have been ignored by others.

To avoid confusion I choose to call my version of the diet the Wellness Diet, and as you will see, my version is quite different from the others. While diet is certainly a necessary element in the health equation, it alone does not appear to be sufficient, which is why there is a large section of The Wellness Project devoted to detoxification. Where possible, in each area of description, I have attempted to list what I consider the "purist" approach as well as some suggestions for those who prefer more leeway in what they eat. While the purist level may seem Spartan in today's world, the purpose of defining it is to establish the baseline for our species – the dividing line between Nature's 2.4 million-year experiment in evolving our species and our follow-on experiments. Without this baseline as a starting point, it is impossible to know with any degree of certainty what effect dietary experiments have had on our species (remember the rat chow experiment). While some might consider the Wellness Diet an experiment, from my point of view what you are presently eating may well be the experiment, with the Wellness Diet representing the truly non-experimental, naturally evolved eating plan for humanity.

Each of us brings to the table a lifetime of following a different diet and lifestyle, and each of us has a different toxin profile that can drastically shape the outcome of our choices. Add to this our individual genetic and other variations and the picture gets more complicated. This is the reason for my purist approach – because we don't have an owner's manual to consult, my goal is to get as close as possible to what Nature intended, in order to maximize the chances that this program will achieve positive results for you. Animal studies seem to bear this out – a particular species rarely experiments with their lifestyle unless compelled to do so by environmental changes, and even then, it is done with great caution. Humans on the other hand have the luxury (or perhaps curse) to experiment upon themselves without caution or even a plan of action. You can get up in the morning and decide to become a vegan, never once having to consider all the implications for your body, which may not be in favor of that decision at all.

Does everyone have to follow this wellness plan to remain healthy? The answer is no. I am convinced that there are folks out there that are disposed to lead a perfectly health life for 100 years eating nothing but cake, ice cream and soda! Are you one of them? I feel confident that I am not. The problem with this view of health is that we only get the answer in hindsight, and since there is no dress rehearsal for life, I for one don't like the odds. I do not mind being a risk-taker in business, but not with my health.

Throughout the book, I will be suggesting literature and websites as reference material for specific issues that I discuss. Many of these references also contain additional information, in many cases regarding diet in general, that conflicts with what is suggested in this book. On the one hand, for those of you interested in comparing and contrasting differing viewpoints on what others consider ancestral diets, this should prove quite instructive. On the other hand, I hope you will find the reasoning put forward in these chapters sufficiently compelling to place The Wellness Diet at the top of your list.

On a last note, viewing The Wellness Project as a change of lifestyle, I urge the reader to consider his/her priorities in life. This, of course, becomes a very esoteric and philosophical exercise that begs the question of why are we here? What is Nature's plan, if any? Reproduction is a clear goal of any living species, but beyond that, I have no answers except as applied to myself, and even those have changed over time. My personal answer is to set happiness as a major goal, which then shifts the inquiry to finding what makes you happy. As it turns out, Weston Price's statement that "life in all its fullness is mother nature obeyed" has rung true for me – I get a great deal of pleasure and satisfaction knowing I am doing the best I can to understand and follow a personal plan evolved by Nature. One purpose of writing this book is to introduce what has given me so much pleasure in the hope that it may do so for others.

# Section Two - Diet

*Thou shouldst eat to live; not live to eat.* Socrates

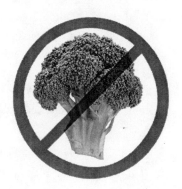 How can you tell the good stuff to eat from the bad? Getting the correct answer to this question is critical to one's health, since I believe that eating foods that are not in accord with your heritage may have the affect of adding toxins to your body at every meal. For many of us, doing that for decades can so burden our defense system that it cannot perform correctly, because either it is overworked, or it can no longer differentiate toxic cells from normal ones in our body, leading to autoimmune issues. If you are in good health, it may be safe to assume that you have made wise food choices, and therefore there is no need to make any dietary changes. In that case, you may want to read this section just as a matter of intellectual curiosity, or you may want to self-experiment with portions of the diet on an occasional basis just for fun.

Most readers of books that contain a diet plan assume, undoubtedly correctly, that the author is attempting to convince them to change their existing food choices and adopt the author's diet. I want to state at the outset that it is not my goal to convince the reader to change anything having to do with their diet or eating habits. My purpose is to define an eating plan that is a baseline, or starting point, defined by Nature, that is safe for anyone to eat, and which has the lowest levels of natural toxins. A reader's decision regarding adopting all or part of this diet should be based on their present level of health and desire to improve it, their heritage, and their interest in experimenting with new food choices.

Knowing the baseline diet, you can also make informed choices such as sticking to it only some of the time, like once a week, and seeing what happens to your health. You may choose to follow it only when you feel under the weather or are under stress (chronic stress is a toxin), the idea being to unburden your defense system from potentially toxic foods so it can deal with other issues. The diet is divided into three tiers of food choices, beginning with the baseline version, Tier One, and ending up with Tier Three, which includes virtually all food choices. One simple way to navigate among these food choices is as a function of your present level of health. If you are healthy, you may wish to continue following your present food choices, narrowing them only in the event you are or become less than fully healthy, all the way to the Tier One diet choices. A lot of information is presented to assist you in making those food choices based on clues from Nature.

Ten different nutritionists may give you ten different answers to the question of what you should eat. As it turns out, they may all be correct, or not. You will see from the following discussion on diet that as our ancestors moved out of Africa and spread around the globe, they adapted to their local food sources (at least the winners did) and over many generations aligned their heritage with their food environment. If we could trace, with a great deal of certainty, our lineage on both sides of our family over many generations to a particular monolithic society somewhere in the world, and we knew their eating habits, it would be quite safe to assume that we could follow their ancestral diet without compromising our health. Since that approach is likely to be limited to only a small segment of the population, another approach is needed. I have taken the following direction. If we go back far enough into our past prior to our ancestors leaving their African roots, we will have in fact traced our common lineage (for all humans) to a single monolithic group in a fixed part of the world. Then, if we could determine their diet at that point in time, my hypothesis is that every one of us could safely eat it, and I would expect it to be very low in toxins. So, my first challenge was to find that very Ancient diet and assess its characteristics. Follow me!

One way to look at Nature in action, at least as it relates to us, is through the perspective of anthropology. That means taking a spin back 2.5 million years ago—about 100,000 generations—to when homo-erectus emerged on the global scene. The description of the human time line below is my personal distillation of many of the theories in the field as to what happened when. Please understand that the best one can do in this area is to piece together a very limited amount of fragmentary evidence and make educated inferences. Some additional information can be gleaned from studies of other primates, particularly chimpanzees, and modern hunter-gatherer societies.

From my point of view, the biggest human experiment of all in our dietary history was the use of fire to heat and/or cook potential sources of food. I will use the word cooking also to refer to merely heating food. There is no consensus among researchers as to when this event may have first occurred. Credible estimates range from 20,000 to about 150,000 years ago (a major variable is the time difference between the ability to make fire and its widespread use in cooking food). As we shall see, the very act of heating or cooking did not have an extreme impact on availability of our animal food sources. It just made it easier to chew and digest these foods, which may have led to a smaller jaw and dental changes, perhaps leaving room for a larger brain. However, cooking had a major impact on our plant sources of food.

Extensive research in this field yields the fact that a majority of potential plant foods available to PA are toxic to humans when consumed raw, and hence were inedible until the development of cooking. Some other plant foods that might not have been extremely toxic were unavailable or impractical for eating, such as certain nuts in extremely hard shells, until heating burst the shells and made the food available. Because I consider cooking a human experiment and I want the Wellness Diet to predate such activity, the purist version of the diet will be looking at plant foods that are safely edible before cooking, whenever that occurred. As you will see, this simple criterion provides some surprising results when compared to other Paleo diet studies.

This is a good point to define "toxic" as we shall use it in the context of foods. The words "toxic" or "toxins" as used in this chapter refers to *natural* substances found in foods that produce a deleterious effect when ingested by humans. It does not refer to human-made toxins that affect food, such as pesticides, genetic modifications, growth hormones, etc., which I will refer to as contamination in this chapter. The natural toxin effect can range from a rapid lethal reaction to much more subtle effects produced only by prolonged ingestion of a given food. In order to assess toxicity, we will look at chemical analyses of food as well as our genetic cousins, the chimpanzees, to observe their food choices in an effort to find Nature's clues regarding what is safest to eat.

An assumption I have made in this study is that the "Out of Africa" theory of human evolution is correct – that is, our ancestors began in Africa and migrated from there to other parts of the world. It is still the major theory in the field, but there are alternative theories such as that our ancestors sprung up independently at various points of the globe and that not all originated from Africa.

The evolutionary theory we will be following begins with Homo erectus evolving onto the scene about 2.5 million years ago (call it 100,000 generations based on a 25-year reproductive cycle). If we assume cooking of food did not appear until somewhere approximately 125,000 years ago, although this date is quite approximate, we have been heating our food in some form only for the last 5,000 generations. So for the first 95,000 or so generations we were hunter/gatherers eating raw meat and plant foods. Cultivation (the planting and eating of grains) and domestication (the raising of cattle and eating dairy products) developed about 10,000 years ago. That's a mere 400 generations back, out of 100,000. The introduction of refined sugar occurred much later. So, what can we infer from this timeline?

In general, changes to diet require genetic or other adaptation. Looking at our food history, aside from cooking, the biggest changes occurred somewhat simultaneously 400 generations ago with the introduction of grains and dairy. Many scholars and alternative health practitioners think that 400 generations is not a long enough time for many people to adapt fully to these new food groups and, in fact, that may be a major factor for the cause of many present day illnesses. We recognize, for instance, that a majority of the world's adult population is lactose intolerant, which, to me, is a clue from Nature that dairy is not a suitable food for many adult humans, the only adult species on Earth known to consume it as a regular part of their diet. We also see gluten intolerance as a common and insidious ailment, which is another clue from Nature regarding the consumption of grains, many of which are the seeds of grasses. The term gluten has many definitions, the usual one defining certain proteins found primarily in wheat, barley, and rye grains. Other grains such as rice, oats, and corn contain different glutinous proteins.

The introduction of agriculture—of grains, dairy, and refined sugars—paved the way for huge population growth, and the evolution of scattered clans and tribes to larger settlements and eventually cities, but many leading anthropologists see this development less as progress but rather as a monumental setback for humankind. UCLA's Jared Diamond, for instance, in an article entitled "The Worst Mistake in the History of the Human Race" [6] [21], asserts that recent discoveries suggest the switch from a hunting/gathering existence to one of agriculture, "supposedly our most decisive step toward a better life, was in many ways a catastrophe from which we have never recovered. With agriculture came the gross social and sexual inequality, the disease, and despotism that curse our existence." Specific to diet, he added that hunter/gatherers enjoyed a very varied diet, while the farmers that replaced them obtained most of their food from a few starchy crops. Cheap calories and poor nutrition were the result.

Diamond puts the timeline in perspective this way: "Hunter-gatherers practiced the most successful and longest-lasting lifestyle in human history. In contrast, we're still struggling with the mess into which agriculture has tumbled us, and it's unclear whether we can solve it. Suppose that an archaeologist who had visited us from outer space were trying to explain human history to his fellow spacelings. He might illustrate the results of his digs by a twenty-four hour clock on which one hour represents 100,000 years of real past time. If the history of the human race began at midnight, then we would now be almost at the end of our first day. We lived as hunter-gatherers for nearly the whole of that day, from midnight through dawn, noon, and sunset. Finally, at 11:54 p.m., we adopted agriculture" [6]. A few field and clinical studies were conducted in the early part of the 20<sup>th</sup> century to determine the effects of diet on physical degeneration in humans and cats. See the side box entitled Physical Degeneration and Dietary Change for more information. I will comment on these studies and their significance below.

The goal in the following section is to define the Wellness Diet that in theory was what our ancestors consumed for most of the 2.5

million years of our heritage, and before human technological intervention, beginning with fire. This would be the baseline diet that all of us have evolved to eat. The format used is to create a food-screening criteria (called the ABC Test™) that will lead to lists of fully acceptable foods and less acceptable foods. The result will be a tiered arrangement of food choices, starting with Tier One foods which represents the purist version of the diet in its most basic form, and happens to be the one I strive to follow because it contains the lowest amount of natural toxins of any fully nutritious diet, and hence has a minimal impact on the defense system. The term "Wellness Diet" as used in this book refers to the diet that is based on Tier One food choices. However, for many people, this purist or baseline version may seem too austere in its simplicity, so there will be a discussion of additional food choices that may be added from Tier Two and Three food categories, where each in turn is farther removed from the baseline version. The Tier One, or Wellness Diet, establishes the starting point upon which to build a diet for modern times, and is the one I have followed for some time. (A patent application has been filed covering certain aspects of the Wellness Diet.) I am now going to go into some detail reviewing the research that went into defining the Wellness Diet.

## Physical Degeneration and Dietary Change

Two inquiring medical minds in the first half of the 20th century exhaustively explored the impact of dietary change on health and found dramatic consequences. The first was Weston A. Price, D.D.S., a Cleveland dentist, who traveled the world during the 1930s to study the causes of dental decay and physical degeneration that he saw on a daily basis in his practice. In his classic book *Nutrition and Physical Degeneration* [1], he reported finding healthy, straight teeth, freedom from decay, robust bodies, and resistance to disease, as common denominators among societies eating traditional diets. In stark contrast, he found rapid and consistent deterioration once native peoples switched to the "impoverished foods of civilization"— sugar, white flour, pasteurized milk, and convenience foods. Dental caries and deformed dental arches, resulting in crowded, crooked teeth and unattractive appearance were signs of physical degeneration, resulting from what he had suspected: nutritional deficiencies.

In a series of experiments with cats during the 1930s and 1940s, Francis M. Pottenger, Jr., M.D., a Los Angeles area physician, clearly demonstrated the power of dietary change. Working with some 900 cats over a ten-year period, he found that diets containing raw meat produced optimal health: good bone structure and density, wide palates with plenty of space for teeth, shiny fur, no parasites or disease, reproductive ease and gentleness. Keep in mind that cats are carnivores and evolved on raw meat.

Cooking the meat or substituting heat-processed milk for raw milk produced reproduction problems and physical degeneration in these cats, increasing with each generation. Vermin, parasites, skin diseases, and allergies increased precipitously and the animals gradually developed degenerative diseases seen in humans, along with adverse personality changes.

The changes Pottenger observed in cats paralleled the human degeneration that Price found among aboriginal peoples who had abandoned traditional diets. It does not require rocket science to see the clear parallel between the commercial, highly cooked, and processed food that we feed our companion animals and ourselves today, and the runaway prevalence of chronic illness besetting humans and pets. We have strayed afar from our evolutionary diet, and forced a similar disconnect on our animal friends, sometimes with disastrous results.

The significance of the research of Price and Pottenger was the inspiration for a California based nonprofit educational organization—called, appropriately The Price-Pottenger Nutrition Foundation (www.ppnf.org)—providing access to modern scientific validation of ancestral wisdom on nutrition, agriculture, and health. The organization's mission is to advance the quality of life through the study, application, research, and dissemination of nutritional and environmental information that can affect health in today's high-tech world. I am pleased to be a member of their Advisory Board.

# Chapter 4 - The Tier One Wellness Diet

As a starting point, there is general agreement among Paleo-anthropologists that raw meat and certain plants were the basic food groups for PA — a diet with about 90,000 generations of history behind it.

Moving closer to the present day in the timeline, added foods become more problematic for many people to eat without some sort of adverse health consequence, such as fish, fowl (it is not clear at what point we domesticated fowl and obtained easy access to eggs), grains, dairy, some cooked plant foods, extracted vegetable oils, and sugars. As we waltz our way through the world of food, keep in mind the "big eight" food categories, as they are affectionately called by allergists, that account for over 90% of the food allergies in the U.S. and tend to be in the top 10 worldwide. They are milk, eggs, peanuts, tree nuts, fish, shellfish, soy, and wheat. Chicken is also high on the list. As you will see, none of these foods formed a part of our Ancestor's original diet. Could this be another clue from MA? In the food group discussions, I will comment on the modern availability of some of the foods, and end with speculation on the relative proportions of each that may have been consumed.

## The ABC Test

In my research to deduce Nature's baseline when it came to food, I used the anthropological record to create what I call an "ABC Test," described in the accompanying side box entitled The ABC Test for Food.

---

# The ABC Test for Food ™

Here is how I apply the **A**vailable **B**efore **C**ivilization Test:

**Available** is somewhat tricky. By this I mean the following:

1) that the food was native to Africa, preferably tropical East Africa, considered the birthplace of our ancestors, and was reachable by a barefoot human; and

2) that no human processing, including heating or cooking, was needed to either gain access to, or digest or derive nutrition from the food in its natural form; and

3) that the food is not toxic if consumed raw.

**Before Civilization** means that the food is not newly hybridized or genetically modified, but is as close as possible to the version that would be available pre-cultivation/domestication and precooking (say more than 125,000 years ago).

---

The acronym stands for: was the food Available Before Civilization? I have used this simple yardstick to determine whether a particular food or food family is likely to be one to which our ancestors naturally adapted, and thus is eligible for inclusion in the Wellness Diet. It has helped guide me in my efforts to make educated decisions on defining the baseline foods to eat, and even lifestyle choices to follow. It's certainly not an infallible guide, but it has worked very well for me.

In my search for Tier One foods, I looked first at where humanity originated in order to find foods common to the heritage of all humans. We know it began in Africa (probably tropical East Africa), so there was one obvious criterion for availability. Is (or was) a particular food or family of foods native to this area? If it is a fruit or vegetable, did it grow in Africa, and if it is a source of meat, did it roam in African climates? If not, the odds are it may not have been an early source of food for humans. Another criterion for the ABC test is how physically easily the food would have been to obtain. Plant foods would also have had to be non-toxic when eaten raw.

An important point of the ABC test that I want to emphasize is that of territory. Although PA began emigration from Africa over a long period of time during the Paleo era, perhaps many hundreds of thousands of years ago, for purposes of our diet discussion, we will initially confine the area of interest to tropical Africa on the presumption that the bulk of our heritage took part in this area of the world. As you will see, this limitation leads to very different conclusions as to food availability, particularly when compared to other Paleo-type diets based on modern hunter-gatherer groups spread around the world. Let's now take a closer look at each of the food categories.

## Animal Foods

In hunter/gatherer societies, the hunter group did their best to find and kill or scavenge what they could with no tools or limited tools. There is speculation that PA was able to stampede herds over cliffs or into canyons even before any tools other than rocks were available. We presume that virtually all edible parts of the animal were ingested, including glands, organs, brains, blood, bone marrow, and the animal's raw intestinal contents, comprising partially digested fermented food, beneficial bacteria, and digestive enzymes. What we do not know is the amounts of the various parts consumed. For example, some carnivorous animals prefer the organs, glands, and fatty parts of their kill to the muscle meat, much of which is left for scavengers.

By examining our present dental and jaw structure, it becomes clear that we are not presently adapted to tear raw meat very efficiently, leading to the assumption of our having adapted to cooked meat. The following are some candidates for sources of animal protein and fat. All meet the ABC test, and in particular could have been eaten raw and without processing, although I personally prefer gently cooking my animal foods.

Cattle are members of the family Bovidae, which include several breeds that are native to Africa. Unfortunately, much of the beef produced in the U.S. is from cattle that are grain fed (mostly corn) in confined quarters, and are also fed or injected with growth hormones and antibiotics. Some are actually fed animal byproducts. For purposes of this baseline, the purist approach to eating beef is to eat only meat from humanely treated organic grass-fed and finished free-range cattle that were never treated with hormones or antibiotics. They are usually labeled as grass-fed. The term Natural as applied to meat is somewhat meaningless, applies to grain fed animals, and does not guarantee anything about the way they are reared. The meat for use on the Baseline diet is available from some health food markets and online suppliers, and usually originates from South America, New Zealand, or small ranches in the Midwest. Cattle are tropical animals not Native to North America, and cannot survive in a winter where the grass is covered by snow. So any cattle raised in the U.S., even grass-fed, needs nutritional support during winters from stored fodder, usually hay as a mixture of dried grasses.

Raising cattle on grain distorts their fatty acid profile, (see the section on essential fatty acids below) and is not what nature intended. The health effect on humans consuming this meat is unknown. A less than purist approach might be occasionally to eat grain-fed beef, but be sure it is organic feed, and that it is hormone- and antibiotic-free, bearing in mind that eating this meat frequently could be a health-risk factor of unknown proportions. For those interested in the grain/grass-fed issues, I suggest visiting the site of the Weston A. Price Foundation [7]. This foundation evolved from the Price-Pottenger Nutrition Foundation [1], both of which are committed to promulgating the teachings of Weston Price.

Buffalo, or bison, is another option, and they also belong to the family Bovidae. American buffalo can be found that has been grass-fed, or sometimes grass-fed and grain-finished. The finishing step takes place before the animals are put on the market, and is used as a last minute effort to fatten them up to yield a higher price. The adverse effect of grain finishing on the health of a human consuming the meat is unknown, but it is likely that these effects are less than those from eating fully grain-fed buffalo. Grass-fed and finished buffalo are available from small U.S. farms and farm cooperatives, including NorthStar Bison [22]. Purist and less than purist approaches discussed above for beef also apply here. The bottom line is that the longer the animal is free-range grass-fed during its lifetime, the closer its meat composition will be to that which was intended by Nature.

Another choice is lamb, the meat of young sheep, also members of the family Bovidae. Much of the lamb on the market is from fully grass-fed sheep, and my favorite is from New Zealand. Goat and other ruminant animals can join the list. Deer, elk, caribou, and moose (from the family Cervidae) do not appear to be native to Africa, but antelope is a candidate, as is goat.

Pork is from swine of the family Suidae, some species of which are native to Africa. For example, the bush pig is a food source for chimpanzees. One of the potential issues with pork meeting the ABC test today is that eating the meat raw can lead to toxic bacterial infections such as trichinosis if the pork is not raised in a natural environment, but this would not have been an issue for PA. If pork is of interest, look for Certified Humane Pork that is hopefully also free-range and organic-fed. While there is a USDA trichinae-free certification program for pork, I am not aware of any pork producers that have implemented it.

I am including ostrich in this category since it passes the ABC test. Although a bird, ostrich is flightless and hence was much easier prey for PA, making it likely as a food source much earlier than winged birds. Ostrich meat is delicious and available from a variety of suppliers, such as Blackwing Meats [23]. The main problem I have with ostrich is its low fat content, which leaves me hungry. Interested readers can do follow-up research of other animal families using the guidelines above.

Regarding the fat content of prey animals, I have concentrated in this section on animal families that are readily accessible to Western cultures, but in fact, there are very many more animal families native to Africa that are now either endangered, extinct, or simply unavailable as food. A simple example is the hippopotamus, distantly related to the whale! If I, as a hunter-gatherer, had a choice between a lean goat or a chunky hippo for dinner, I would choose the hippo just based on the larger amount of fat present in bigger animals (not factoring in the difficulty of obtaining that dinner!).

Some Paleo diet studies have concluded that while PA would certainly have preferred the fattiest part of animals, he/she would actually have had a relatively low animal fat dietary intake. This is based on their analysis of, for example the animal fat content of caribou and its seasonal variations (higher fat content in the fall and winter). Caribou, related to reindeer, is not native to tropical Africa, and is unlikely to have been a PA food until their emigration to the Northern climates in later periods. Also, traditional seasons do not exist in the tropics of PA, where the weather is either wet or dry, but there is no fall or winter. Other Paleo diets are based on studies of modern hunter-gatherers such as the Inuit, who are certainly not representative of life in the tropical Paleo era. Thus, it is easy to come to very different "ancient" diet conclusions if these distinctions are not clearly established. Of course, it is difficult to intuit what did take place more than 10,000 years ago in tropical Africa, but that is what this section is attempting to do.

Now, let's take a look at what portions of the meat were eaten. I prefer fatty cuts of meat because of their taste and because they are very satiating. Some studies have shown that hunter-gatherers universally sought out animal fat. In many cases, it is not easy to find high-fat cuts, so I supplement my diet with additional animal fat. I use my gut feelings to tell me when I have had enough – I feel full. Our ancestors are very likely to have eaten the animal glands and other organs, and there is evidence from studies of Inuit and American Indian groups that the intestinal contents of the animals were also consumed [24]. In the case of ruminants, this would include fermented or partially fermented grasses, along with the enzymes and bacteria from the animal gut. I discuss a particular group of those bacteria called spore-formers in the dirt section below.

Many folks do not like to eat animal glands and other organs or find them difficult to obtain. Toxicity is another potential deterrent created by modern farming and ranch practices, particularly related to consuming brain and liver tissue. An unknown issue is whether glands and other organs need to be eaten raw to derive all of their nutritional benefits. As an alternative, one can take various food supplements with each meal, discussed further below. The intestinal contents of prey would be even harder to come by in today's markets, so I suggest in later sections ways of either adding some fermented foods to the diet as a substitute, or supplementing with some of the healthy spore-forming bacteria found in animal intestines. There is also evidence that our Ancestors broke apart the bones of the animals and ate the marrow, which is filled with nutrients such as gelatin. To fill this gap, you might consider obtaining marrowbones from your butcher and using them to make soup. Recipes can be found in the book *Nourishing Traditions* by Sally Fallon [25]. More information on gelatin can be found in the supplement section below.

In his travels, Weston Price found that the Masai tribe in Africa drank cow's blood as part of their diet, and reading this bit of information led me to a fascinating bit of sleuthing. I remembered as a young kid recovering from diphtheria that our doctor recommended I be fed "beef tea" to speed my recovery. My mother made it by boiling meat for a long time and collecting the juice, which I devoured. I vividly remember how salty it was, and visually it reminded me of blood. Well, one of the pieces of the puzzle that had been bothering me for some time was the salt content of the PA diet. Most of the Paleo diet gurus have come to the conclusion that such diets were very low in salt, which seemed incongruous with the electrolyte needs of a hunter-gatherer running around in tropical Africa, coupled the fact that MA has provided us with salt taste buds. Just ask any marathon runner how long he/she would last on a low salt diet.

So I decided to look into the salt content of blood, and the results were quite shocking. My analysis went something like this: the sodium chloride content of blood is estimated to be about 0.9%, or about 9 grams per liter, which is also the ratio used to make isotonic salt solutions for intravenous use in hospitals. Most mammals have a whole blood volume in milliliters that is about 5-7% of the weight of the animal in kilograms. A typical cow, depending on her size, contains somewhere between 25 and 40 liters of blood, which yields between 225 and 360 grams of salt! That is an enormous amount – between a half and three quarters of a pound of salt just in the blood of a cow [26]. Imagine a hippo or a mammoth – they would be virtual salt farms.

Well, it is not rocket science for me to jump to the conclusion that PA had all the salt he/she could possibly desire, just from the blood of their prey. As a sanity check, I ran my analysis by one of my local university biology professor friends, who approached the analysis differently but came up with the same answers. Salt is an important part of the Wellness Diet, and I discuss it more thoroughly in later sections of the book. It also turns out that many modern cultures throughout the world do consume animal blood, but tend to disguise it with names like black pudding, and other names for what is really blood sausage.

Excluded from the animal category for the Wellness Diet are any prepared forms of meat, such as sausages or cured meats. In the event you are interested in obtaining the acceptable animal products mentioned in this section, many of them, including glands and other organs, and bone stock are available from US Wellness Meats [27].

For those concerned with cholesterol, saturated fats, and heart disease, see the box entitled Cholesterol Commentary for additional insights. Here is the short form. Can saturated fat contribute to heart disease? Yes, but not for any of the reasons put forth by the medical community.

Can elevated cholesterol be a marker for heart disease? Again, yes, but not for any of the reasons put forth by the medical community. From my research, the medical community reasonings regarding saturated fat and cholesterol are further examples of faulty experiments where there is no controlled baseline, where necessary and sufficient causes are mixed up, and where correlation is confused with causation. Basically, a repeat of the rat chow experiment. Here is how I approached these issues.

# Cholesterol Commentary

I am sure the reader is aware of the saturated fat/cholesterol/heart disease information ingrained in our culture. Even some of those favoring Paleo diets seem to shy away from the saturated animal fat issue. There are studies showing the typical fatty acid composition of various animals in an effort to try to fit a Paleo diet into the politically correct saturated fat theory. Of course, having an animal analyzed in this way does not lead to the conclusion that our ancestor's fat intake mimicked the analysis, since we do not know what and how much of each part of the animal was eaten.

The first inkling I got that the saturated fat theory needed further investigation was when I ran a self-experiment that clearly demonstrated the more saturated animal fat I ate (while following the Wellness Diet), the lower my total cholesterol. In fact, my entire lipid profile "improved," as this term is defined by the cardiology/pharmaceutical industry. Well, that launched me (pun intended) into an investigation of the whole saturated fat/cholesterol theory of heart disease and, as you will read, magnesium deficiency surfaced as the culprit.

I presume my dismissal of the saturated fat/cholesterol issue will not satisfy those readers concerned about heart disease and/or who have a family history of such disease. I have such a family history. On my father's side, I am the longest living male in three generations (I am 66 as I write this book) – all succumbed earlier to cardiovascular illnesses. So, here is what I did to allay my fears.

Putting on my engineering cap, my first task was to check the actual condition of my arteries. The medical community would have everyone believe that a lipid profile (cholesterol profile and triglyceride blood tests) accomplishes that task. Science and common sense say that one should not measure something indirectly if it can be easily and accurately measured directly. Actually, I don't consider a lipid profile to be a test of anything reliable when it comes to the condition of my arteries, but it may be an indication of magnesium deficiency, which is related to cardiovascular health - see the magnesium factor section below.

Direct testing of artery health took me into the world of medical testing and lo and behold, there are many non-invasive, inexpensive, and accurate tests to determine directly the condition of one's arteries. The first is the carotid ultrasound test, which takes only a few minutes and displays on a computer screen a nice picture of the large arteries leading from the heart to the brain, along with real-time blood flow color-coded for velocity. Some in the medical community say this is not good enough. What about the peripheral arteries in the lower part of the body, they ask? Okay, how about a do-it-yourself free test for that? Measure the reclining blood pressure at your arm and then at your ankle (a helper comes in handy). A reading of 90% or greater (the ratio of leg to arm) is considered a good indication of unclogged peripheral arteries. This test is sometimes referred to as an ABI test (ankle/brachial pressure index).

Still others in the medical community said that ultrasound does not reliably pick up calcium deposits in the arteries. Okay, onward to a body scan. I am not a fan of x-rays because they may cause cancer, but I make an exception for a body scan, done, say, every ten years, because the potential payoff is so great. One should opt for the latest equipment, which has the lowest x-ray levels. This test is excellent for determining an arterial calcium score (the goal is zero). Lastly, I was again taken to task because I had not gotten any information about the possibility of microvascular disease – clogging of the very small arteries throughout the body. Well, I found some anecdotal evidence showing that your friendly eye doctor can give you a clue by looking at the tiny arteries and veins in the retina, which is actually easy to do as part of a regular eye exam at no additional cost. Trained doctors can give you a valuable opinion based on their findings. Lastly, I added a stress echocardiogram to the list, although I did not feel it was necessary.

So, how did I do? When I had these tests performed, I had been on the Wellness Diet for anywhere from 15 to 20 years, eating no grains, dairy, sugars or extracted vegetable oils. Instead, I ate meat at every meal, and if still hungry, I would down up to three egg yolks per day. Of course, I took magnesium supplements. My carotid ultrasound results were a rousing success – wide-open arteries, excellent blood flow. The peripheral blood pressure test yielded a reading of 113% (90% or better is desirable), which shocked the technician. My body scan calcium score was zero, and the radiologist confessed that his was not that low. He cautioned me that I should not take that reading as a license to go out and eat hamburgers, which is exactly what I did (no bun, no cheese, and no sauce). The eye doctor gave me a green light at my eye exam, not only for the condition of my micro arteries, but also for my eye health in general. The stress test yielded excellent results.

I have gone to some length to cover this topic because the saturated fat/cholesterol/heart disease theory is very ingrained in our cultural psyche. I will add that my wife, who is much less of a purist than I, and who had been on the Wellness Diet in one form or another for about 10 years, underwent the same tests and scored perfectly as well. While some radiology labs require a prescription to do a carotid ultrasound, several companies are now doing them quite inexpensively along with some of the other tests like the ABI, without that requirement. An example is Life Line Screening [28]. Full body scans can be somewhat expensive, but the long-term consequences of not knowing the condition of your arteries can be a lot more expensive!

I made a list of items that are *suspected* causes of cardiovascular disease, and saturated fat and cholesterol are on that list. I say suspected because it is clear from the research that you can have elevated cholesterol and eat lots of saturated fat and not have heart disease, and the reverse is also true [29] [30] [31] [32]. I then made a list of items that are *known* causes of cardiovascular disease, meaning that if this item is present, you have or will develop cardiovascular disease. There is only one item on that list – *magnesium deficiency*. Are you surprised? My guess is that many in the field of heart health would also be surprised, but they shouldn't be. There is plenty of research on the subject, and I go into more depth on it in the food supplement section below [33] [34, 35].

Once I had these two lists along with reams of data on magnesium, the likely correlation between saturated fat, cholesterol, and cardiovascular disease became clear to me. Virtually everyone on the SAD diet is deficient in the essential mineral magnesium, obtainable from food and mineral water. This deficiency is highly correlated with every facet of cardiovascular disease, from angina, arrhythmias, clogged arteries, strokes, to sudden death. Well, it just so happens that saturated fat binds with magnesium in the gut, forming compounds that reduce assimilation of the mineral. So, if you are already deficient in magnesium and increase your saturated fat intake, you will become more deficient, further increasing your chances of heart disease. Is the solution to reduce saturated fat intake? Of course not. The solution is to cure the magnesium deficiency.

What about cholesterol? Well, magnesium deficiency can cause elevated cholesterol in some people, so a high cholesterol level can be a marker of magnesium deficiency, not a direct cause of heart disease. In fact, magnesium lowers cholesterol in the same way as statin drugs, but without the side effects [36]. It is well known that cholesterol is a necessary element to life itself – without an adequate amount, we would be sick indeed, if not dead. We need it, just as we need sunlight. The analogy between the cholesterol theory and the skin cancer theory described earlier is compelling. In each case there is an element (sunlight and cholesterol) supposedly contributing to the illness, but that element is also necessary to the overall health of the body. In each case, the medical/pharma establishment has glommed on to suppression of these essential elements, leading to huge profits in the sunscreen and statin drug businesses, but also leading to a litany of other illnesses that will plague the patient in years to come. We have yet to see the devastating effects of chronic use of sunscreens and statins. Just as I believe artificially reducing sunlight is a dangerous game, so is artificially reducing cholesterol.

Cholesterol elevation can be caused by many factors. When it is an indicator of magnesium deficiency, it is at most an indirect and unreliable marker for the real cause of heart disease, and that is what we see from the research. There are an enormous number of people with supposedly elevated cholesterol levels (say above 200 mg/dl) that do not develop heart disease. There are likewise an enormous number of people with levels below 200 mg/dl that do. In fact, the largest study of its kind, the famous Framingham Study, produced results showing that those with total cholesterol below 200 mg/dl had a higher incidence of heart disease than those with levels above 200 mg/dl. If you read some of the references I listed above on cholesterol, you will find from an analysis of the major studies on the subject that the cholesterol limits which *minimize* mortality from all causes are as follows: total cholesterol in excess of 226 mg/dl, and LDL levels in excess of 144 mg/dl!

My position regarding the prevention of heart disease is to have a sufficient magnesium level in your body. Saturated fat and cholesterol are merely warning lights for the real problem. Magnesium will reappear throughout this book along with iodine as two of our mineral champions in The Wellness Project.

A discussion of animal products would not be complete without some mention of insects, which are a part of the chimpanzee and many modern hunter-gatherer diets. PA would certainly have consumed them in small quantities in eating fruit. At the risk of losing my audience, I would like to explore this subject a bit further.

Entomophagy is the practice of eating insects as food, and there is some fossil evidence that PA did so intentionally. From his research of modern indigenous tribes around the globe, Weston Price found that all but one tribe ate insects as part of their diet. Insects are not only a very nutritious food; they are also at least four times more efficient than mammals in converting plant matter into protein and fat, and if their fast breeding rates are factored in, they have true conversion efficiency close to twenty times that of beef. There are enormous ecological advantages to harvesting insects for food, not the least of which is the elimination of the need for insecticides, one of the major sources of toxins on our planet. The high conversion efficiency might provide an answer to worldwide starvation. Traditionally, insects have been a part of the diet in some Central and South American, African, Asian and Australian cultures, but are considered taboo in most Western societies [37]. As to whether insects pass the ABC test, the issue is one of toxicity. There have been reports of allergic reactions to various insects and their larvae, but research in this area is so sparse that it is hard to draw any firm conclusions. So, for now we will put insects on the wait-and-see list for the Wellness Diet.

## Plant Foods

Unlike animal foods, plant foods present a variety of difficult issues relating to human diet that have been the subject of much debate in the scientific community. Remarkably, the majority of research on components of Paleo diets has been conducted for animal products, with virtually nothing on plant availability during this time period. I funded research in the Department of Ecology, Evolution, and Marine Biology at the University of California, Santa Barbara to assist me in uncovering whatever data was available in this area, which is not very much.

As you will see, this is one major area where clues from Nature become paramount in discerning what comprise acceptable plant foods. Here is the generally accepted theory, which makes great sense to me. Unlike animals that can move, run, and hide from predators to increase their chances of survival, plants are immobile. Thus, in an evolutionary sense, they were under continuous pressure to solve their survival problems by chemical means. They produce what are called secondary compounds or substances that do not contribute to their metabolism, but are designed to repel or discourage predators, ranging from other invading plants, to insects, to animals including humans [38] [39]. Basically, this is a part of the plant's defense system.

Many of these secondary compounds are toxic in a variety of ways, some of which we have yet to uncover. The ones that produce relatively immediate signs of toxicity, such as vomiting or rashes, are easy to spot. Others are much more subtle and represent a challenge to the medical community. One reason is the long period of time that may have elapsed before symptoms of toxicity become evident. These toxic substances cover a wide range of chemical compounds that produce toxic effects in very different ways. They include enzyme inhibitors, physiological irritants, allergens, and hormone disrupters. Within each of these categories are a vast number of compounds distributed throughout the plant community, and I feel confident there are many more yet to be discovered [40]. Interestingly, several insect, bird, and animal species have adapted to a few of these plant toxins and developed a synergistic relationship with specific plants that would otherwise be toxic, and I discuss this more thoroughly in the probiotics section below. There is no room in this book to delve into all of Nature's protective plant mechanisms and the wide range of ill effects they can cause on humans, and there are many books on the subject. However, I want to emphasize the importance of this clue from Nature because I believe that ignoring it has been one major cause of illness today.

When I became aware of this toxic plant issue and researched it more thoroughly, a fascinating pattern became clear. First, not all plants contain toxins, or only contain them for a portion of their growth cycle. Many fruits fall into this category, and the Darwinian rationale is as follows. The fruits with the lowest or no toxicity seem to be those that have a sweet fleshy layer covering seeds within. One objective in plant reproduction is to disseminate seeds at a distance from the parent, to increase chances of survival and reduce the competition for nutrients that would occur if a plant simply dropped its seeds. One of Nature's plans for dissemination (there are many including wind, sticking to animal hides, etc.) appears to be to package these seeds (themselves indigestible raw) in an attractive sweet outer layer to *attract* animals to consume them. The seeds pass through the intestinal tract undigested and are returned to earth along with fecal matter (a great fertilizer) some distance from the parent plant. Voila! The reproductive cycle is completed.

This is the positive side of the Darwinian analysis (plant foods naturally designed *to be* eaten), and it contains a valuable hint. Note that the seeds of the fruit are designed not to be digested, and for insurance they contain relatively strong hulls that survive gastric juices. As it turns out, if the seeds were eaten in the sense of biting through the shells, they could lead to health problems for the eater because they contain some of the toxins I referred to above. Some of these seeds can be in the form of what we call nuts or pits or stones. Just to give you some idea of the kinds of seed toxins we are talking about, does cyanide get your attention? It is in the seeds of such fruit as apples, cherries, peaches, and apricots. Swallowing these seeds raw is no problem (except for the size of some pits!) because the outer hull protects the user from the toxins.

To complete the picture for fruits, Nature has gone one step further to increase the chances of successful plant reproduction. The sweet outer shell ripens at about the same rate that the seeds inside are developing toward the point of supporting germination, so the ideal time for consumption from the plant's perspective is when the fruit is ripe. This also coincides with the point where the fruit becomes sweet. If consumed too early in an unripe state, the fruit is bitter and may be toxic at this stage.

Two of our five groups of taste buds are designed to sense sweet and bitter tastes. Is this coincidence? More likely, it is yet another clue from Nature to avoid eating bitter-tasting fruit. This is particularly true for berries, some of which are toxic. From my research, these toxic berries are universally bitter in taste, and are Nature's clue to stay away.

An attempt to compile a list of typical fruits that meet the ABC test turned out to be quite a frustrating experience. Determining what fruits are or were native to tropical East Africa, as opposed to those that were introduced later, was the first hurdle. It turns out that most of this knowledge is lost. The next problem, from what I could glean of native fruits, was to find something equivalent that could be readily obtained in Western markets. This was a problem because most of these fruits simply are not harvested to any degree anywhere (having been replaced by the fruits with which we are now familiar). The bottom line is that the list is embarrassingly short, prompting me to propose a compromise to the ABC test for this food category, which is discussed below. Keep in mind that all of the fruits you eat should be organically grown to minimize human-made chemical contamination.

Fortunately, as I was writing this book, the National Academies Press finally published a reference that has been in the making for several years. Entitled *Lost Crops of Africa, Volume III, Fruits*, it is a summary of a limited number of both wild and cultivated fruits of Africa, with much background information [41]. The list of fruits chosen for review was biased toward those that could have a material impact on the African economy, but it is nevertheless of great interest and contains information that was not previously publicly available. An additional research aid was the reference *Edible Wild Plants of Sub-Saharan Africa* by Peters, et al. [42] Here is a summary of those fruits for which I was able to find a related fruit somewhat widely available.

Custard Apples from the Annonaceae family are related to the fruit called cherimoya. Ebony from the genus Diospyros is related to persimmon. Gingerbread Plums from the family Chrysobalanaceae, and Carissa from the family Apocynaceae appear to be similar to conventional plums. Imbe of the Garcinia family is related to mangosteen, sometimes referred to as the world's most delicious fruit. Medlars of the family Rubiaceae are related to the noni berry. Monkey Orange of the family

Strychnaceae tastes like orange, banana, and apricot. Star Apples, which look like plums, are available in some specialty markets, as are tamarinds and sugarplums, which look like giant purple grapes. Balanites from the family Balanitaceae resemble dates, and butterfruit is said to resemble the mango. Virtually all of the melons in the family Cucurbitaceae are on the list, including watermelon, honeydew, cantaloupe, and others.

Figs, from the Ficus genus of trees, pass the ABC test. I prefer fresh figs as opposed to dried, which are quite high in concentrated sugars. Fresh figs also appear to be a favorite chimp food. Watermelon, mentioned above, has a water content that is so high it is used as a source of drinking water during droughts in Africa. The fruit has a diuretic effect, which can act as an excellent kidney cleanse. I have found that the more congested the kidneys, the stronger the diuretic effect. Persimmons, also mentioned above, should not be eaten unripe, since they can form an obstruction in the stomach. In addition, I avoid any that are bitter or very astringent. Use your taste buds – if it is not sweet or it is very astringent (usually due to excessive tannins), do not eat it. Jujubes, from the genus Ziziphus, passes the ABC test, but are not easy to find. Let's summarize for a moment: we are looking for ripe, sweet, non-astringent, non-bitter organically-grown fruit with seeds.

We are now going to assess the possibility of broadening the fruit category beyond the few choices resulting from the ABC test. Because eating fruit seems to be in the best interest of the plants and is in keeping with Nature's plan (as evidenced by the very low toxin profiles of all sweet fruit), I am encouraged to expand our horizons in this arena without fear of compromising health. One simple variation of the ABC test is to open up the territory from Africa to the nearest area of emigration, the Middle East. As it turns out, this change adds a lot more choices in this category. Fresh dates from date palms become available. While some ripe dates fall to the ground, others require climbing skills, and for those who have visited tropical climates, it becomes obvious that even small children easily acquire such skills. Eat dates fresh, not dried, which overly concentrates the sugar. Next is citrus, including grapefruit, orange, lemon and lime. Remember not to deliberately eat (bite) large quantities of the seeds (swallowing them whole is okay) or any bitter parts such as the rind. Juicing should be avoided for reasons discussed below. If the fruit has a thin skin as opposed to a thick rind, and it is not bitter, it can be eaten.

If the assumption is correct that MA wants us to eat her sweet fruit wherever it is grown, then the fruit category can be further opened up to include virtually all of the popular sweet fruits with which we are familiar, including sweet berries like raspberries and blackberries (bitter berries can be toxic). Many people love fruits because of their sweetness, which of course is Nature's plan, and it is actually fun to discover and use our sweet and bitter taste buds. I make sure all fruit is ripe before eating and I prefer those that contain seeds or a pit, as MA intended.

Tropical fruits are likely to have been in PA's diet the longest, so you may wish to choose those first. In particular, pineapple is high in enzymes useful in the digestion of protein, and I discuss this more fully in the digestive rehabilitation section below. Papaya is also high in enzyme activity but, unfortunately, a significant portion of the papaya now grown is a genetically modified variety to provide immunity to the ringspot virus and the results of such genetic manipulation on humans is unknown. I avoid any genetically modified foods, and it concerns me greatly that this activity has begun with respect to fruits.

Most of the commercially grown fruit, even organic, contain human-made contaminants on the surface, so a cleaning step is a good idea before cutting or eating. Soaking for long periods is not a good idea because this could leech out important nutrients. Using toxic chemicals to clean fruits, such as chlorine, is also counterproductive. The method I prefer is scrubbing with clean water having a few drops of iodine in it (see the section on iodine below). You can also wash the fruit using soap nuts, a fruit described in detail in the lifestyle section [43]. Where possible, use glass containers in the cleaning process.

I avoid the juicing of fruits for several reasons. First, the very act of juicing heats the fruit to a temperature that is dependent on the construction of the juicer and the speed of juicing, but in any case, this heating effect may destroy valuable nutrients including vitamins and enzymes. Further, in most juicers, the pulp is discarded, which contains very valuable parts of the fruit, not the least of which is fiber. Therefore, what is left is something akin to sugar water. Finally, juicing can crush the seeds, allowing their toxins to be released. There are many juice bars serving this sugar water under the guise of a healthy drink, but I think not. If you ate all of the whole fruit that goes into these drinks, you would surely get the runs or a serious stomachache. To add further to the injury, pre-bottled fruit juices are practically all pasteurized (sometimes disguised as "flash" pasteurized), which definitely destroys valuable nutrients. I eat the fruit as MA intended – raw, whole, sweet, and ripe.

Nature's clues relating to fruit consumption provide valuable pointers for our next investigation into the other, or negative side of the Darwinian analysis (plant foods naturally designed *not to be* eaten). From the above, it seems obvious that, as part of their defense system, plants have developed methods of deterring activities that interfere with or detract from their successful reproduction. Since there is substantially more plant life than animal life on our planet, these methods are clearly effective. I want to state at the outset that this animal/plant tension has played out over millions of years and continues to do so in a very clever, very adaptive, and very complicated manner. From my research, for other than fruit, it appears that the goal of MA is to allow certain animals to eat certain parts of certain plants in certain amounts. This is a careful balancing act so that (barring human intervention) plant species do not become extinct because of animal/insect predator activity, and animals do not become extinct for lack of plant foods. If this sounds complicated it is, and I will try to provide several examples to show how some of it works.

Let's start with an investigation of how potentially edible plants reproduce, starting with the plant itself. Anything done to outright kill the plant, like uprooting it, is certainly detrimental to its reproduction. Here, we are talking about foods in the form of roots and tubers, which grow underground and require plant destruction (yanking the plant out of the ground or eating it from underneath) to obtain them. A tuber is a thickened part of the plant that is located at or below the soil line and is used by the plant to store nutrients to further its propagation. A potato is one example. Well, if our Darwinian model is correct, roots and tubers would contain some nasty stuff for most animals, including humans.

Wait a minute, you say, everybody knows that rabbits devour carrot roots, and so do humans, clearly killing the carrot plant. However, what you see in a modern garden or farm is far from what nature intended. If we take a closer look at carrots, we find out that the ancestor of our cultivated carrot is the wild carrot plant (also called Queen Anne's Lace). As found in nature, it contains carotatoxin (also referred to as falcarinol), a neurotoxin related to hemlock. As many rabbit lovers know, this plant will sicken or kill a rabbit, so, unbelievably, rabbits do not naturally eat carrots in the wild. Somewhere in the last few thousand years, humans selectively bred the raw carrot to minimize the levels of these toxins, resulting in the modern carrot, which rabbits and humans do eat. The potential problem with this is that even the modern carrot contains some amount of these toxins, which appear to have anti-cancer properties at one dose, and are neurotoxic at another dose. There is virtually no research on these issues, and I have no idea who, if anyone, is watching the store when it comes to the natural toxin levels in ordinary carrots. I do not know of anyone exhibiting immediate symptoms of toxicity from eating carrots, and I feel confident that many of us have a defense system that can deal with it. The point I want to make is that eating a plant part that MA did not intend to be eaten requires that our defense system deal with natural toxins, leaving less capacity for it to deal with all of the other human-made toxins that we are subjected to in our modern lifestyle, and thus increasing the chances of illness.

Yams and potatoes are also toxic if eaten raw. In particular, potatoes, in the nightshade family, native to South America and first cultivated about 5000 years ago, contain solanine and chaconine, poisons capable of killing animals and people, and these toxins are not eliminated by cooking [44]. Like carrots, potatoes were and are specially bred by humans to ensure toxin content is below some established threshold of acceptable toxicity [45] [46] [47]. As a result of the seriousness of these toxins, there is a monitoring program in place by the USDA to check different varieties for toxin levels, based on levels that have been chosen somewhat arbitrarily as safe. MA has really outdone herself when it comes to protecting potatoes from predators. Even when the potato is out of the ground, exposing it to light or even bruising it can increase its toxin concentration.

Sure, zillions of potatoes have been eaten over the years with few deaths. All potatoes contain these toxins, and the real question, which has no answer, is: what is the long-term effect of eating potatoes on a regular basis? Clearly, our defense system is responsible for handling the toxin load, potentially reducing our immunity to more serious toxins, many of which are described in detail in the detox section. It is interesting that anthropology studies show that if our ancestors were to eat a raw potato, they probably also ate clay to assist in detoxification [48]. As you will see shortly, clay plays an important role in the Wellness Diet. The nightshade family also includes tomatoes (native to South America), eggplant (native to India), and chili peppers (native to the Americas). To some extent, they all share the toxin heritage of the nightshade family. We could go on and on regarding roots, tubers, and toxins, but I presume you get the picture. I tend to avoid these plant parts as nutritionally unnecessary in the Wellness Diet, and a toxic burden on my defense system. Let's move on to seeds.

Another way to interfere with plant reproduction is to destroy the seeds of those plants that reproduce from seeds. As was stated earlier, seeds can take the form of nuts, as well as beans and peas. From a review of the literature, raw seeds, beans, and peas contain a wide range of compounds toxic to humans including protease inhibitors, lectins, glucosinolates and other goitrogens, cyanogens, saponins, gossypol pigments, lathrogens, carcinogens, and other hormone disruptors. The range of illnesses that can be caused by these toxins extends from a stomachache to neurological damage, cardiovascular damage, hormonal issues of all kinds, and nutrient deficiencies that can lead to many illnesses, and even death. In fact, virtually all pharmaceuticals began their life as a plant toxin, from aspirin to statin drugs. Plant toxins can have an upside if the plan is to kill or disable something in your body in the hope that it will cure some ailment without killing or disabling you, which is how drugs work.

About 80% of the world's present human population lives on a diet based on plant seeds, roots and tubers, so how did we get here? Enter technology in the form of fire. It is well accepted in the nutrition community that when humans learned to cook plants, this *supposedly* either destroyed or rendered harmless the toxins they contain. Add to this the additional technologies of seed milling, fermenting, sprouting, soaking, and plant cultivation in general, and we now have a world dependant on those portions of plants that it would seem Nature would prefer we did not eat.

This is one of the biggest nutritional experiments in the history of humanity, and has been going on since fire was used for cooking (say

5,000 generations ago), but really took off about 400 generations ago with the cultivation of grains (grass seeds). In my opinion, for a substantial portion of the population, it has been a faulty experiment leading to illness. Of course, one could argue that except for having access to these plant foods, a substantial portion of our world population would not have sufficient food. That argument raises ethical, philosophical, and global ecological issues way beyond the scope of this book, the purpose of which is to investigate ways of maintaining the health of those of us who are fortunate to have a wide range of choices for the foods we eat. The reason the experiment of eating grains, tubers and other plant parts may lead to illness is that heating, milling, fermenting, sprouting, and soaking do not always destroy or render harmless the toxins in these foods. In some cases, such as with fermentation, this process may even *increase* the concentration of plant toxins, and we have yet to accurately identify or measure them all. Couple this with the fact that, for some of us, our heritage did not prepare our defense system to handle these toxins on a daily basis, and you have the potential for illness. The bottom line here is that we have employed technology to fool with MA by trying to defeat her plant safeguards, creating the illusion that everyone can eat foods, without any adverse consequences, that many of us are not evolutionarily designed to eat.

A classical example is wheat, made from grass seed. A growing portion of our population is being identified as intolerant of the gluten in wheat, rye and barley. Proteins in wheat can cause an autoimmune intestinal disorder in individuals who are susceptible, causing damage to the mucosal surface of the small intestine by a toxic reaction to the ingestion of gluten, which interferes with the absorption of nutrients. Attempts have been made to totally eliminate the gluten by sprouting or fermenting, but to no avail. Of course, other grains, even if gluten free, all derive from seeds and hence contain cocktails of other toxins in keeping with Nature's plan.

Nuts and beans are another example. Soaking supposedly renders harmless some of the toxins in these foods, such as phytates, which interfere with mineral absorption in the body, but tests show that phytates are not completely eliminated by this means, and in fact may only be reduced by a small amount. Cooking does not do the job either.

Brassica is a genus of plants in the mustard family that includes cabbage, broccoli, cauliflower, Brussels sprouts, turnips, and radishes. Their seeds include mustard and rapeseed, the source of canola oil. While none of these are native to Africa, it is instructive to see Nature in action in the composition of these "healthful" plants. Broccoli and cauliflower, known as cruciferous vegetables, are the unopened flowers and stems of the plant before it has had a chance to bloom. Removal of these parts of the plant prevents or delays reproduction, so let's see what Nature has in store for those who partake. Virtually all of these vegetables are classified as goitrogens, meaning they contain compounds that interfere with the production of thyroid hormones, primarily the uptake of iodine, which could lead to goiter and hypothyroidism, among many other problems.

The amount of animal research in this area is really enormous, reporting somewhat devastating effects of Brassica family vegetables on the thyroid health of animals. I discuss the importance of iodine in some detail in the halogen problem section of Chapter 17, and show why (in particular in today's toxic environment), anything interfering with its uptake is a very bad idea. As you will see in that section, iodine is critical to the health of the entire body, not just the thyroid. It is particularly critical for maintaining breast and ovarian health in women. Considering the near epidemic proportions of thyroid conditions, particularly in women, which include hypothyroidism and Hashimoto's disease, I predict that cruciferous and other goitrogenic vegetable consumption will be found in the future to be a leading cause of many of these problems.

An excellent report on the negative and positive health characteristics of cruciferous vegetables is *Bearers of the Cross: Crucifers in the Context of Traditional Diets and Modern Science* by Chris Masterjohn, published in Wise Traditions by the Weston A. Price Foundation, Summer 2007, pp. 34-45 [7]. Steaming these vegetables reduces the goitrogens somewhat, boiling reduces them even more, but fermentation appears to increase the goitrogenic effect, leading to a potential problem with products such as sauerkraut. Raw cabbage and radishes can be as potent as prescription anti-thyroid drugs in shutting down the thyroid. Of course, we have all heard about the anti-cancer properties of cruciferous vegetables, which seem to be connected with phytonutrients, sometimes more accurately called phytochemicals (phyto means plant).

Actually, the bulk of the phytonutrients du jour, such as carotenoids, anthocyanins, and resveratrol, are primarily found in fruit.

In the cruciferous group, the phytochemicals proffered are the very ones identified as toxins that interfere with or disable natural human processes. How can we reconcile this? Well, I think all we have to do is wait, and eventually MA's message to leave her plants alone will be heard. Here is just one example. The nutritional gurus isolated from these vegetables a compound called indole-3-carbinol (I3C), which was hailed as a breakthrough in breast cancer prevention, and women were taking it by the handful as a testament to the power of broccoli, so for a while it looked like nutritionists=1 and MA=0. Uh-Oh. A study in rats has shown increased colon tumors in chemically treated rats given I3C as a dietary supplement [49]. It turns out that some nasty stuff resembling dioxin (a poison) is produced by I3C, which causes DNA damage and can lead to mutations and cancer [50]. Well, at this point the score is MA=1, nutritionists =0. Not to be outdone, the nutritionists then came up with diindolyl-methane (DIM), which is formed from I3C, but you would have to eat a boatload of vegetables to get a good dose, so they have conveniently made up potent doses of the stuff. As they say in the legal biz, the jury is still out, but I am betting on MA. I am personally confident that following Nature's blueprint has all of the anti-cancer properties I need. I would also like to predict that at some time in the future, it will be obvious that, for some people, eating plants that MA does not want to be eaten is equivalent to undergoing chemotherapy at every meal, with all of the dangers, side effects, and occasional benefits connected therewith.

What about leaf vegetables? Eating a major portion of a plant leaf can destroy or interfere with plant propagation, especially if it is a small plant. The list of toxic leaf vegetables is quite long, including such innocents as spinach and wild lettuce. There are probably non-toxic leaf vegetables out there, but I for one do not feel comfortable guessing which ones are in this category. Chimps eat leaves, but unlike humans, their large hindguts are designed to digest very high fiber plants that we cannot, and perhaps this difference in anatomy also aids chimps in detoxifying some plant species that we cannot, but all of this is speculation.

How about eating sprouts? Sprouting is sometimes touted as a healthy way of eating seeds, but in fact, many sprouts have the potential of being quite toxic when eaten raw, not surprising since this is a very delicate point in the reproductive cycle of a plant. Kidney bean sprouts, buckwheat sprouts and alfalfa sprouts are some examples. I could go on and on as to attempts that have been made to remove known plant toxins from food, but the results are quite poor. Compound that with the fact that we have yet to *identify* many of the toxins in these foods and we do not know what the safe levels of ingestion are for humans over the long term, and you get the picture that we really don't know what we are doing in this area. So, for the Tier One Wellness Diet, designed to closely follow Nature's clues, we will not fool with her plan and, thus, we leave out seeds, nuts, beans, peas, roots, tubers, and flowers.

This decision did not come lightly. After all, this is a significant portion of the vegetable category of plant foods. So, I decided to do some "sanity checks," as follows. First, I scoured the literature to see if anyone had reached a similar conclusion for the pre-cooking human diet. In "Toxic Substances in Plants and the Food Habits of Early Man." Science 176: p.513, the authors concluded [38]:

> "Some archeologists have suggested that the importance of vegetable foods used by early man may have been grossly underestimated because vegetable materials would not persist in archeological remains. Recognition of the widespread occurrence of toxic substances might make the opposite argument more tenable; if one makes comparisons with present-day hunter-gatherer tribes, all of which possess cooking skills, the importance of vegetable foods to evolving man may have been overestimated."

This article spurred a flurry of activity in the anthropology community to address the issue of what pre-cooking hominids may have eaten, based on fossil evidence; a study of plants indigenous to tropical East Africa; and further investigation into the diets of other primates, including chimpanzees and baboons [38-40, 51-55]. There is much disagreement as to what constitutes the plant portion of a pre-fire hominid diet, but some interesting findings are that fruit was for the most part the largest category of plant food consumed by PA, with leaves and shoots supposedly a close second, very similar to the chimpanzee diet. Nuts and seeds are also on the list (chimps can use rocks to crack some nuts), but in smaller amounts. Most wild primates do not feed on grasses, grass seeds, or underground storage organs (tubers or roots) [56].

Next in my diligence study came a check against the current most prevalent foods for allergic reactions, listed earlier, which came up with peanuts (a bean), tree nuts, soy (a bean), and wheat (a seed), which would indicate late evolutionary adoption by our ancestors, leaving less time for adaptation. All in all, when factoring in what appears to be MA's plan for her plants, I am comfortable with my decision as it applies to the Tier One Wellness Diet.

So, who does eat plants? Herbivores, many of which are ruminant animals, meaning they have multi-chambered stomachs and a very involved digestive system evolutionarily evolved for the express purpose of eating plant material such as grass. These animals, left to their natural environment (un-tampered with by humans), have learned which plants and which parts of each plant to eat and which to avoid to maximize their survival (if only we were that smart). This takes us full circle in MA's plan, because these are the very animals we eat to maximize *our* survival. Another way to answer the question of who eats plants is that *we* do, but the animals we eat first process them, and thus we indirectly derive nutritional benefit from plants in this manner. Ah, but this is only part of the answer to who eats plants. Insects eat plants and appear to possess unique detoxification systems to deal with plant toxins. As discussed above, insects may prove to be a big missing link in our diets and another way for us to partake of plants indirectly as food.

Before leaving this plant discussion for the moment (it is continued in the section of Tier Three foods), you may well raise the question that if MA's plan is to protect the survival of species, what possible protection can be afforded to, say, buffalo, by having them hunted and killed? Here is my personal theory as to how it works, trying to second-guess MA with the help of Darwin. When animals are chased and killed, by either humans or other animals, the ones most likely to be caught are the old and infirmed who are probably beyond reproductive age, and thus have already contributed offspring to the continuance of the species. It is also likely that the overall genetic pool of the species is strengthened in general by culling those that are not the fittest, which are the ones that are easy to catch. So even if some easy to catch animals are of reproductive age, they are likely to be genetically weaker and their lineage will be eliminated, leading to stronger offspring of others that are harder to catch, improving the overall survival of the species. Perhaps this may be considered cruel in a human frame of reference, but it is obviously effective.

## Water

Water is an essential part of the diet, and the kind to drink is fresh high-mineral water as found in Nature, such as spring water and the water naturally found in fruit. There is very little information available regarding PA and water, so I will have to make some hopefully educated guesses. In the tropics during the rainy season, rainwater would have collected in virtually every depression, including tree trunks and rocks, as well as in flowing streams. This water would have absorbed a high concentration of dissolved solids, particularly when found in rock pools and mountain streams, and would thus have provided an important source of minerals to the diet, such as calcium and magnesium. It would also have contained organic acids such as fulvic and humic acids, and certain healthy bacteria, all discussed in detail in the next section. I avoid highly carbonated water, as it is rarely found in natural form. As far as water containers go, cupped hands, folded leaves (chimps use this), and hollowed out plant parts, such as a watermelon shell, might have been used. Considering the climate and need for a lot of physical activity while hunting/gathering, I would assume PA sweated quite a bit and needed frequent fluid replenishment. I view water as perhaps the major source of calcium and magnesium for PA.

I do not drink water chilled or iced, and preferably not any colder than spring water, and I do not ingest ice at any time. For the gut to work correctly, it needs to be close to body temperature, which is where enzymes and other reactions work best. Pouring cold water on this process is likely to disrupt digestion, leading to future health problems. Modern water containers should be made of uncolored glass or ceramic, not plastics or metals. Ideally, only limited amounts of water should be consumed during a meal because it can dilute stomach acid, among other things, which also disturbs digestion. Drinking hot liquids with a meal, such as soups (like bone broth) or non-caffeinated fruit teas, can actually help maintain gut temperature. As far as how much water to drink each day, I use urine color as a gauge, and try to maintain it a very pale yellow, almost colorless. Below is a discussion of water filters and containers.

## Hard water vs. soft water

Many people do not like so-called hard water, which is what is delivered by most municipalities. It is high in calcium and magnesium, which cause a white film on surfaces, reduce the sudsing effect of soap and detergents, and leave a plaque-like "scale" on the inside of pipes and water heaters that can eventually reduce efficiency and block lines.

Consumer discontent spawned the water-softening industry, where the customer pays for a service that replaces the calcium and magnesium with a sodium or potassium salt. Potassium and sodium are needed electrolytes in the body that are plentiful in the Wellness Diet, but we also need the other two electrolytes, calcium and, more importantly, magnesium (see section on magnesium below). The resultant soft water is super-sudsing slimy stuff that rarely exists in nature. While my shower door might look better and my appliances work better, what about my body? My priority is to my health. While I can always clean and replace appliances, I only have one body, so the trade-off for me is a no-brainer, meaning no soft water. I regard softened water as Frankenwater and there are dozens of studies worldwide that show a strong inverse correlation between the hardness (mineral content) of water and cardiovascular disease, primarily due to a deficiency of magnesium in soft water [57] [58]. A website containing a wealth of research on the subject is www.mgwater.com [59]. I would not bathe in soft water, let alone drink it. By the way, I will be using various terms like Frankenfood to describe a food or other product that has been so messed with by human technology that, in my opinion, it is no longer something I want to put in or on my body.

Before we continue with the hard/soft water discussion, I want to clarify some terms. Hard water usually refers to water with a high content of calcium and/or magnesium, generally in the form of bicarbonates. Healthy hard water, as shown in the research, is one that contains substantial amounts of magnesium as well as calcium. As you will see later, my view of the ideal is to have a level of magnesium that is at least fifty percent of the level of calcium. These are the waters that contribute to low levels of cardiovascular disease.

Concerning water softeners, new models of dishwashers have the option for a built in water softener to which you add salt, and I have no problem with this limited use. I know of some unscrupulous soft water marketers who scare people into thinking that the minerals that clog copper pipes will also clog one's arteries and need to be removed, an absurd bit of twisted logic. Without access to the copper-pipe-clogging minerals calcium and magnesium, a person would have no bone strength and/or be dead. In my house, I go to great pains to add lots of additional minerals back into the filtered water. From a water analysis, I get close to 3 mg of calcium and 1.5 mg of magnesium per ounce of high-mineral water, making available to me about 250 mg of calcium and 125 mg of magnesium per day just from drinking water. My assumption is that the water that PA drank contained even more of these critical minerals, so mineral supplementation becomes important, and is dealt with further below. There are many laboratories available to test home water and I encourage such testing [60].

## Water filters

In today's world of contaminated drinking water, various filtering techniques are in wide use to eliminate toxins, but many of them also remove important essential minerals, or otherwise add unhealthy compounds. I avoid distilled water (I don't think it exists in Nature), reverse osmosis (RO) treated water (similar to distilled), and soft water (rarely found in Nature). Virtually all of the drinking water available to us today does require filtering to eliminate toxins.

Many healthy indigenous groups have had access to spring water packed with minerals collected on the way down from mountain heights, and sterilized by ultraviolet light from the sun. I do not think it is a coincidence that some of the longest lived groups live in mountainous areas close to free-flowing streams. In modern times, the water that reaches your home usually starts its journey from a reservoir, then goes through one or more treatment plants that add toxins such as chlorine and fluorine, then perhaps travels through an aqueduct before going underground through a pipe system. The pipes may be made of iron, plastic, copper, or ceramic, and the water picks up some of the particles of these materials. Alternatively, you may be using well water, which picks up all of the groundwater toxins that have percolated into it from human-made sources.

In order to protect consumers against bacterial buildup, since 1908, municipalities have been treating with chlorine the water they sell to consumers. Unfortunately, this element is toxic not just to bacteria but to humans as well. When chlorine reacts with organic substances, it forms compounds called chloramines, which are known carcinogens. Chlorine itself is a neurotoxin and interferes with certain hormonal processes, as discussed further in the detox section. Municipal water may also include variable trace levels of nasty substances such as runoff residuals of fertilizers, pesticides, herbicides, and fungicides, heavy metals, cysts, viruses, fungi, bacteria, industrial wastes, rocket fuel, and prescription drugs such as antibiotics and hormones.

Drinking, showering or bathing in this stuff is a good way to add toxins to the body. In a shower the hot water opens pores and we can inhale and absorb large amounts of the bad stuff (spas, hot, tubs, and pools add to the toxin problem with their use of chlorine, bromine, and algaecides; this is dealt with separately in the halogen portion of the detox section). Therefore, water filtering is a necessary part of the Wellness Diet, with the goal of matching the healthy characteristics of fresh mountain stream water as closely as possible.

One option is the reverse osmosis system (RO) system, commonly used in under-the-counter kitchen filters. The problem with this method is that it removes not just the bad impurities but a lot of the good stuff as well, namely minerals. Plumbers installing RO (and distillation) filters take care to be sure that the water from the filter does not run through a copper pipe to the drinking spout. The instructions for such systems, in fact, caution not to use copper (or any metal) for this purpose. That's because RO (and distilled) water will suck the copper right out of the pipe.

For those using an RO or distillation system, there are a number of re-mineralizer systems on the market that claim to add back some of the missing minerals, primarily calcium and magnesium, and they may be worth an investigation. Another approach is to take a mineral supplement along with RO or distilled water. It seems to me that an important part of the mineral content of mountain spring water comes from the rocks over and through which the water flows as it travels down to the ocean. A very common type of such rock is a form of limestone known as dolomite. It has a high concentration of calcium and magnesium carbonate in approximately a 1.7 to 1 ratio. Carbonate forms of minerals have been dismissed by the mineral supplement industry on the basis that they have a low percentage of assimilation in the human gut. If that was in fact true, all mineral waters would seem to be useless, and they are not. Calcium and magnesium in natural mineral water appear in the form of soluble bicarbonates, which are produced when the carbonate forms of the minerals, such as in dolomite, are combined with carbon dioxide in the water.

I would rather listen to MA than the supplement industry, and I use a dolomite supplement to replicate closely the mineral content of spring water. A few years ago, dolomite supplements had a bad name because some brands contained high levels of lead. I have found a source of dolomite from a supplier who indicates they derive their dolomite from deeply buried ancient mineral deposits free of toxic metals. They test their product for lead, with a limit of ten parts per billion, a very low level [61]. While there is no safe level for lead, magnesium acts to displace and replace it in the body, so the high levels of magnesium in dolomite mitigate against even these small amounts of lead as being troublesome. One dolomite tablet with each glass of water (not with meals because it can neutralize stomach acid), up to four tablets per day (a total of 630 mg of calcium and 360 mg of magnesium), would seem to restore a good part of the natural calcium and magnesium missing from RO or distilled water. I will be discussing dolomite further in the mineral section below, but I want to emphasize its importance as a completely natural compound, undoubtedly loaded with essential trace minerals. A fascinating book discussing the health benefits of dolomite was written decades ago by Jerome Rodale, a pioneer in the health field [62].

Although I am not a fan of plastic pipes, in the case of RO or distilled water systems they are definitely required. Copper toxicity is a much-overlooked contributor to health problems including rheumatoid and osteoarthritis, bone fractures, decreased libido, panic attacks, hair loss, fatigue, and childhood hyperactivity and learning disorders. These types of filtered water should not pass through any kind of metal, including metal water bottles or cooking utensils, as the water may absorb components of the metal itself. An issue I have with many RO and distiller systems is that the drinking faucet may be made of copper or brass, so the water sitting in contact with the faucet may well be leaching metals from the faucet into the water. Copper is an important mineral for health but only in very small amounts, beyond which it is toxic [63].

Unfortunately, RO and distilled water may also absorb toxins from the plastic pipes. Why is this so? As many of you recall from science class, water is the universal solvent, and acts to dissolve solids up to the point where it is fully saturated. Well, distilled and RO water contain virtually no dissolved solids, so they act very aggressively to dissolve whatever it is they are in contact with. Opposed to this is water with a high desirable mineral content, which is close to or at saturation, and hence has very little affinity for dissolving unwanted substances, like copper and plastic from pipes and containers. This is not rocket science. Which brings up stainless steel.

Most water distillation filters use a stainless steel tank (hopefully food grade) to heat and hold the water. Stainless steel is used everywhere in the food industry, from raw ingredient containers to cooking utensils to eating utensils, as well as in medical and dental instruments. Stainless steel is the name given to iron based alloys containing at least 10% chromium. I am not a metallurgist, but I took my share of metallurgy courses in college, and it is well known that all iron alloys exposed to water and oxygen will corrode, and a popular industry spec for stainless steel allows for 0.1 mm of surface corrosion per year. So-called food-grade stainless alloys include Type 304, which contains chromium, nickel, carbon, and manganese, and is known as 18/8 stainless. Type 316 has higher corrosion resistance, and further includes molybdenum. Stainless steel is also used in water heaters and water filters. Since it is virtually impossible to avoid stainless steel, my point is to raise the possibility that small amounts of iron, chromium, nickel and molybdenum may be leaching into the food and water chain, increasing the importance of having a filter that removes metals. This corrosion factor is another reason I do not use stainless steel (or any other metal) for water containers.

Here are my filter suggestions. Starting with the simplest, for drinking water I have used under-counter (and counter-top) filters made by Doulton, a British company, and sold by many distributors [64]. The main filter uses a ceramic cartridge impregnated with silver. Many other cartridges are available for specific filter requirements, such as eliminating fluoride, and the model HIP-320 is a good choice. In a way, using ceramic mimics MA's natural rock filtration system. By the way, the bibliography section and Appendix C at the end of this book contains many website references to potential sources of information and/or products.

For a shower filter, I have used the Shower Soft Filter by Hydro-Flow Filtration Systems [1], and it is easily installed in most showers just behind the showerhead. It uses KDF, a filter medium that works well in cold or hot water to remove chlorine and many organic toxins, so your shower (and you) will no longer have a chlorine odor. For those who like to take baths, the tub can be filled with water from the shower.

One of the most intriguing water filters on the market is called the Wellness Filter, a Japanese product line ranging from showerheads to whole-house systems that is designed to replicate mountain stream water [65]. The filters not only remove most of the bad stuff (fluoride is an exception), many models re-insert into the water desirable minerals mined from various volcanic mountain locations in Japan which have been studied for millennia for their healing properties. They mine the rock from those locations, pulverized it, and layer it into their filters, which also include carbon, KDF, and magnetics. Apparently, Japanese hospitals and some of their Olympic teams are using these filters, and high-end American restaurants have started to install them as well. I have a whole-house version of the filter that works well. It is programmed to backwash weekly, and no media (filter element) replacement is required for many years.

For communities that have fluoridated water, the filter problem is substantially more complicated. Eliminating fluoride requires either RO, or distillation, or a special media filter, so for those unlucky enough to be in a community that fluoridates its water, one of these filters would be useful wherever there is a drinking water spout. The media filter uses aluminum oxide, so there should be a KDF and carbon filter following it to remove any aluminum oxide that may leach into the water. The

Doulton filter does the job with the right selection of filter elements. Users of the whole house Wellness filter, which does not remove fluoride, may need to include a Doulton unit at drinking stations. I do not know of any whole house system for removing fluoride, leaving one vulnerable to shower inhalation and absorption of this potentially toxic mineral. Alternatives are to petition local government to get the fluoride out of the water (it is a nasty toxin), or to move (I moved). I cover the fluoride problem in more depth in the detox section, where I also discuss water filters for hot tubs, spas, and swimming pools.

## Water Bottles

The plastic water bottle is everywhere, and it is difficult to pick a starting point to discuss its toxicity because the playing field is rapidly expanding. Let's begin with the most popular plastic, polyethylene terephthalate (PET), shown as a #1 inside a triangle on the bottle bottom, and used by virtually all brands of bottled water. A somewhat recent study showed elevated levels of the metal antimony leaching from these bottles into the water [66]. Antimony is nasty stuff, and while the amounts measured were below the supposedly acceptable level, they were hundreds of times higher than levels normally found in drinking water, not surprising since antimony trioxide is used in the production of PET. There is almost no information on the hazards of oral ingestion of antimony, but it is a cumulative metal with a long half-life, and it is rated as carcinogenic. It also appears in breast milk, crosses the placenta, and may be a cause of miscarriages. Compound this with the fact that much of the bottled water is made using the RO process, so it is in a state where it can aggressively absorb bad stuff, like antimony. Over thirty years ago, it was reported that plants watered with water stored in PET bottles did not grow as well as those watered without using plastic [67], which raises all sorts of issues as to the impact on plant foods of plastic used in irrigation systems.

Moving on to polycarbonate bottles, these are the hard plastic ones that sometimes come in colors, or have a bluish cast in a semitransparent style, with a #7 on the bottom in a triangle. They leach bisphenol-A (BPA) into the water, and this chemical, which is also found in soup and soda can liners, is an estrogen mimic that can cause hormone havoc. It had been found in baby bottles, pacifiers and other toys, and because it can be particularly devastating to children, its use has been banned in many of these products [68]. Washing these bottles with a detergent can worsen the situation. I have seen people at the market line up with their re-usable # 7 water containers and put money into a machine that generates RO water from tap water. Here again, putting mineral-free RO water into plastic is not a great idea, and I wonder if there is any real health benefit for their efforts. So far, plastic containers labeled #2, #4 or #5 have escaped the toxic tide, but my guess would be it is only a matter of time before they too meet the fate of #1 and #7. This is not rocket science. All plastic containers are toxic.

Many health-minded people are switching to metal bottles, and stainless steel is becoming the vogue. I already covered the issues I have with stainless, and I would not drink from them or cook in metal. Other fashion bottles claim to have inert liners of one sort or another, such as epoxy. Most common epoxy resins are produced from a reaction between epichlorohydrin and bisphenol-A. We dealt with bisphenol-A above, and epichlorohydrin is a known reproductive toxin. Many epoxies are FDA approved for contact with foods, and they may be somewhat inert until scratched or otherwise abraded. Those who insist upon metal might want to consider drinking out of a sterling silver goblet (see side box below).

## A Non-Toxic Plastic Water Bottle?

Many folks know of the potential toxicity of plastic water bottles, but are not willing to lug around a heavy glass one. I will be commenting further about the unique properties of silver, and certainly one could safely drink out of a silver cup. I came up with the idea of combining silver and a plastic such as polycarbonate with two objectives in mind. First is to use the silver to bind with the toxic components in the plastic to prevent them from being leached into the water. Second is to provide a source of silver ions on the inside and outside surface of the container to disinfect the water in the container, and to disinfect the hands of the user on the outside of the container, in an effort to avoid the spread of nasty bacterial infections such as MRSA (methicillin resistant staphylococcus aureus). I have filed a patent application covering the concept in the hope of attracting a company to commercialize it.

So what's left to drink out of? How about good old glass? Yes, it can break on impact, and it's a lot heavier than plastic but it's the best and safest choice, along with uncolored ceramic. Some flat mineral water products are sold in glass bottles, such as Evian, and they can be reused. Alternatively, glass bottles of all shapes and sizes can be purchased online from a variety of sources [69]. I particularly like swing-top locking flask designs. Cloth water bottle holders with straps are available to minimize the chances of breakage, and can also be used to make a fashion statement!

## Dirt

By dirt, I mean soil, but the word dirt is so much more dramatic! Is dirt an acceptable food? Few people appreciate the fact that soil itself is a form of food. It is unlikely that PA washed off what she/he ate, and so ingested some soil with fruit, animal prey, and drinking water. Surprisingly, soil contains many beneficial bacteria, amino acids, and trace minerals, as well as other compounds that we have yet to identify. From my research, there appear to be four separate groups of soil materials that contribute to health both for animals (including humans), and plants.

The first group is in the form of acids named fulvic and humic acids, which are major constituents of what you may be familiar with as potting soil, humus, or peat moss. This material is the accumulation of partially decayed vegetable matter, before it turns into coal or oil. It is great for plant growth, and some interesting research has been conducted regarding the beneficial effects from human consumption [70]. What becomes clear from this research is the importance of starting with very clean soil, free of toxins. Put another way, if you ingest toxic soil, it will toxify you, which appears to have happened on at least some occasions [71]. My approach was to find suppliers who have been providing these soil components as supplements for human consumption for a decade or more. In the U.S., the predominant source of soil for these supplements is known as the Fruitland Formation, located in Northwestern New Mexico. This shale formation from which the soil is taken is the remains of an ancient shallow fresh-water sea dating from about 80 million years ago. Several companies have been mining the soil from it for decades for use as soil conditioners as well as for animal and human use [72] [73]. Some of the cited human benefits include improved mineral utilization, and antiviral properties. These soil acids also bind with heavy metals so they can pass out of the body, and act as an immune system stimulant.

One of several companies that have been offering soil products for human use for some time is Morningstar Minerals [74], who offer capsules and liquids containing high concentrations of fulvic and humic acids. The products I use are those with minimal processing, referred to as Immune Boost 77 (capsules) and Vitality Boost HA (liquid). It seems to me that PA would have ingested a daily dose of these acids by drinking water found in tree and rock depressions, and even in flowing stream water that picks up soil along the way. I add one capsule or one ounce of the liquid each day to my drinking water as a way of more closely duplicating PA's diet. There is a more thorough discussion of humic and fulvic acids in the detox section below. Note that the high carbon content of these supplements may cause darkening of the water and the stool.

The second group of materials from soil is bacteria, and they turn out to be an important component of the Wellness Diet, as well as an important part of the detox protocols. These bacteria, sometimes inaccurately referred to as soil based organisms (SBOs), are quite different from the conventional probiotics most of us are familiar with, such as acidophilus, so to avoid confusion I will not refer to them as probiotics. While these organisms are certainly found in great quantity in soil, it really is not clear where they might have originated. In addition to soil, they are found throughout nature in water, dust, air, and in the intestines of animals, insects, and sea life, but they are not native to the human gut and do not take up permanent residence there, unlike conventional probiotics. They survive stomach acid, thrive in an oxygen environment, have the ability to form spores (actually endospores) and can bind with toxins.

The ability to form spores has resulted in the name *spore-formers* being used to describe these bacteria, and I will refer to them as such. I will be going into some detail in this section because I believe they are a very important missing ingredient in our diets that can have a profound positive effect on our health. Some of the reasons they are missing include the widespread use of fungicides and pesticides in the soil, and the use of disinfectants such as chlorine in our water supplies, all of which can prevent spore-formers from proliferating.

There is research being performed on spore-formers in the belief that they may eventually replace conventional antibiotics, which are rapidly becoming obsolete due to bacterial resistance. Spore-formers could have appeared in PA's diet from dirt or dust on fruit, in drinking water, and from the intestinal contents of their animal prey, discussed in the probiotics section below.

For some of my comments, I will be drawing from an excellent review of the subject entitled *The Use of Bacterial Spore Formers as Probiotics* by H. Hong, et al. [75]. One simplified way to understand spore-forming bacteria is to use a seed analogy. Just like a plant seed that has a strong coating protecting the embryo, the spore-formers have a strong coating protecting an endospore. They can lie dormant for years until germinated by being placed in a suitable environment, which usually includes a liquid. The human gut is an ideal environment for many of these species to germinate. As we have seen, plant seeds do not find our gut hospitable for germination and, of course, they contain all of the natural toxins discussed earlier. I like to think of the spore-formers as MA's way of providing us with "friendly seeds" designed to grow for a short time in the "soil" of our intestines and provide great health benefits. Having said that, there are spore-formers that are quite nasty, such as anthrax, so it behooves us to tread with care in this area.

Although research is still in its infancy as it applies to humans, the potential benefits that can be derived from these bacteria are somewhat overwhelming. From what is known, immune system stimulation and the generation of unique antimicrobials are just two areas of great interest. A third benefit is that of competitive exclusion (CE), where the spore-formers take up temporary residence, and through a variety of poorly understood mechanisms, exclude pathogens from adhering to the gut wall. At one time, I thought that conventional probiotics could fill this role, but from my experience, they cannot hold a candle to the spore-formers in the pathogen exclusion arena. Yet another area of interest for spore-formers is that of cardiovascular disease. A fermented soy product called natto (and nattokinase) has been touted as preventing heart attacks and cancer, among other benefits. Well, natto is made by fermenting soy with bacillus subtilis, a spore-former, so it is certainly possible that it is the subtilis, not the soy, which is responsible for the benefits.

Reading between the lines of some of the research studies [76], I ponder the following. If ingesting a somewhat continuous supply of spore-formers with our food (they tend to last less than 30 days in the human gut) can effectively exclude pathogens from taking up residence, could they be a preventive for a whole host of bad guys such as salmonella, C. difficile, H. pylori, MRSA, anthrax, and the bacteria responsible for malaria and Lyme disease? In the fungal arena, there is a great deal of evidence that spore-formers can exclude Candida and other fungi from the gut and this will be covered in more depth in the detox section. Spore-formers are also known bioinsecticides, opening up a fertile area of research into a natural form of mosquito control [77]. By now, you may be sensing a great deal of excitement on my part for the goodies described in this dirt section of the diet, and at one point I thought of naming the Wellness Diet "The Dirt Diet™," but well-meaning friends suggested I reserve it as an alternate title.

Here is how I use spore-formers as part of the diet. My approach, as in the case of the humic and fulvic acid products, is to find suppliers that have been providing spore-formers for human use for a decade or more. Several species of the *bacillus* genus of spore formers have seen extensive use in human supplements worldwide, and they include b. subtilis, b. licheniformis, b. megaterium, b. clausii, b. coagulans, and b. laterosporus. After some research, I have chosen two species that have a long history of non-pathogenic use and favorable symptom relief. The first is bacillus coagulans, which is also called (somewhat incorrectly) lactobacillus sporogenes. It is supplied as capsules under the lactobacillus sporogenes name by both Thorne Research [78] and Pure Encapsulations [79]. The second species is bacillus laterosporus, strain BOD [80], which is widely distributed by O'Donnell Formulas under the names Flora Balance and Latero-Flora as capsules and powder. These supplements can be purchased at many supplement retailers [81]. Because they are found in soil and water in their natural environment, I take them with drinking water along with the humic-fulvic acid supplements. For a maintenance dose, I use one capsule per day, or an equivalent dose of the powder.

Although not a normal dietary component, other very valuable forms of dirt -known as clays- have always been used in the animal kingdom and among humans as a detoxifying agent, and form the third group of materials that make up dirt. I have devoted an entire section to the health benefits of clay in Chapter 16. As you will see in that discussion, before cooking allowed PA to experiment with eating plants that are toxic when raw, if it was necessary to eat these foods or face starvation, PA sought out certain clays to eat with the food. These acted to either adsorb or otherwise detoxify the toxic compounds in the plant food. Although we avoid these naturally toxic foods in the Wellness Diet, we can use clay to assist in removing a variety of other toxins from our body, and as a digestive aid for those wanting to switch diets.

The fourth component of dirt for purposes of our discussion is dolomite, which was discussed in the section on water. Dolomite, a rock that is a form of limestone, is widely found on and in the Earth's surface as stone formations and as natural sediment in the soil. It is discussed further in the mineral section below.

In summary, there are four components to dirt as it is defined for the Wellness Diet: humic/fulvic acids, spore-forming bacteria, clay, and dolomite. We will visit this combination again in the detox section.

## Chapter 5 - Summary of The Tier One Diet

This completes the analysis section defining acceptable foods for the Tier One Wellness (and purist) diet of our Paleo Ancestors, to the extent I have been able to glean information from my research. Table 2 summarizes these findings. Recall that the purpose of this diet study was to establish a baseline set of foods that most closely resembled those of our ancient pre-fire ancestors before any tampering by human technology.

The premise is these foods most closely align with our nutritional heritage, they can be eaten by all humans without harm, and will provide nutritional support for a healthy life, as demonstrated by 90,000 past generations. I am not proposing that everyone must follow the Wellness Diet to remain healthy. I am proposing it as a tool for use in the field of nutrition as a standard of comparison against which other foods and diets can be compared. This is based on my conclusion that The Wellness Diet contains the lowest amount of natural toxins (phytates, oxalates, trypsin and other protease inhibitors, lectins, glucosinolates and other goitrogens, cyanogens, tannins, saponins, gossypol pigments, lathyrogens, carcinogens, and various other hormone disruptors) and has an enormously successful evolutionary history behind it.

---

### Table 2
### The Tier One Wellness Diet

Here are the general food categories for the Tier One Wellness Diet. Within each category, the ABC test can be applied to a specific food to get an idea of its suitability:

- Animal protein and fat, including glands and other organs, bone marrow, blood, and intestinal contents from free-range hormone/antibiotic-free animals that eat their natural diet
- Non-Bitter Ripe Fruit - organically grown
- Soil: humic/fulvic acids and spore-forming bacteria
- Mineral-rich water with a high content of magnesium

---

In the following sections, I examine the food groups excluded from Tier One in light of what I have learned from the baseline diet. I attempt to make educated guesses as to what foods might be added, in the framework of a cost/benefit analysis as it applies to the possible detrimental effects on our health.

Before moving past the Tier One Wellness Diet, let's complete the discussion by looking at how much animal food vs. plant food might be consumed. One way to answer the question is to look at the potential macronutrients derived from each category versus what is generally accepted as the minimum required in a human diet. Clearly, there is very little fat or protein in fruit compared to animal products, which are low in carbohydrates. From my personal experience, the most critical macronutrient component of the Wellness Diet is *animal fat*. Unless there is enough fat in the diet, it will not prove satisfying, and can even lead to annoying symptoms such as fatigue and diarrhea. I am not the first to have come to this conclusion in connection with ancestral diets.

Vilhjalmur Stefansson was an anthropologist and Arctic explorer who spent many years living with the Eskimos and Indians of Northern

Canada. He reported that wild male ruminants like elk and caribou carry a large slab of back fat, weighing as much as 40 to 50 pounds. The Indians and Eskimo hunted older male animals preferentially because they wanted this back-slab fat, as well as the highly saturated fat found around the kidneys. In his book *The Fat of the Land*, he wrote:

"The groups that depend on the blubber animals are the most fortunate in the hunting way of life, for they never suffer from fat-hunger. This trouble is worst, so far as North America is concerned, among those forest Indians who depend at times on rabbits, the leanest animal in the North, and who develop the extreme fat-hunger known as rabbit-starvation. Rabbit eaters, if they have no fat from another source—beaver, moose, fish—will develop diarrhea in about a week, with headache, lassitude, a vague discomfort. If there are enough rabbits, the people eat till their stomachs are distended; but no matter how much they eat they feel unsatisfied" [82].

Stefansson is unique in having taken part in a fascinating experiment in which he and a colleague undertook a physician-supervised one-year program in 1929 where they ate nothing but meat, attempting to duplicate the diet they had followed in the Arctic years earlier. The fat content was increased early in the experiment based on the participant's requests. A March 31, 1930, article in *Time* magazine reported on the experiment:

"Last August four physicians of the Russell Sage Institute at Bellevue Hospital, New York, announced after three months deliberation that Vilhjalmur Stefansson and Karsten Anderson, Arctic explorers, had not harmed themselves by living on an all-meat diet for one year and ten days. Said the physicians: "In general, white men, after they have become accustomed to the omission of other foods from their diet, may subsist on an exclusive meat diet in a temperate climate without damage to health or efficiency." Said Meat-Eater Stefansson: "I am wide awake and am more aggressive in my work than I was before I started this test. . . .""

With the exception of cooking my meat, I personally have followed the Wellness Diet in one form or another for many years, while also experimenting with adding other food categories. I feel best when I stick closely to the Wellness Diet. The average macronutrient ratios that seem to work best for me as a somewhat sedentary researcher are one part carbohydrate to two parts protein to between three and four parts fat, by weight. For a 2,000 calorie per day diet, this yields ten to fifteen percent of calories from carbohydrates (50 to 75 grams), twenty to thirty percent of calories from protein (100 to 150 grams) and sixty to seventy percent of calories from fats (133 to 155 grams).

Most of the research in the field of pre-agriculture hominid diets centers on post-fire modern hunter-gatherer nutrient intake, which is not relevant to this Baseline study and produces very different results. One example is the Kalahari Bushmen, mostly a gatherer society, who learned to use fire to open the hard shells of mongongo nuts. The heat also probably reduces the toxin load of the nut. Our PA had no such luxury and, consequently, a dietary comparison would be somewhat meaningless. Still other research uses indigenous populations that have developed skills and tools not found in our area of interest, such as fishing and some domestication or cultivation.

I do have a personal theory, however, as to what might have taken place in PA's time, based on my experiments. Lots of studies place an optimum dietary protein content in the 20-30% range, where larger amounts can overtax the digestive system and even lead to rabbit starvation, and lower amounts are insufficient to support energy needs. That leaves 70-80% to be divided between carbs and fats. Well, I presume PA's diet was quite opportunistic, depending on the fat content of the animal prey and the availability of fruit. So, perhaps one day (or week) PA's diet might have been mostly fat if a large animal was caught, or mostly fruit and protein from small animals if not. How that averaged out is anyone's guess, but if it was me, I'd go for the fat to the extent it was available, before grabbing the fruit.

Put another way, trying to assign macronutrient ratios to PA's diet is not realistic. PA did not have the luxury of plucking foods from a supermarket, but instead took advantage of what was available. The closest we can figure is that animal protein was probably readily available, even if it had to come from small lean animals at times, so the real variables were carbs and fat. As far as how often to eat, three times per day works for me.

Using a 2000-calorie diet as an example, with a carbohydrate allowance of 50 to 75 grams, let's see how extensively we can indulge ourselves with fruit. How about this: a half grapefruit with breakfast (12 gm), a large wedge of watermelon with lunch (21 gm), and a bowl of fresh raspberries with dinner (10 gm), leaving three fresh figs (30 gm), or three passion fruit (15 gm) available with snacks (USDA database). Hardly a spartan diet.

I don't know if PA ate snacks, but here is a suggestion that works well with the Wellness Diet but does not strictly meet the ABC test. Pemmican is a modern food believed to have been developed by the American Indians. It consists of dried pulverized meat, animal fat, and occasionally some dried berries, and meets the ABC test if we allow for a minimal amount of processing (drying). Many recipes are available for do-it-yourselfers, but be sure to use grass-fed animals for the protein and fat, and I would stay away from sugars other than berries or similar fruit. Plain jerky (dried meat) is another possibility, but I find it to be too low in fat, and so do not use it. Pre-made pemmican is available from some online meat suppliers such as US Wellness Meats, mentioned previously [27].

I have not mentioned caloric intake in the discussion of the Wellness Diet for a number of reasons. First, the eating program is not about losing weight, it is about getting and staying healthy. Second, it is difficult to overeat on this diet because of the satiating effect of animal fat. Of course, if the amount of energy your body derived from your food intake exceeds your energy expenditure, the excess will accumulate, generally as body fat. Regarding derived energy from food, if your body was a perfect energy-converting machine, in theory it could derive from food its entire caloric value, which is the maximum amount of potential energy contained in the food, sort of like the BTU (British Thermal Units) rating of automobile fuel. The energy conversion takes place in the digestive system, and requires a whole symphony of processes to be successful, which are dependent on enzyme reactions, bacterial fermentations, fat emulsification, and some we have yet to figure out.

Assuming your gut is less than perfect, which I fear is mostly the case these days, then the energy derived from food will be less that the caloric maximum, and can vary based on the type of food. For example, for those who no longer have their gall bladder, chances are they digest fats inefficiently because of a bile acid deficit (correctable by supplementation as described below). So some of those who follow the Wellness Diet may experience a weight loss because of the high fat content. Where does the unconverted energy go? Well, let's use a car as an example. If your car is in need of a tune-up, it will most likely not burn fuel efficiently, wasting a portion of the potential energy of the fuel, and your MPG (miles per gallon) will suffer. Where does the unburned fuel go? Look at what comes out the tailpipe. The same with people – look in the toilet bowl. Poor fat-converters often exhibit steatorrhea, or fatty foul-smelling floating stools. Chronic diarrhea or constipation can also be clues to malabsorption, where a portion of food passes through you undigested. This really is not rocket science, yet I have seen a great deal of puzzlement in the nutrition field as to how, for some people, an equal number of food calories ingested can produce different results in that person as a function of the macronutrient composition, and all kinds of exotic theories have been concocted to explain it. This mystery has even been given the name Metabolic Advantage, when in fact it is a metabolic *disadvantage*. One of the goals of The Wellness Project is to get the gut into fine shape so that it can derive the maximum energy benefit from foods, regardless of the composition of your diet.

From years of studying the natural toxicity of foods, I feel comfortable saying that the Tier One Wellness Diet is the lowest in natural toxins, having virtually eliminated phytates, oxalates, trypsin and other protease inhibitors, lectins, glucosinolates and other goitrogens, cyanogens, tannins, saponins, gossypol pigments, lathyrogens, carcinogens, and other hormone disruptors. The chances of having a true allergic reaction to meat or fruit are close to zero. However, those who have a digestive system in disarray as a result of toxins may well experience a reaction to these foods, and this is further dealt with in the digestive rehabilitation and detox sections. Additionally, when beginning the Wellness Diet after following a SAD diet, some may think they are having an allergic reaction to the new foods, but it is more likely their gut is going through shock in attempting a return to its natural state. More on this later.

Some people that suffer from hypoglycemia (low blood sugar) might have a problem eating large amounts of fruit, which causes their blood sugar to dip. It has been my experience that hypoglycemia results from an endocrine system disorder, usually relating to pituitary, adrenal and/or thyroid issues, discussed below in various detox sections. Until this condition can be dealt with, eating fruit along with even a small amount of animal fat and/or protein, such as some pemmican or even a few desiccated liver tablets (described below in the supplement section) should temporarily eliminate the low blood sugar problem.

Fasting has no place in the Wellness Diet, but for those eating any other diet, such as the SAD diet, I would certainly encourage it. Remember the rat chow experiment? Anything that decreases the intake of toxic foods is certain to improve health, which is probably why some folks eating the wrong foods report that they feel better when they fast. In fact, I have often wondered if fasting could be used as a test to see if a person is eating incompatible foods. For those who fast and feel better, my guess would be that they are eating incorrectly, so not poisoning themselves three time a day is a definite improvement. This is yet another case of the diet gurus defining something (fasting) as healthy. But healthy as compared to what (eating the SAD diet)? In the case of the Wellness Diet, because it is naturally toxin free, fasting is counterproductive and certainly not what MA had in mind. For PA, food deprivation for any but a short length of time would be fatal, and it seems to me that fasting would put the body into a major state of stress.

# Chapter 6 - Deviating From the Tier One Diet

In this section, we will look at communities around the world that deviate in one way or another from the Tier One Wellness Diet and yet live a very healthy life. The objective is to derive some clues to this phenomenon that may be applicable to our own lives, as well as assessing the potential health risks involved.

We all know people who seem to be able to eat "anything" and remain healthy, and they were referred to as the *winners* in the introduction section of this book. How are they able to do this? We can glimpse the answer by reviewing the findings of Weston Price as he went around the globe in the 1930s visiting indigenous tribes in an effort to determine how they stayed healthy. His conclusion was they ate local foods, the ones Nature had provided, which had been consumed in that same area by their ancestors for generations. Note, however, that these so-called primitive tribes were nowhere near as primitive as our PA. They all had the use of fire for cooking, and most had learned to fish, cultivate crops, and/or domesticate animals. By our definition, they certainly were not Ancient, and ate non-Wellness Diet foods while remaining healthy.

The diets of each of the healthy groups Price studied were all quite different. In the Swiss village where Price began his investigations, the inhabitants lived on whole rye bread and cheese, eaten with fresh milk of goats or cows. Meat was eaten about once a week, along with bone broth soups and a few vegetables they could cultivate during the short summer months. They were all healthy and had near perfect dentition, which was one of Price's yardsticks for determining health. Hearty Gallic fishermen (and presumably women) living off the coast of Scotland consumed no dairy products, and fish formed the mainstay of their diet, along with oats made into porridge and oatcakes. The Eskimo diet was composed largely of fish, roe, and marine animals, including seal oil and blubber.

Hunter-gatherers in Canada, the Everglades, the Amazon, Australia and Africa consumed game animals, particularly the parts that we tend to avoid, such as organ meats, blood, and marrow along with a variety of grains, tubers, vegetables and fruits that were available. African cattle-keeping tribes like the Masai consumed no plant foods at all--just meat, blood, and milk. South-sea islanders and the Maori of New Zealand ate lots of seafood along with pork meat and fat, and a variety of plant foods including coconut, cooked cassava root, and fruit. Insects were another common food in all regions except the Arctic. In sum, the range of foods that enabled the people he visited to remain healthy covered the gamut including meat with its fat, organ meats, whole milk products, fish, insects, whole grains, tubers, vegetables and fruit. How can this be reconciled with the relatively spartan Wellness Diet?

Enter Darwin. Let's start with the Swiss village Price first visited, which had about 2000 inhabitants at that time. The village was in a remote area of the Alps known as the Loetschental Valley, about a mile above sea level. We can safely imagine that these folks did not magically appear here, but migrated from lower, more populated areas of Switzerland. The fact that they had mastered grain cultivation, milling, and bread baking, along with animal domestication and milking practices would indicate quite a recent legacy, say within the last four thousand years. This is based on an estimate of the time of migration of grain eating from the Middle East (about 10,000 years ago) to its appearance in Western Europe some time in the Bronze Age. The valley had limited grazing area so it is unlikely it could have supported sufficient grazing animals to feed 2000 people on a meat diet, and the short growing season severely curtailed the availability of edible plants such as fresh fruit. Therefore, in order to survive, animal milking (as opposed to slaughter) would have been the intelligent approach, along with grain storage (to tide them over in the winter months).

Now, let us suppose that among the pioneering group that trekked into the valley generations ago was a group (or a family) that was intolerant of casein (a major milk protein) and/or gliadin (a major rye protein). How long do you think they would last on a milk/rye diet? This is where evolution takes over, and the survival of the fittest (those who, through evolution, can best fit into the environment) is the rule. The bottom line is that only those who, through evolution since the time of the Wellness Diet, acquired the ability to assimilate safely dairy and glutinous grains, and thus survived in this valley. All of the others died out.

Because of the isolation of the valley, there would have been considerable interbreeding, further enhancing the gene pool necessary to survive in this environment. What Price encountered was a group that had evolved to eat a dairy/grain diet, and hence thrived on it. It is very important to distinguish this conclusion from one that infers his discovery meant that a raw dairy/whole-grain diet is healthy for *all*. Many others and I can tell you from first hand experience that it most certainly is not and, if a person's heritage is not aligned with these foods, they can make one very ill indeed. In the case of the unlucky Swiss group, certain families became extinct. We can go down the list of every group that Price visited, and draw the same conclusions, with the only variable being the foods they ate, which were the ones necessary for survival in that particular environment.

Now, let's look at how this analysis translates into variations on the Wellness Diet. Clearly, since leaving Africa over a long period of emigration (guesses range from 50,000 to more than 1,000,000 years ago), PA was subjected to all sorts of environmental pressures that, over many generations of evolutionary variations, shaped the diet of his/her descendants to one that, out of necessity, may have been quite different from the Wellness Diet. This brings us to the present conundrum of finding the diet variations that each of us has acquired. If we knew that both sides of our family tree were direct descendants of the Loetschental Valley Swiss, we could decide with reasonable certainty that dairy and rye (and undoubtedly mountain spring water full of minerals) are healthy for us to eat and drink. Unfortunately, for most of us in the melting pot that represents a good part of modern Western civilization, it is rare that such a monolithic ancestry is the case.

Nutritionists have struggled with this question for a very long time, and from their efforts has emerged what can best be described as a hodge-podge of dietary advice based on such diverse personal characteristics as one's blood type, body type, metabolic type, genotype, Ayurvedic type, etc. I heard a skeptic in the field predict the development of a nutritional program based on one's social security number! As an avid experimenter, I enthusiastically and personally evaluated as many of these diets as I could find before deciding that I did not intend to place my future health in the hands of any of these programs. As Mark Twain so eloquently put it, be careful about reading health books– you may die of a misprint. The basis of most of these programs is that there is not one diet that fits all, but of course, I disagree. From my research, the Wellness Diet originally (and still does) fit all, and then some became acclimated to variations thereof, but none of us lost the ability to thrive on the original diet, which is quite a different conclusion.

Can we find any clues from MA on this subject? Well, from a look at the animal kingdom, it seems clear that virtually every other mammalian species on the planet has one natural diet that fits all, regardless of their location. Felines, from tigers to house cats, are natural obligate carnivores, whether in California or Africa, and they have three different blood types. Canines, from dogs to wolves, have at least 13 blood types, but all are natural carnivores. In the case of cattle, (where it seems that each distinct animal has its own blood type!), they are all naturally grass eating, whether in India or Indiana. I want to make the point that the above diets are those found in a *natural* environment.

Could we artificially breed a vegan dog? Sure, and it might even be healthier than one fed the typical canned cooked dog Frankenfood. The same is true for humans. As omnivores, we can eat almost anything, and some of us do. At the risk of being redundant, I want to point out again that the Wellness Diet has been derived as the original one, *but not the only one*, for all humans, as designed by Nature. Individuals can modify or ignore it to their heart's content, with varying degrees of success, from perfect health to illness. I follow it for the simple reason that I do not like the odds of experimenting with other diets where my evolutionary compatibility with them is unknown, as is their impact on my health.

Ah, you may ask, isn't it possible that as a result of evolutionary adaptation to various diets, the Wellness Diet may no longer work for some of us? Can we lose our ability to assimilate animal foods and fruits? There are examples where nature has removed from us the ability to produce or properly assimilate certain foods or nutrients when it became evolutionarily unnecessary or inefficient to do so. One example is the ability to make Vitamin C, which we and other primates lack, presumably because we get enough from our diet. It is estimated that we lost this ability several million years ago, and it is not reversible. Lactose intolerance is caused by the loss of a digestive enzyme, lactase, as we reach adulthood, but there is some evidence that this intolerance may be reversible for some with prolonged ingestion of milk products. Although not related to food, our ability to make melanin in our skin decreased over many generations as we acclimated to sunlight-reduced environments far from the Equator, and this is not easily reversible (I have some interesting observations and suggestions on sunlight in the lifestyle section below.)

The pattern here seems to be one of "use it or eventually lose it," with the unknown factor being the definition of "eventually." I do not know of any studies directed to answering the question of how long is long enough for permanent digestive changes, so let's see if we can get any clues from MA in this area. We will start by looking at the probability that humans can lose the ability to digest meat, say because they have lived a vegan lifestyle. Permanent genetic changes of the type we are talking about do not occur within a lifetime, but take many generations, so now we need to look at the possibility of multigenerational veganism.

From the research that Price conducted, virtually all of the native tribes he visited around the world were meat eaters, at least for a part of their diet. Some modern African tribes such as the Kikuyu and Wakamba were multi-generational agriculturists and their diet consisted of sweet potatoes, corn, beans, bananas, millet, or sorghum. However, there is also evidence that these tribes did consume large amounts of insects including flies, bees, wasps, beetles, butterflies, moths, crickets, dragonflies and termites, most of which are rich in the fat soluble factors found in blood, organ meats, fish and butterfat, which may have kept their digestive system attuned to animal protein and fats. Nevertheless, it is possible that if a person's heritage is from either of these tribes, or they know that both sides of their family have been healthy vegans for many generations, they theoretically may have lost the ability to digest properly animal fats and proteins, and perhaps should continue with a vegan lifestyle. Otherwise, it would seem that most of us have not been distanced from animal products for a sufficient period of time (multiple generations) that would permanently compromise our ability to digest them if we chose to do so.

I occasionally meet people that tell me they have a hard time digesting meat. It feels like it is sitting in their stomachs as a lump or is constipating, and makes them feel uncomfortable. Many of them assume that meat is just not a healthy food for them, which seems to be in conflict with the Wellness Diet. I will not be so arrogant as to state that everyone must eat meat to stay healthy, but I will present here a very analogous situation with our furry friends, our domesticated cats and dogs, as a possible lesson from Nature regarding the eating of meat.

My wife and I love cats, and as I write this book, we have two beautiful Tonkinese in-house cats that are tenth-generation raised eating raw animal food (meat, glands and other organs, and bones) and a very small amount of vegetable matter (from the guts of their prey) to match closely their native diet as carnivores. The breeder of these cats, Celeste Yarnall, has undertaken the task of raising cats on this diet in place of commercial pet food to demonstrate the health benefits for domesticated animals raised on a natural diet [83]. Considering the explosion of medical specialties in the veterinarian community (oncologists, dermatologists, radiologists, endocrinologists, etc.), and how it mirrors the human illness maintenance industry, her work is most timely. It also provides some interesting insights into issues we, who are also domesticated animals, may face in converting from a prepared food diet to a natural one.

Commercial cat food is filled with ingredients no undomesticated cat would normally ever eat, and it is then cooked, which destroys amino acids necessary for cat survival, such as taurine, which are added back in synthetic form. Remarkably, cats raised on this stuff no longer recognize or are attracted to their natural diet. Certainly, cats can survive for many years and reproduce on this Frankenfood, thanks to the miracles of science, but look at the illnesses they accumulate along the way, just like with humans.

Let us say you were given a cat that had been raised (perhaps for many generations) on commercial food and the task was to reintroduce her/him to their natural diet. (A vet once confided in me the obvious: the perfect food for a cat is a rat.) Well, it turns out this is no simple task. If you merely switch one food for another, the cat may stop eating and get quite ill. If you put the cat in the garden to catch a mouse, she/he may catch one and merely play with it, not knowing how to eat it. (This is traditionally learned from a hunting mother.) If you try force-feeding the cat, it may regurgitate the food or develop diarrhea. Some human companions might give up at this point, and conclude that the cat has lost its ability to eat its native diet. However, those dedicated to the task have found this is just not so. While it may be that certain digestive processes have gone into hibernation as unnecessary for the digestion of the commercial stuff, all is not lost. The trick that works is to start introducing the natural food in very small quantities along with the junk food, and slowly increase the amount, weaning the animal back to Nature, which could take some time, perhaps months. The effort is worth it – a cat on its way to leading a healthy natural life.

Sure, humans are not cats, but I presume the analogy to the above is now obvious; for those who want to experiment with meat but are concerned about the ability to digest it, one approach is to follow the cat program with a slow introduction. In a later section, I will also discuss some supplements that can be taken during the transition period to support the gut.

Finally, I would like to make a prediction for our modern society, based on Price's work. Using the theory postulated above that a society will, through selection, distill or cull its heritage to match its environment, including food, it would seem self-evident that the same culling is going on as you read this book. In other words, the health crises we are seeing today are in some part due to adaptation to the SAD diet. Those not evolved to handle it are in fact dying out, just like what happened in the Swiss village. That leaves those who, through the luck of heritage, are able to use these foods and will be the final victors in the health arena. This dying out process is taking the form of many of the chronic illnesses ravaging society, spurred on by our contaminated environment. Thanks to the miracles of medicine, we are able to stay alive, and hence able to reproduce more evolutionary losers (among whom I include myself), so this selection process is taking a very long time.

This presents an interesting race to see who will win – medical technology or MA. If history is any guide, MA always wins, leading to the result that future generations will be those adapted to eat cake, soda, candy, and French fries, and they will live long and healthy lives. In the meantime, in spite of the pressures from the food industry and the health community to fit into an environment for which I am not adapted, I am doing what I can to live a lifestyle that is in concert with the ancient heritage of my species, which of course, is the foundation of The Wellness Project.

# Chapter 7 - Foods Excluded From Tier One

The objective of this section is to look at the major food categories that were excluded from the Tier One Wellness Diet, in the context of the rationales for their exclusion. We will also try to estimate the degree of risk associated with adding a category into the diet.  Table 3 is a list of the Tier Two and Three categories to be examined.

Anyone can add some or all of these foods to the Baseline diet to form for themselves a custom diet.  I am presenting some of the criteria that a reader might want to consider in making such choices.  As I have mentioned several times earlier in the book, each of us is responsible for our own food choices.  Knowing the Wellness Diet and MA's plans can go a long way in making those choices informed ones.

| Table 3 |
| :-- |
| **Tier Two and Tier Three Food Groups** |
| **Tier Two Foods** |
| • Fish |
| • Fowl |
| • Eggs |
| **Tier Three Foods** |
| • Dairy |
| • Plant Parts Other Than Fruit (Seeds, Beans, Nuts, Tubers, Roots, Flowers, Leaves) |
| • Sugars (natural or artificial) |
| • Extracted Vegetable Oils |
| • Liquids Other Than Mineral/Spring Water |

## Chapter 8 - Tier Two Foods

The foods in this category were chosen because they would have passed the ABC test except that it is believed they were either not introduced until after cooking was available or not introduced until after the end of or very late in the Paleo era, primarily because of the physical difficulty in obtaining them.  When they became available to PA, no significant processing was required, and they could be eaten raw.

## Fish

The estimates for the introduction of fishing into our heritage range from about 125,000 to 20,000 years ago. It seems logical that shellfish would have been introduced into the diet first for those PA's near the sea, followed by the development of fishing. Note that both fish and shellfish are on the list of the most prevalent allergenic foods, which may be because of their late introduction into the diet.

Fish is a wonderful food nutritionally, and I would heartily suggest including it into an expanded Wellness Diet, except for the contamination issues. As most of you are aware, fish have become the leading source of environmental exposure to mercury. They absorb the toxic mineral from water as it passes over their gills and from eating other marine organisms. Large predator fish get an even higher dose from their prey – other fish. Mercury binds tightly to proteins in fish tissue, including muscle and, over time, it builds up in a process called bioaccumulation. Fish also accumulate toxic organic compounds such as PCBs (polychlorinated biphenyls), as do shellfish, which accumulate mercury at slightly lower levels than finfish. Compounding the organic toxin problem, in the halogen portion of the detox section below, it will become apparent that brominated flame-retardants known as PBDEs are everywhere and are quite toxic to humans. A study has shown that the neurotoxic effects of PBDEs are enhanced when combined with PCBs, such as found in fish [84].

Cooking fish does not reduce the toxin content, but does bring up another issue. One of the reported nutritional benefits of fish is the omega-3 fatty acid content. This fatty acid group is polyunsaturated and easily degraded by light, heat, and air (see the section below on essential fatty acids). Therefore, the ideal way to eat fish, for those who are going to eat it, is raw - sushi and sashimi are examples.

Eating fish is a Catch-22, and as we shall see in the section on detoxification, the contaminants in fish are the very ones that many of us need to evict from our body to ensure health. The FDA has tried to define safe limits, but from my studies and hands-on experience in the world of detoxification, these limits are somewhat meaningless, arbitrary, and driven by industry. In the case of mercury alone, there is no test to measure total body burden in a human, and when you consider the added mercury burden from vaccinations and amalgam fillings, eating fish raises definite risks.

Now, let's look at the benefits of eating fish. The one most often referenced is the high content of omega-3 fatty acids, which are essential to the body. Comparing the omega-3 content of salmon with *grass-fed* beef yields a surprising result. Beef, on average, has slightly more omega-3 fatty acids by weight than fish (2% vs. 1.2%). It is also well known that the critical factor in essential fatty acids for humans is the ratio of omega-6 to omega-3 fatty acids. The ideal ratio is somewhere between 1:1 and 4:1, but for the SAD diet, the ratio can be over 20:1 due to an omega-6 overload. In the Wellness Diet, virtually the entire omega-6 overload has been eliminated, so that eating grass-fed meat easily achieves the desired fatty acid ratio without the need to consume any fish. Well, what about cholesterol – isn't the level in fish lower than that in meat? No, it is not, another surprise. The cholesterol level by weight for salmon is slightly higher than that for beef (as I previously indicated, the whole cholesterol issue is a *red herring* as far as I am concerned). Want more omega-3s? Eat organic grass-fed beef or lamb liver, which is loaded with good stuff [85].

Those who want to eat fish might want to concentrate on the smaller variety, because the smaller the fish the less contamination. As an example, sardines have a lower level of mercury than the large predators, but most commercially prepared sardines are canned, which is a less than healthy way of preparing fish. To meet health department requirements, canned fish must be essentially sterilized in the can to destroy all bacteria, which is why they last so long on the shelf. The time/temperature settings for this sterilization vary somewhat but are usually higher than the boiling point of water for many minutes. All of this takes place in a sealed metal can that may outgas its own toxins at these temperatures. As mentioned above, fragile omega-3 fats are easily damaged by heat, even though most of the air is evacuated from the can prior to heating. Thus, I cannot get too excited over a diet that includes canned fish (or canned anything, for that matter). Canning allows a product to sit on a shelf for years, which is good for the product's shelf life, but what about the shelf life of the consumer - does it contribute to their health and longevity? There are sources of salmon and other fish on the market that are selected for a lower than average mercury content, such as Vital Choice Wild Seafood [86].

This is a good place to mention other foods from the sea, such as algae in the form of seaweeds like kelp. Most of these are heavily contaminated with mercury, arsenic, and chemical toxins. The arsenic level in certain seaweed has gotten so high that there have been cases of arsenic poisoning in those eating large quantities [87]. Allergic reactions to fish can manifest as hives or swelling, or can be so serious that they are life-threatening. Fish proteins cause some of the symptoms, and worms or algae-based toxins cause others. As is the case for most allergic reactions to animal products, the symptoms appear very soon after eating the offending food. Fish oils and fish liver oils are discussed below in the section on essential fatty acids.

It is with a great deal of sadness that I take the position that until we can clean up the oceans, lakes, and rivers, I am staying away from anything presently living in these bodies of water. I take full responsibility for any personal bias in this decision, resulting from my own horrific mercury toxicity experience, due in part to my love of fish. I am not suggesting that all others follow suit. I feel quite confident that there are many people that can ingest loads of mercury and PCBs without health consequences. As a guide to individual health risks in eating fish, I suggest reading the detoxification sections below, which presents an in-depth review of the mercury and pesticide issues.

## Fowl

Somewhere along the timeline—we don't know quite when—humans learned how to catch and eat birds. Chickens are a domesticated bird descended from the red junglefowl, or guineafowl, related to the pheasant, of which there is an African variety. The flesh can be safely eaten raw, assuming the fowl is truly free range, and organically fed. The best guess as to domestication is about 1500 BCE by the Egyptians, which is extremely recent. The modern turkey is not related to chickens, and it appears to be native to North or Central America. Other flying birds native to Africa are duck and goose, and for the non-purist, these would be my first choices for experimental additions to the Wellness Diet because of their high fat content. As a caution, chicken is high on the list of allergens, perhaps due to its more recent introduction into our diet.

Symptoms of bird allergy usually show up very soon after eating and may include rashes, stomachache, fatigue, headache, and respiratory problems. I personally love duck and eat it on occasion. For those who are fowl lovers, I strongly recommend selecting organically fed free-range birds, which are readily available in health food markets.

## Eggs

Eggs might fit closer to the acceptable time-line category simply because hunter-gatherers could easily climb up trees to a certain height and raid nests, so eggs would have been available earlier than the birds themselves (who were much harder to catch). Ostrich eggs may have been the earliest obtained as food in this category, since ostrich nests are in the ground.

Nutritionally, eggs are a great food choice, especially if eaten raw, assuming they are from organically- fed free-range birds. Raw retains the full, undamaged value of the fatty acids and prevents oxidation of the cholesterol in the yolk. While salmonella is a concern, statistics show that such contamination is very rare. A strong defense system (which is a goal of The Wellness Project) is intended to handle the bacteria with perhaps a stomachache or the runs as the toxins are eliminated. If raw is not appealing (it does not appeal to me), cook eggs as gently as possible, boiling or poaching them to protect the fatty acids. The temperatures involved in frying are much higher than boiling and likely to cause fatty acid damage in ways we have yet to determine.

Some people, including me, are allergic to egg albumen, which is part of the white of the egg. A simple saliva test can sometimes pick up antibodies to albumen, and taking one may be worth it for those who choose to add eggs to the Wellness Diet [88]. Allergic symptoms to eggs are very similar to those of chicken allergy. In my case, I toss the whites and only eat the yolks, without any symptoms. Actually, I would discourage eating egg whites without the yolks, particularly if the whites are raw. The whites contain avidin, a protein that bind up biotin, an important vitamin. On the other hand, egg yolks are very rich in biotin, and I do not know of any adverse effects of eating only the yolks. Personally, I love medium-boiled egg yolks and eat them often. I choose high omega-3 eggs from organically fed free-range birds fed high omega-3 natural foods such as flax seeds. There is more detail on this topic in the essential fatty acid section below.

Now, onward to a discussion of the Tier Three foods.

# Chapter 9 - Tier Three Foods

The Tier Three foods are the ones that were excluded from the Wellness Diet because of potentially high levels of natural toxins. Aside from dairy, all of the other foods in this group are in the plant kingdom. There is no question in my mind that there are large numbers of people that can safely ingest many of these foods without compromising their health. The problem, of course, is the lack of knowledge as to which person fits which food. While I am very comfortable suggesting Tier One Foods, and also quite comfortable suggesting Tier Two foods (other than fish), because my research supports these food categories, I will not be so arrogant as to presume to have the answers when it comes to the Tier Three food category. At the end of this section, I will propose an approach that may lessen the impact of these foods on the defense system of those who wish to continue eating large amounts of Tier Three foods.

I have already suggested some pointers that might be of use in food selection, such as knowledge of one's dietary heritage over several generations of healthy ancestors on both sides of the family. Other pointers that may be of use come from our chimpanzee cousins. We know that at times when fruit was not readily available, those chimps with the intelligence to break open the shells of nuts did so and ate them as a source of nutrition, so freshly shelled raw nuts might be a category to investigate. On the other hand, roots and tubers seem to have exceedingly high levels of natural toxins, and chimpanzees are not known to eat much from this plant category.

Of course, cooking methods can have a great effect on natural toxins (increasing or decreasing them), so this is another variable to consider. For detailed discussions of various cooking methods and how they may relate to toxins, I want to again recommend the book *Nourishing Traditions* by Sally Fallon, as well as the food-related articles that appear on the Weston A. Price website [25] [7].

Another factor that can have a major impact on Tier Three food choices is the present nutritional status of the individual. As an example, it is one thing to eat plant foods that tend to bind minerals and prevent their absorption when you already have high minerals levels.  The health impact of occasionally eating these foods would likely be minimal.  On the other hand, if your present nutritional status is such that you are already mineral deficient, eating these same foods could have a substantial impact on health.  As you will see from a reading of the detox chapter, unnatural toxins in the body have a strong impact on nutritional status, which is why I do not believe one can separate diet from detoxification in any meaningful way on the road to health.  Therefore, I think it is prudent for the reader to become familiar with the toxin issues discussed in the next section before deciding on dietary choices.

Most tests for food incompatibilities look for some immune system response to ingesting the proteins or other compounds in these foods.  The result of such testing is often a false negative (indicating you are not intolerant, when you really are), based on a number of variables.  One is when you last ate that food.  Another is the total length of time you have been eating that food, and finally there is the condition of your immune system to consider.  If you have not eaten the suspected food lately, there may be no measurable immune system response.  If you have been eating that food for a very long time, the immune system may no longer respond to its toxic compounds, and this also can be the case if your immune system is in a weakened state.  I know of people who tested negative for a variety of foods, yet when they eliminated them from their diet as a trial, their health improved.  This indicates to me that an elimination diet, where potentially incompatible foods are not eaten for, say, a few months, may be the best way to make some food choices.  Armed with the information in this section, it would be easy to use the Tier One diet as the baseline, eliminating Tier Two and Tier Three foods in a planned manner and noting the result.  This approach can work well for those foods where the negative response (or its absence) is easy to detect and occurs in a reasonable time period.  Other than the above, I do not know of any foolproof way to evaluate food choices, which is why I take the easy way out and stick mostly to the Tier One foods.

As I now go through each of the categories of foods in Tier Three, I will attempt to suggest approaches that may be of assistance in the food consumption decision-making process.

## Dairy

Humans are the only mammals that routinely drink the milk of another mammal, and do so into adulthood. I don't presume to know Nature's plans, but this sure does not sound like one of them. The introduction of milking would have taken place some time after cattle domestication, believed to have begun about 10-12,000 years ago in the Middle East. The economic advantages are obvious. You can get a lot more protein and fat from a cow by milking it for as long as possible as opposed to killing it for food, and this undoubtedly was the original motivation for consuming dairy. It is interesting that some indigenous African tribes visited by Weston Price had developed an alternate approach to this problem by drinking small amounts of cow blood over time, while keeping the cow alive.

Assuming we are not under the environmental pressure of having to drink milk or starve, let us look at the pros and cons of dairy as an addition to the Wellness Diet. Referring now to unpasteurized and non-homogenized milk as it comes from a free-range organically grown grass-fed cow that has been spared hormones and antibiotics, the pros are that it is a good source of animal protein and fat, as well as fat-soluble vitamins. While milk is supposedly a good source of calcium, most of it is not very available to the bones because of missing co-factors, including magnesium, and this calcium can build up in the arteries unless there is enough magnesium present. I regard magnesium deficiency as a major factor in the near-epidemic osteoporosis scare among women, and it is covered in detail in the magnesium factor section below. Milk can be fermented and otherwise processed into a variety of foods such as cheese, yogurt, and kefir, some of which are high in supposedly healthy bacteria, and it can be churned into butter. For those readers who are fortunate enough to have a heritage that is compatible with dairy, as long as sufficient magnesium is in the diet, dairy is a reasonably good food source. For the rest of us, it is not.

Well, how does a person know if they are dairy compatible? Going back to the groups visited by Price as an example, he found several that thrived on dairy, including our Swiss friends, who needed it to support their population. Once again, for those who know their heritage on both sides for many generations, and it fits one of these indigenous populations, I would say their chances of dairy compatibility are high. There is also some evidence that portions of Northern European countries have subsisted for generations on dairy (for the same reasons of survival), and this may be a clue that you can include dairy in your diet if that is your heritage. Tests have shown that the majority of the adult populations in these areas are still able to produce lactase, an enzyme necessary to break down the milk sugar lactose.

However, estimates are that 70-80% of the world's adult population is lactose intolerant, having lost the lactase enzyme on the way to adulthood (it is needed in children to digest breast milk). Well, I can take a hint from MA, and to me this is a big one. There are a variety of tests that can be performed to see if a person is lactose intolerant, and for some people it is obvious from the bloated feeling in their gut when they consume dairy. If no immediate adverse effects occur, does that mean compatibility? No. If tests show lactose tolerance, does that mean dairy tolerance? No. In addition to the sugar lactose, there are at least two animal proteins in milk that have been identified as troublesome to many humans, casein and whey, and there are some tests for intolerance to these as well.

Are there additional troublesome compounds in milk? Researchers are still trying to figure out what is in milk (human and otherwise), which is no easy task because it is filled with a multitude of compounds. Ignorance in this area has produced some embarrassing (and sometimes fatal) results in the infant formula business, where manufacturers periodically realize they have left something out that is critical to the health of a baby. What is known is that cow's milk is different from human milk, and is undoubtedly the perfect food for a calf. Some of the relatively immediate symptoms that an intolerant or allergic person might experience from dairy include nausea, diarrhea, bloating, flatulence, itchy skin, gastrointestinal upsets, excess mucus, and respiratory disturbances.

Of course, those that have a problem with dairy can try to fool Mother Nature by getting lactose-free milk or by taking enzymes, and some of the obvious symptoms may abate. From my perspective, fooling with MA is a risky business. I know people who stopped dairy and their respiratory problems and arthritic pain disappeared very quickly. There isn't a clear explanation, but dairy seems to stir up inflammatory responses in the body that disappear when the dairy disappears.

For those who want to experiment with dairy, I strongly suggest getting products that most closely resemble what Nature intended, not an easy task. A starting point is to avoid pasteurization, homogenization, reduced-fat products, growth-hormones, antibiotics, grain-fed animals, and vitamin D2 supplementation, all of which turn milk into Frankenmilk. This leaves a precious few family-run dairies that avoid all of these pitfalls and sell raw milk and milk products. Unfortunately, they periodically run afoul of regulatory agencies that want to put them out of business, ostensibly for selling an unhealthy product! Their concern is that the milk will be contaminated with bacteria because it is not pasteurized, and I address this issue below. A grass-roots effort has been underway to lobby regulatory agencies to try to keep alive the right to access raw milk [89]. For those who are tolerant of dairy, this is an important project to support. In any case, I suggest that dairy eaters supplement with magnesium to avoid an overload of unusable and potentially harmful calcium. Note that the synthetic vitamin D2 supplementation added to some dairy products interferes with magnesium absorption (vitamin D3 is the correct form to use).

This is probably a good place to discuss pasteurization. What we know from a nutritional standpoint is that pasteurizing milk (or any other food) is not a good idea. The bulk of commercial dairy available in the world is pasteurized, a process that unfortunately creates toxicity. Dairy food requires the very bacteria that pasteurization kills to make it digestible for those who can digest it, and to suppress other bacteria toxic to humans. Pasteurization actually renders milk more toxic with time because it no longer contains the beneficial bacteria needed to control overgrowth of toxins. At least one of these bacteria is of the spore-forming type discussed earlier.

The reasons we have pasteurization have to do with money. The first reason is that the supply chain from cow to consumer is filthy, and it costs money to clean it up. By filthy, I mean it is contaminated with bacteria and other pathogens that can make one sick. The problem begins with the cows themselves. In most dairies, they are kept in unnaturally close quarters, and given antibiotics in their feed along with growth hormones. The result is a chemical cow with disturbed gut flora. The cow problem is so bad that cow dung is now toxic, and when it is used intentionally or unintentionally to fertilize vegetables (like spinach), they too become toxic with pathogens such as E.coli. This may surprise some readers, but cow dung from healthy cows (free-range, grass-fed, no hormones or antibiotics) has antibiotic properties and is an insect repellant! In India, it is used topically as part of Ayurvedic medicine to treat skin problems. It is also used as a floor liner to repel insects, particularly mosquitoes, and of course, it is a great fertilizer [90].

The second reason for pasteurization also has to do with money. By destroying much of the beneficial bacteria and enzymes, pasteurization extends the shelf life of products dramatically, resulting in significant cost savings compared to raw products. Virtually all liquid foods in a can or bottle and many in sealed boxes are pasteurized, which causes a loss of vitamins and enzymes, resulting in Frankendrinks.

The pasteurization process was popularized by Pasteur, as was the germ theory and vaccinations, although according to several historians, he did not develop any of these himself. During his lifetime, the Germ Theory (germs cause disease, leading to the conclusion that they need to be killed to stop disease) was in competition with what is called the Terrain Theory, which taught that defects in the internal environment of the body permit germs to cause illness, and that strengthening this internal environment is the key to health. I discuss this competition of theories and its consequences in much more detail in the bacterial problem portion of the detox section.

Returning to the dairy discussion, some people that have an adverse reaction to Frankenmilk feel better with raw milk products from properly treated range-fed cows, and others feel better using fermented dairy products such as yogurt or kefir. In fact, there are isolated communities that thrive on these products, such as those in mountainous areas of Eastern Europe, including Bulgaria and the CaucasES, and they live very long and healthy lives. Once again, if a person's heritage is well known, they might feel confident enough to add these products to their diet. I personally do not feel good eating any raw dairy, fermented or not, which is too bad because I really love cheese. Although it would be helpful if I could enumerate all of the adverse long and short-term effects of eating dairy if it is not in a person's evolutionary makeup to do so, there is insufficient information for a comprehensive list. One problem is the long time lapse between ingestion and symptoms, leading to a cause-effect disconnect.

Some relevant information may be gleaned from a study performed in China where rural Chinese people who consumed dairy foods high in the protein casein developed major illnesses over time. The Chinese people have a long history of not eating dairy, so the outcome of this study is no surprise, and clearly shows the long-term effects of a dietary evolution/environment mismatch. The author of the study came to the conclusion that the solution to the problem is to adopt a vegan diet, discounting the possibility that eating the proper animal foods (i.e. the Wellness Diet) might produce the best overall health result [91].

On a personal note, I went through an experimental phase a few years ago where I introduced a lot of raw cheese into my diet. After several weeks, I developed heel pain that was quite annoying, and which I never had experienced before. Upon stopping the cheese, it resolved in about a week. Months later, I repeated the experiment (I am sometimes a glutton for punishment) with the same result. I thought at the time that the high calcium content of the cheese was somehow causing my problem by displacing magnesium. More recently, while running some experiments with various mineral combinations, I was able to reproduce the heel pain whenever I took high doses of calcium without offsetting it with similarly high doses of magnesium. I now feel comfortable stating that excessive intake of calcium, as may happen with a high dietary intake of dairy, can be a cause of bone spurs if it is accompanied by a magnesium deficiency. As discussed at length in the mineral section below, magnesium deficiency may arise in those people leading a chronically stressful life, because stress rapidly depletes magnesium. This leads me to the conclusion that those modern societies that do well on a high dairy intake in their diet also must have a reliable source of dietary magnesium, and a lifestyle that is low in chronic stress. One source of magnesium could be mineral water, or maybe people in these societies have developed the ability to extract magnesium from plant parts such as nuts and seeds, somehow overcoming the natural toxins such as phytates and oxalates that interfere with mineral assimilation for many of us.

That brings me to a discussion of calcium, considered by the dairy industry as one of the important ingredients in milk products, particularly for bone health. Further, we are all told by mainstream and alternative health communities and the government RDA (Recommended Daily Allowance) charts that we need at least 1000 mg of calcium daily. Since the Wellness Diet (and that of our ancestors for 99,600 generations) does not include dairy, let's check in with MA to see if she can shed any light on the subject. From ancient skeletons and teeth, we know that PA had excellent bone strength, on average better that modern man. From a survival point of view, this would make sense since a hunter-gatherer with a broken bone was probably a goner. Of course, these skeletons were all from a period where animals had not yet been domesticated (a recent event), and hence dairy was not part of our ancestral diet for about 2.45 million years. So, where did PA get his supposedly "necessary" 1000 mg of calcium?

Before we try to answer this question, let's take a look at the RDAs for nutrients, since many diet plans use the RDA as a standard. The RDA is put together by a governmental committee, and is supposed to be based on averages derived from "healthy people." It is not updated very often. As previously defined, *healthy* is certainly a relative term, but you can be assured it is based on people who eat the SAD diet, including all of the categories of foods not included in the Wellness Diet. The Tier Three plant foods in particular contain anti-nutrients such as phytates (in grains, nuts and seeds) that are known to interfere with the assimilation of minerals, including calcium and magnesium. Oxalate is another plant anti-nutrient found in such vegetables as spinach and rhubarb and in most grains, and it also binds calcium and magnesium [92]. Therefore, one can conclude that a person eating foods high in these and other anti-nutrients would end up requiring a much higher mineral intake than one on an anti-nutrient-free diet like the Wellness Diet.

If that were the case, the RDA of 1000 mg might be reduced to, say, 600 mg for those on the Wellness Diet. I give this example to illustrate that the RDA system presently in place is likely to be largely irrelevant for our purposes, and in fact, I do not know of any studies to determine what the "real" numbers are. To compound the problem, it is also very difficult even to determine the micronutrient nutritional value of the Wellness Diet as it would have appeared to PA. This is because the nutritional values we presently use, generated by the USDA, reflect present-day food products, which in many instances are vastly different (lower) than the nutritional content of those foods in the time of PA because of soil depletion and other modern agricultural issues.

From my review of the literature, most of the plant nutrient falloff between PA's time and today has occurred in the vegetable category as opposed to fruit, but there is no good database that I am aware of that tracks this information. Of course, much of it is lost because we have no record of the composition of most ancient plant products. The point is, we may have to add food supplements in certain categories, somewhat based on guesswork, with the goal in mind of restoring the Wellness Diet to its original nutritional value. As you will see in a later discussion, it is my opinion that PA obtained a major portion of his/her dietary calcium (and magnesium) intake from natural mineral water, which you will recall is an important element of the Wellness Diet. Animal blood is another source. There are about 5 grams of calcium in the blood alone of a typical cow [26], along with about 750 mg of magnesium [93].

A discussion of calcium usually brings up the topic of osteoporosis (porous bone), which today is the major driving force behind high-dose calcium. Let's start with defining the goal in the "war against osteoporosis," which is the prevention of bone fragility that can lead to frequent fractures. In other words, we want *strong* bones. What does bone strength have to do with osteoporosis? In many instances, nothing. I remember taking a course in school called Strength of Materials, where we learned early on that there in not necessarily a direct correlation between material strength and its density, or its porosity, or its hardness. A key factor for strength is the crystal structure of the material.

Bone mineral density is typically measured using dual-energy x-ray absorptiometry, known as the DEXA test. It is supposed to yield a measure of osteoporosis, a term that seems to have many definitions, but the objective of the test is to determine risk of fracture. In fact, however, one can test as having osteoporosis, yet have very strong bones that are not at all likely to fracture. On the other hand, one can test as having excellent bone density, yet have fragile bones very prone to fracture. So, what good is the test? Well, it sells a lot of drugs called bisphosphonates, which do increase bone density, so you pass the DEXA test, but unfortunately they can make your bones more fragile, whereby you are very prone to fracture [94]. In some very sad cases, the drugs actually cause bone disintegration, particularly of the jaw, which is somewhat impossible to repair [95].

On the other side of the coin, Inuits, who subsist on a diet of animal food that seems very low in calcium, test as having a high rate of osteoporosis, yet they have very low fracture rates, which puzzles the researchers [96]. In other words, they have a diet low in calcium, would fail the DEXA test, but have very strong bones. As you can imagine, for their lifestyle, frequent bone fractures would be catastrophic. As we will see later, this supposed puzzlement also occurs among menopausal Mayan women.

What can we make of this dilemma? The only way to definitively measure bone strength that I know of is destructive – testing how much force it takes to break the bone - so let's leave that out. What remains is a wait-and-see type of destructive test based on accidents – in other words, wait until you fall and see what happens. I do not like those odds, so I am betting that the Wellness Diet, tested by 99,000 generations will work for me. So far, so good. I have had some nasty spills over the last 20 years, but have never broken anything - yet. Note that some of the factors that have a positive influence on healthy bone are magnesium, vitamin D, and vitamin K. These nutrients are further discussed in the food supplement section. The effectiveness of calcium used alone as a supplement to strengthen bones has been discredited [97].

A discussion of dairy would not be complete without a discussion of infant formula. In theory, human milk is the ideal food for human babies and, of course, is in keeping with MA's design. I say in theory because it all depends on the health of the mother. In some instances, because of a lousy diet, the mother is deficient in important nutrients that are then also lacking in her milk. Another scenario is that the mother's body is loaded with toxins that pass through to her milk, toxifying the baby. One of the most insidious of these is mercury from amalgam fillings, vaccinations, fish, or all of the above (discussed in the detox section below). For these and other reasons, it is sometimes necessary to find an alternative to mother's milk, which is no easy task, especially since we have yet to define all of its components. What is clear is that the composition of the milk of a different species (cow, goat, etc.) is different in many respects, and we really do not know what the long-term effects are on the health of a person raised on these products. Under any conditions, the substitute milk used should be raw, from grass-fed animals that are hormone and antibiotic free. Valiant efforts have been made by the alternative health community to try to design a human milk substitute, and examples can be found on the Weston Price Foundation website previously referenced [7].

Let's see if we can get any clues from MA. First, of course, it is important that a woman intending to get pregnant should first clean up her body with the right diet and detoxification protocols (enter The Wellness Project). If problems remain in breastfeeding, the natural solution, which has been around for ages, is to substitute the human milk of another nursing mother either who has excess milk or who has weaned her baby but decided to act as a "wet nurse" to aid other mothers. There are many examples of this in the animal kingdom, where a nearby adult female sustains abandoned cubs, or even cubs of another species. There are several caveats to implementing this solution for humans. The first is that the surrogate must also be in good health with respect to diet and toxins. The second is how to get fresh human milk from one distant location to another without contamination or other damage. The last thing you want to do is to pasteurize the milk, which would kill a lot of the good stuff. Freezing may be a possibility. Well, these are not easy problems to solve, and very few people are working on them for the classic reason that there is really no money in it as compared to selling canned infant formula in the supermarket. Besides, it is inconvenient, so the Western world continues to fool with Mother Nature, with unknown consequences.

I want to bring up another and in my view more elegant, solution to this problem that is also ancient, which I will call the "grandmother solution." It is well known that non-pregnant women (even those in or post-menopause) can induce lactation through repeated nipple stimulation, either by placing a suckling child to the breast repeatedly or by using mechanical means. I consider this a very important clue from MA. Assuming one or more healthy grandmothers are locally available, this to me is a wonderful and natural solution to breast feeding problems, which would, incidentally, form strong baby-grandmother ties. For the adventurous grandmas out there, here is an interesting experiment right out of a rocket scientist's bag of tricks. There are a variety of electrically powered breast pumps on the market for nursing mothers [98]. The experiment I have in mind would be to hook one of those up to a willing participant as a nipple stimulator, using it on a daily basis to see if it can indeed induce lactation. By the way, fellows, MA has also provided men with the ability to lactate in response to nipple stimulation, so keep that in mind when your nursing wife is tired!

If you think about it, this is really a gift from MA to assist in the continuation of our species. One can imagine in the time of PA that many nursing mothers died for the typical reasons of starvation, predators, or accidents, and the ability of others in the family to continue breastfeeding the child would be in concert with the survival of the species. Modernly, it allows mothers of adopted children also to experience the wonders of breastfeeding. The La Leche League website has some discussions on inducing lactation [99].

This naturally brings me to the topic of menopause. Yes, menopause. If menopause is truly a natural phenomenon as opposed to one that is environmental in origin, its purpose remains one of MA's great mysteries. While I doubt that menopause should be characterized as an illness, its origins are quite unusual and it occurs rarely in other mammals. The two simplified explanations are that menopause is meant to protect the older female from the rigors of childbirth, and that animals don't live long enough to experience menopause. Maybe, but these are just guesses.

Here is what we presume to know from research, filtered by my personal interpretation. Each woman is born with a set number of eggs, apparently predetermined before birth, and it is believed that this pool of eggs is never replenished, which may or may not be the case. At around 16-20 weeks of gestation, a female fetus will have the greatest number of eggs (about 6-7 million). For unknown reasons, at birth, this number decreases to about 2 million, and by puberty to about 300,000. This process of decline continues throughout life until menopause, and does not seem to be interrupted by birth control pills, pregnancy, or ovulation. From this reservoir of eggs, fewer than 500 will ovulate during a woman's reproductive years, until they run out at menopause.

What does menopause have to do with dairy? Well, in the search for a reason for menopause, one colorful theory that has emerged is called the "grandmother hypothesis," and it goes something like this [100]. It is conceivable that during our evolutionary history, older mothers who lost their fertility were able to spend more of their time helping, protecting, and teaching their children and grandchildren. Experiments and observation have shown that those animals that have had time invested in them by family members, in the form of protection and education, are much more likely to live to the age at which they are able to reproduce, certainly a Natural goal. The reason I am bringing this up here is that the ability to induce lactation, even in a menopausal woman, may favor this theory just on the basis that it allows grandmothers to nurture, even years after the loss of fertility.

While on the subject of menopause, an interesting question to ponder is whether aligning one's heritage with one's lifestyle (particularly diet) would obviate the annoying symptoms of menopause without the need for hormone therapy. I can find two studies relating to the issue, both concerning Mayan women. The first study of a small group of Mayan women in the Yucatan found that none could recall any of the typical symptoms of menopause so prevalent in our society, such as hot flashes. Even though tests showed they had the typical menopausal decreases in bone density and estrogen, there was no increase in fractures or decrease in height [101]. A later study of Mayan women in the highlands of Guatemala found a higher incidence of reporting menopausal symptoms. The clearly puzzled author concluded that "symptoms in women in the years around menopause must be interpreted in geographical, nutritional, biological, psychological and cultural context" [102]. Other ethnic studies have also found puzzling differences between cultures. For example, there is no word for hot flashes in the Japanese language [103].

While I would like to think the Wellness Diet could have a major impact on menopause symptoms, I have only one case study – my wife. She is in menopause, uses no hormone therapy, and when she sticks somewhat closely to the Wellness Diet, she is symptom free. If she starts to deviate too much, hot flashes appear. She can control them to some extent by taking clay, which would indicate there is a toxin connection to some menopausal symptoms. Since it seems clear that PA favored animal glands and other organs, I wonder if the ovaries from prey animals were reserved for the women in the family. For adventuresome female readers with menopausal symptoms, an additional food supplement to the Wellness Diet might be an ovary glandular, such as Cytozyme-O by Biotics Research [104]. The bottom line for me regarding dairy is to avoid or minimize its consumption on the basis that the benefits of eating other-species dairy (if there are any) do not outweigh the risks.

For those who want to experiment with dairy and yet are unsure of their level of intolerance, gelatin, found in bone broth, has been found to improve the digestion of milk and milk products, particularly casein. Gelatin is discussed in detail in the food supplement section below.

## Plant Parts Other Than Fruit

In this section, we are going to discuss seeds (grains), beans, nuts, tubers, roots, stems, flowers, and leaves. In many instances, I will be referring to human attempts to eliminate natural plant toxins by the use of heat, soaking, fermenting, etc., and the lack of efficacy of such attempts. While there are dozens of supporting references on the subject, a particularly useful one in this area is *Toxic Constituents of Plant Foodstuffs*, edited by Irvin Liener [40].

### Grains

In the Wellness Diet discussion, we covered the basics of why portions of plants other than sweet fruit are not included. Here, we will look at a risk/benefit analysis for a variety of excluded plant products to evaluate the prudence of adding any of them to the Wellness Diet.

The glutinous grains (seeds) such as wheat, barley and rye have the most notoriety with respect to allergies and intolerances that may lead to delayed illnesses, ranging from aching joints, gastrointestinal disorders, depression, eczema, low blood iron levels, and an increased risk of diabetes, bowel cancer, anemia, and osteoporosis. Celiac disease is a gluten-related intestinal illness that interferes with the absorption of nutrients from food. This condition damages or destroys the tiny, fingerlike protrusions lining the intestines through which nutrients are absorbed into the bloodstream. While there are some gliadin antibody tests that might uncover this problem, I know of many cases of what seem to be false negatives, based on the fact that stopping the intake of grains for these people yielded great health improvements regardless of negative test results for grain intolerance.

From Price's research, we know that several modern indigenous groups in Western Europe have incorporated grains into their diet, such as the Swiss group (rye) and the Scottish group (oats). Starting about 10,000 years ago, the spread of grain consumption form the Middle East to Western Europe is estimated to have taken several thousand years. Therefore, in areas such as Switzerland and Scotland, grains are an even more recent crop, being incorporated into the diet say about 4000 years or about 160 generations ago. What this indicates to me is how quickly environmental pressure can cause evolutionary "selection" in monolithic communities, whereby those who by heritage are not able to accommodate the available foods die off, and the remainder thrives. As I indicated above, if a person can trace their heritage to these specific groups, their chances of compatibility to these respective grains may be quite good. However, as a caution, the modern populations of far Western Europe, particularly the British Isles, such as the Irish, British and Scottish, have an extremely high incidence of gluten intolerance, most likely because of the short period of adaptation [105]. Note that oats do not naturally contain gluten, but may become contaminated with it during harvesting and processing.

About 80% of the world's human population subsists on grains for want of other food sources, and their individual genetic heritage will undoubtedly determine their health outcome. Some of the non-glutinous grains in wide use are corn and rice, and there has been resurgence in the use of some ancient gluten-free grains, or pseudo-grains, such as the seeds and leaves of quinoa and amaranth. Quinoa contains saponins and is toxic raw (birds will not eat it). Amaranth, also toxic raw, is high in oxalates and the leaves are high in nitrates that can convert to toxic nitrites during heating. This is just more of the same story that Nature does not want us tampering with her seeds. For those of us fortunate enough not to need to eat seeds for sustenance, there is no nutritional benefit to adding them to the Wellness Diet.

I love wheat, and as a kid, I could eat a loaf of rye bread and wash it down with a box of pretzels. What I did not know at that time was that wheat feeds Candida (discussed in detail in the next section), and I already had a severe overgrowth of this fungus as a result of frequent antibiotic use. The bottom line for me: other than some brown rice occasionally, I won't go near any of this stuff. We have not even scratched the surface in identifying the toxins in these portions of plants, and I for one do not want to be a guinea pig in this arena when there is no health benefit.

For those who wish to have grains as part of their diet, I suggest avoiding the glutinous variety, as in wheat, rye, and barley, and concentrating instead on whole grain versions of brown rice, quinoa, and amaranth. You can experiment with fermentation and sprouting to try to lower the natural toxin content. Because virtually all corn is GMO, I avoid it. Presoaking oats can reduce its toxin levels somewhat. Sally Fallon's book *Nourishing Traditions* has lots of information in this area [25]. Another approach is the use of gelatin, found in bone broth, which has been found to improve the digestibility of the proteins in grains other than corn [106]. Gelatin is discussed in detail in the food supplement section below.

## Beans

Beans are like seeds and Nature has taken great pains to protect them because they represent the reproductive potential for plants. Detoxifying efforts have been made, such as sprouting them, fermenting them, soaking them, and heating them, but none have been completely successful, which just adds to the clues from MA – stay away.

Most of us have participated in the jokes regarding eating beans and large volumes of intestinal gas, caused by complex sugar molecules called oligosaccharides that are broken down by the large intestine into carbon dioxide and hydrogen. The end result (pun intended) is gas, which I view as yet another graphic clue from MA that most of us are not adapted to digesting them as a result of a missing enzyme, very much like lactose intolerance for dairy. Sure, you can resort to Beano® and try to fool Mother Nature, but I don't know if you really are, and neither does anybody else.

A classic example of bean toxicity is soy, supposedly a health food, at least in the minds of the soy industry. I invite soy lovers to read the book *The Whole Soy Story*, by Kaayla Daniel [107]. I have yet to find a soy eater who has read this book and continued to eat any soy products. A wealth of information can also be found on the Weston Price Foundation website [7]. They have posted online a brochure called *Soy Alert!* that should do the trick. Reading the above literature will also give one great insight into the supposed love affair between the Asian culture and soy (historically, on average they eat about two teaspoons per day of naturally fermented soy as a condiment).

Because there is so much great information out there on the dangers of soy, I will not spend a lot of time on it here, except to hit a few highlights. The phytoestrogens in soy can disrupt the endocrine system, leading to testicular problems for young boys and early puberty in young girls, so using it in infant formula is really bad news (it travels in breast milk), and it can also contribute to breast cancer and infertility. High levels of phytic acid interfere with mineral assimilation, including calcium, possibly contributing to bone fractures. Trypsin inhibitors interfere with protein digestion and may cause pancreatic disorders. Goitrogens can cause hypothyroidism, autoimmune thyroid disease, and possibly thyroid cancer. The processing of soy to make the Frankenfoods you see in the market contributes to the production of highly carcinogenic nitrosamines.

For me, soy is a poster child as to why you do not want to fool with MA, at least in the bean category, which also includes peanuts. Peanuts are not a nut and are variously referred to as a bean, or a legume, or a pod, or a pulse, depending on a nightmare of definitions in this field, and are one of the most allergenic of foods.

Flax seed has become popular as a plant source of omega-3 fatty acids. Like most seeds, it must be processed to yield any nutritional value, since the whole seed would go right through your digestive system (as MA intended). Because of the fragile oil profile, once milled, it must be consumed quickly, and to avoid rancidity, never heated. Flaxseed contains some interesting anti-nutrients including very high levels of phytate, the mineral binder, and ones that interfere with vitamins B6 and B1.

For those who want to include beans in their diet, I would avoid soy unless it is traditionally fermented in the Japanese style, and then only eat it in small quantities. I would also favor those beans that can be eaten raw with minimal discomfort, such as snap and green beans. As in the case of grains, gelatin has been shown to increase the digestibility of the proteins in beans [106].

## Nuts

One of the most popular nuts in Africa is the mongongo nut, which is a favorite of elephants because of its sweet fruit covering. The elephants are drawn to the sweet fruit, the nuts survive their digestive tract, and end up in heaps around the forest floor along with a pile of fertilizer, just as MA intended. Modern foragers harvest them from the heaps and heat them to open the very hard shells and get at the nut. If one can trace their heritage to Kalahari Bushmen, perhaps cooked mongongo nuts are right for them. Other than that, nuts suffer the same fate as seeds, where a variety of processing methods have been tried to reduce toxicity, with limited success. Some, such as the apricot kernel and bitter almond, are sufficiently toxic that their compounds are used as a drug (laetrile) in an attempt to kill cancer cells (some even suggest they cause cancer). They contain amygdalins, which produce cyanide. While I am certainly not suggesting that eating nuts will kill people, my point is that they contain toxins, many of which we have not yet identified or studied, and for which the long-term effects of ingestion are unknown.

Some of what we commonly refer to as nuts are also sometimes classified as fruits. One example is the almond, which in its wild form contains the glycoside amygdalin, which becomes transformed into deadly prussic acid (hydrogen cyanide) after crushing, chewing, or any other injury to the seed. The only way wild almonds could have been eaten was if they were processed by leaching or roasting to remove their toxicity, so they clearly were not a food of either PA or the chimpanzee. Selective breeding resulted in today's domesticated almond, but it is unknown and uncontrolled as to the remaining toxins or their concentration.

Cashews are a classical example of the nightmare of terminology in the botanical world. What appears to be the fruit of the cashew tree is an oval shaped *pseudo-fruit* called the cashew apple. It ripens into a yellow and/or red structure that is edible, and has a sweet smell and a sweet taste. What is referred to as the *true fruit* of the cashew tree is a kidney shaped hard shell within which is a single *seed*, called the cashew *nut*. The hard double shell contains a resin, urushiol, which is a potent skin irritant also found in botanically related poison ivy, leaving in doubt its use as an Ancient food.

What is the upside of eating nuts? They are a source of protein, but on the Wellness Diet, who needs more protein? They are supposedly a good source of minerals such as selenium, zinc, and magnesium, but paradoxically they contain anti-nutrients that bind minerals so that they are mostly unavailable. People have tried soaking and heating nuts to reduce the anti-effects sufficiently to make their mineral content available, but who knows. What we do know is that heating nuts damages the fragile polyunsaturated oils they contain (mostly omega-6), as does shelling them and leaving them exposed to light and air.

Brazil nuts are high in selenium, but as their name implies, they certainly were not native to Africa. Let's look at the Wellness Diet with respect to some of these minerals. Starting with selenium, research shows that the largest and most bioavailable proportion of human selenium intake is from meat, particularly beef. Plant forms of selenium are less available [108]. For zinc, research also shows that the largest and most bioavailable proportion of human zinc intake is from meat as opposed to plants [109]. With respect to magnesium, fresh fruit is a source, and contains no anti-nutrients to interfere with absorption.

The mineral water in the Wellness Diet adds significant minerals to the mix, including magnesium and calcium. This fact is often completely overlooked in the nutritional analyses of Paleo diets. As I stated above, applying nutrient RDA values to the PA diet makes little sense as they are based on the SAD diet, so the only benchmark we have for the Wellness Diet is 99,600 generations of accumulated data. I discuss the inadvisability of using nut and seed oils in a later section on cooking oils.

Coconut deserves some special consideration. The origins of the coconut, particularly in relation to Africa, are somewhat muddy, with conflicting opinions, including the claim that Polynesians brought them to Africa, or that they were indigenous to East Africa. The two closest botanical relatives to the coconut are found in southern Africa and Madagascar [110], which may have some bearing on early native African existence of coconut palms. Coconuts are not the easiest food to retrieve, but it is certainly doable by the nimble, and a large, sharp rock is sufficient to get at the goodies. Ripe coconuts are also known to drop on you unexpectedly. Unlike other nuts, coconut pulp and water, assuming it is not from a tree growing in polluted soil, has a very low toxin profile, but there have been some rare cases of people having allergic reactions to the pulp, and even the oil. Coconut water has actually been used intravenously as a rehydration fluid in emergencies [111].

As to why MA would leave the coconut more vulnerable than other nuts, my best guess is its size and tough shell, which makes it somewhat indestructible to all but clever humans late in the evolutionary history of palm trees. Having said all this, while its medium-chain fatty acid profile might be useful for people eating a SAD diet, I see no compelling nutritional reason to add coconut to the Wellness Diet. Small amounts could be tried as a snack if you are not sensitive to walnuts or almonds. As you are probably aware, tropical oils such as coconut and palm have been demonized because they are high in saturated vegetable fat, raising the heart-unhealthy arguments. From my research, this is nonsense, but I still do not encourage the use of any extracted oils in cooking.

For those non-purists who wish to eat some nuts, I would advise eating them raw, right out of the shell - there are many quality nutcrackers on the market. They should be stored in the refrigerator until shelled. Most nuts are rich in polyunsaturated oils, and out of their shells, the oils they contain can become readily rancid, since they are easily damaged by heat, air, and light. In their original natural packaging, the likelihood of damage is reduced. Of course, one still has the natural toxins to contend with, and raw nuts can be hard to digest (another clue from MA). Coconut, hazelnut, and macadamia nuts are low in phytates, and might make good choices for raw eating.

## Roots, Stems and Leaves

It is interesting that most herbal medicinal preparations are derived from plant roots, stems, and leaves. What is going on here is that the toxins in these plant parts are being used medicinally to alleviate various symptoms. These are the same plant parts (including bark) that have been used by the pharmaceutical industry to derive drugs, all of which are also toxic. Why would you want to eat drugs as a regular part of your diet?

For those who wish to eat some vegetables, my best suggestion would be leaves or stems of very large plants such as trees. Presumably, MA would be less concerned about damage to a large plant from leaf or stem removal, and hence lessen the toxic load in these. There is some research to show that leaves in the upper reaches of trees have fewer toxins than those easily reachable, which makes sense as an evolutionary survival tactic [9]. There is every indication that the long neck of the giraffe evolved for the very purpose of reaching the less-toxic upper leaves of trees.

Remarkably, plants communicate with each other by giving off volatile compounds when under attack by a predator. Nearby plants react to the signal by quickly increasing the level of toxins they produce, in an attempt to ward off the predators. On the other hand, some animals have learned this trick, so they do not feed on adjacent plants, but move far enough away to find plants that did not get the warning signals. If only humans had not lost this intuition, perhaps we would be able to know the what, when, and how much answers as to which of the toxic parts of plants are safe to eat.

## Sugars

Fruit is the main source of natural sugars in the Wellness Diet, and as previously indicated, I believe they should be eaten raw and not juiced. If sweet and edible, the skin has many nutrients as well as good fiber. The process of making sugar by evaporating juice from sugarcane first developed in India around 2,500 years ago. From there, sugar became a prized trading commodity, and eventually a huge cash crop throughout the world as a staple of cooking and dessert. The story of sugar refinement has been a horror story for humans, and along with it came dental caries, diabetes, and many other health problems. As far as artificial sweeteners are concerned, in my opinion (and those of others) they are all toxic, including the neurotoxins aspartame, and sucralose (a chlorine derivative) [112]. Strangely, from my research of the popular artificial sweeteners, saccharine is by far the least toxic. Stevia, a popular alternative sweetener, is derived from a leaf, hence not part of the Wellness Diet, and there have been some reports of its toxicity.

Honey, an insect product, is not on the Wellness Diet list for a few reasons. First, taking it from the hive interrupts the reproductive cycle of the bees (notwithstanding their considerable defenses), so I consider it doubtful MA would approve. Further, honey takes on the toxic properties of the flowers from which it was made, and there have been cases of life-threatening allergic and other toxic reactions as a result. Considering the fruit content of the Wellness Diet, there should be no need to supplement the diet with additional sugars. It is not rocket science that picking fruit it is a lot more fun than sticking a hand into a beehive, and the tropical African climate is conducive to year-round fruit availability.

Now for some potentially good news in the sweetener arena. Brazzein, a relatively new plant-based sweetener will soon be hitting the market [113]. Lo and behold, it is made from an African fruit! Assuming the sweetener is extracted from the fruit pulp or edible peel, as opposed to the seed, it should be an acceptable product in small quantities.

## Extracted Oils

Extracted vegetable oils (from seeds) are a very recent addition to the SAD diet, and while they look clean and bright on the grocer's shelves, I cannot think of any reason to consume them. Of course, we have already eliminated seeds from the Wellness Diet, but I want to drive home the point with respect to seed oils so that there is no mistake as to my feelings on the subject. I am referring to seed oils like safflower, sunflower, cottonseed, corn, sesame, peanut, walnut, pumpkin, canola, and the like. Oil processing begins with the extraction of crude vegetable oils from the seeds, a process that requires high temperatures and pressures, and sometimes involves a chemical solvent. Some of the steps involved in processing include caustic refining, bleaching, deodorizing, filtering, and removing saturates to make the oils more liquid. This has created a whole family of Frankenfats and dietary oils with unnatural molecular patterns, such as trans-fats, hydrogenated oils, cyclic fatty acid derivatives, cross-linked fatty acid chains, dimers, polymers, cross-linked triglycerides, and body-shifted molecules.

In the future, I expect we will uncover all kinds of additional molecular disturbances and toxic effects from oil that is heated. As one toxic byproduct after another is brought to the attention of the public (e.g. hydrogenated oils and trans-fats), in the vegetable oil industry, the lipid chemists go to work "eliminating" it, but from what I can see, they are merely creating others that for the moment remain hidden from the public eye. There is a lot of profit-driven creativity out there because these oils play a big role in the SAD diet. For instance, scientists have apparently figured out how to heat a vegetable oil and not produce a measurable trans-fatty compound. They have engineered soybean and other vegetable oils into forms that can be heated all day. They test for trans-fats and there aren't any, but this is just another attempt to fool MA, and nobody knows the long-term effects.

For years, "Mediterranean diet" studies have made a nutritional celebrity out of olive oil. This oil is unique in that it is extracted from a fruit, the olive, as opposed to a seed, so perhaps it is a candidate for addition to the Wellness Diet. Well, the olive fruit straight from the tree is a very bitter one, and quite unpalatable raw unless processed in chemical solutions or fermented, so it does not qualify as a Wellness Diet fruit. Olive oil is high in oleic acid, a monounsaturated omega-9 fatty acid that our body does not need from foods, since it can make its own. So why has olive oil been singled out as very *healthy* (remember that this is a comparative term)? Well, when compared to the other oils sitting on the shelf, it is less unhealthy for the very reason that it is monounsaturated. Virtually all of the other oils are naturally high in omega-6 polyunsaturated fatty acids, which are more fragile and easily damaged by light, air, and heat, so many of them are rancid as they sit on the shelf. Therefore, olive oil wins by default, since omega-9 is more stable than omega-6 and, hence, less damaged by processing.

Canola oil (Canadian Oil) has become another favorite, thanks to a major marketing effort. It is made from a genetically modified form of rapeseed which, in its natural form, is toxic to humans and some animals [114]. Its fatty acid profile is similar to olive, and it contains some omega-3 fatty acids, which may well have been damaged by the many processing steps involved in production. A great deal of additional information on this oil can be found on the Weston Price Foundation website.

Fortunately, no processed or extracted oils are needed in the Wellness Diet. I personally would not go near any of these oils, and would certainly not heat or otherwise cook with any poly- or monounsaturated oil. For anyone wanting to be a guinea pig and put their health in the hands of lipid chemists, the only oils that I could even suggest heating would be those high in saturated fats, such as coconut or palm oils, or animal fats such as beef, lamb and pork fat.

## Liquids other than mineral/spring water

Liquids such as juices, teas, coffee, alcoholic beverages, sodas, sports drinks, dairy, and anything in a plastic or paper container are not a part of the Wellness Diet, with the following exceptions.

Fruit teas can be made by cutting and mashing some fresh fruit and adding it to hot water to make a drink. The so-called fruit teas on the market are not made with the fruit but are usually made with the leaves of the plant, which contain natural toxins. Examples are raspberry tea, which is actually made with raspberry leaf, not the fruit, and watermelon tea, which is actually made with watermelon seeds, not the fruit. I do not know of any commercial tea made with fruit pulp, but here is a way to make some that is somewhat easier than mashing fruit. One fruit farm, Brownwood Acres, produces a liquid fruit product that includes the acceptable parts of the fruit, namely the pulp and the skin. Presently, it is available using cherries, pomegranates, and a berry mix. This company identifies these products as liquid fruit supplements (as opposed to their concentrates, which are just the fruit juice) [115]. A teaspoon in hot water is plenty to make a fruit tea.

While I do not suggest it, fruit could be juiced using a slow speed, low temperature juicer, but the pulp should be put back into the glass. Also, the seeds or pits should be completely removed before juicing to avoid those toxins. Most commercial fruit juices are pasteurized, usually include additional sweeteners, and are devoid of the pulp.

This competes the discussion of the Tier Three food group. Before going on to the food preparation section, I would like to make a suggestion of how some of the Tier Three foods might be added to a Tier One/Two diet in a manner to moderate the impact they may have on the body defense system. Essentially, the idea would be to eat foods from only one subcategory on any one day. The subcategories are dairy, grains, beans, nuts, roots (and tubers), stems, leaves, sugars and extracted oils. My preference would be to avoid completely the sugar and extracted oil subcategories, and then choose foods from among the other seven subcategories on a rotation basis. For example, on one day add to the Tier One/Two foods some dairy food such as raw cheese, but no foods from any of the other Tier Three subcategories. On the next day, replace the dairy with some grain such as rice. On the next day, replace the grain with some nuts, and so on. The intent is to moderate the toxic load on the defense system by limiting the Tier Three subcategories to only one per day, and then rotate them. Perhaps a particular Tier Three subcategory would not be repeated more than once per week. While I have no evidence to back up my supposition regarding the moderating effect on the toxic load, I have to believe this approach will be an improvement over eating multiple Tier Three categories as a substantial part of the diet on a daily basis, which is the case with the SAD diet. To the extent you know you are allergic to or incompatible with a food subcategory, obviously avoid those foods.

# Chapter 10 - Food Preparation

In this section, I will comment on various food preparation methods, and how they might, or might not, apply to the Wellness Diet. In general, I do not heat any of the fruit on the diet, but I do gently bake the meats that I eat, trying to keep them somewhat on the rare side.

Fermentation as practiced by humans is a relatively modern technique to try to make toxic plant foods and some dairy foods either less toxic or more nutritious. As stated previously, this sometimes backfires, and in the case of cruciferous vegetables such as cabbage, fermentation can actually increase the concentration of toxins. On the other hand, it is more than likely that PA would occasionally come across a piece of fermented fruit that had dropped from the parent plant, over-ripened and broken open, and been colonized by some yeast in the neighborhood, perhaps floating in the air. Some fermented fruit is known to have an alcohol content of ten percent or more, providing PA with an opportunity to become inebriated. Animals (and even insects) have been known to get totally wiped out on naturally fermented fruit, but it certainly has its disadvantages when there are predators hiding in the bushes. So, the supposition is that PA's binges would be few and far between, just based on survival instinct [9]. For the adventuresome reader, feel free to ferment a piece of allowable fruit on occasion. Let it not be said that you could not occasionally get buzzed on the Wellness Diet. Of course, wine is a fermented fruit (grapes), so I leave it to the reader regarding experimentation in this area. Note that for those with a Candida overgrowth problem (discussed in the detox section) alcohol greatly aggravates this condition.

From a review of some of the modern hunter-gatherer societies such as the Inuit and the American Indian, as well as from studying the behavior of carnivorous animals, it is clear that the intestinal contents of herbivorous prey animals were also consumed. This would consist of fermented or partially fermented plant products such as grass for a ruminant like a buffalo, or plankton in the case of a seal [24], and would contain the valuable spore-forming bacteria discussed earlier. In our modern diet, it would be hard to come by this delicacy. The nearest commercial product I can think of is raw sauerkraut or Kim chi, but neither the vegetables used nor the fermenting medium match up with what we are after, and they contain natural toxins. So, out of a sense of frustration, I set about devising a way that we could reproduce healthy fermented food (see the side box entitled An Artificial Cow Gut).

Until the actual cow gut contents or a synthesized version become available, very small amounts of raw (unpasteurized) sauerkraut might be ingested on occasion, with the caveat that it contains thyroid hormone disrupters. Spore forming bacteria supplements can also be used to supplement the diet, which will at least represent a portion of the bacterial component of animal gut contents. The interesting thing about this component of the Wellness Diet is that it brings vegetables into it, but in a form that nature intended, that is, preprocessed by the gut of an herbivore that Nature designed to eat the stuff.

## An Artificial Cow Gut

In an effort to mass-produce the fermented intestinal contents of, say, a cow, I proposed the following. In a suitably heated container (heated to the temperature of a functioning cow gut), mix together the typical natural foods of a cow (grass, clover, etc.) with the bacteria and enzymes normally found in a healthy cow gut, which were extracted in a humane manner. Stir and heat until fermentation takes place in the container, then remove a portion for consumption. Add more grass to continue the process indefinitely. Wouldn't it be great to turn the grass from your newly mowed (chemical free) lawn into a dinner side dish? I have filed a patent application covering the making of this food using this method, in the hope that it will interest a forward-thinking food producer to give it a try.

Previously, I stated that I bake my animal foods but try to keep the cooking time and temperature to a minimum because heat damages food, and the more you heat, the more you damage. Pasteurization is a classical example. At the far extreme is frying, which is cooking food surrounded by a fat or oil that is heated to a very high temperature. We have already discussed the dangers of heating fats or oils other than those that are mainly saturated, because their chemical structure resists heat damage better than the unsaturates. I do not believe PA would have been using frying to cook animal products. The lowest temperature method of cooking meat would be boiling it in water, which ensures that no portion of the meat exceeds the boiling point of water. Archeological evidence seems to point to the use of hearth-like structures that may have been used to indirectly heat the food, say, by using a bed of clay or one or more heated rocks in a manner similar to baking, which is the method I use. I prefer electric heat as opposed to gas, because of the potentially toxic byproducts of burning gas, and the likelihood that they will be absorbed into the food. A convection-type oven works well, eliminates oven hot spots, and speeds up the cooking process. An example of an inexpensive counter-top convection oven is widely sold under the Aroma Housewares Aeromatic brand.

I do not use microwave cooking. The debate on the dangers of microwaving food has been going on for years, but independent research is limited. Who's going to pay to study it? Certainly not the microwave industry, which ranges from the device manufacturers themselves to the companies that produce instant, microwavable food. There is no real money in proving that microwaves are toxic. A few studies have been done and they tend to be negative enough for me, so for that reason, I don't use a microwave [116]. In particular, one study showed that microwave heating converts the amino acid l-proline to d-proline. They write, "The conversion of *trans* to *cis* forms could be hazardous because when *cis*-amino acids are incorporated into peptides and proteins instead of their *trans* isomers, this can lead to structural, functional and immunological changes." They further note that "d-proline is neurotoxic and we have reported nephrotoxic and heptatotoxic effects of this compound [117]. Proline is found in large quantities in gelatin, an integral part of animal foods. So, one can assume that when animal foods are heated in the microwave, they may become toxic to the liver, kidneys and nervous system.

It is now well-recognized that microwaving food in plastic containers is a very bad idea because the heated plastic (and other materials) can outgas toxic substances into the food [118]. Even the use of so-called microwavable plastics is not part of an experiment I want to participate in because we have yet to identify all of the toxins in the various plastics, let alone the safe levels of each, if there are any.

As far as cooking utensils go, I cook in glass dishes and do not let the food come in contact with metal racks, some of which are chrome or nickel-plated and may tend to flake off. Even stainless steel is not impervious to outgassing, and it contains chromium and nickel, both toxic in large quantities. Aluminum is a neurotoxin, so I avoid any aluminum-containing cookware, and I also avoid coated products, even porcelain. The bright colors are provided by metal pigments of unknown origin. Teflon-coated cookware has been in the news of late because when heated, some of the compounds in Teflon become extremely toxic and potentially carcinogenic.

Uncolored glass is the way to go for me, and brands such as Pyrex® are inexpensive and come in every possible shape you might need, some with handles. I cook with Pyrex and use it for storage; it is available with plastic tops but they do not come in direct contact with the food.

The beauty of glass is that you can take it right out of the refrigerator, cook it in the same container, and know it is safe.

For serving pieces, I opt for uncolored glass or ceramic. For silverware, my suggestion is real silver, not stainless. The ideal is sterling silver, which is an alloy of silver and very small amounts of a metal such as copper, zinc or platinum. Yes, you may take out the "special-occasion-only" sterling flatware and use it every day – aren't you entitled to it? Silver will be covered more fully in the detox section, but it is a somewhat unique heavy metal in its interactions with the body. It has antibacterial, antifungal, and antiviral properties, yet in very small quantities it does not appear to have toxic effects. In large quantities, it can discolor the skin gray (argyria) somewhat permanently and can be neurotoxic. I do not foresee a problem using silver as flatware, but I would not cook in it or use it for hot drink containers. Modernly, silver is available in colloidal form and as nanoparticles for use as a supplement. It is gaining wide acceptance in the medical instrument field as a coating, and is also available in bandages for its antiseptic properties. Silver plate is another option for flatware, but a concern is that the plate will either wear or chip off, exposing the base metal.

# Chapter 11 - Food Supplements

You might wonder how I can make a pitch for supplements when I'm advocating a natural, prehistoric type of diet? Unfortunately, for a variety of reasons, it is somewhat impossible to reproduce nutritionally in its entirety the Wellness Diet or even some of the other indigenous diets. One reason is that some of the foods are simply not available, such as a hippo, or a mammoth, or some of the exotic African fruits. Another reason is that, even if available, we have not developed a taste for some of the important animal parts such as the various organs, blood and marrow, or there is fear of human-made contamination. Yet another reason, particularly in the fruit category, is that modern cultivation practices are yielding produce that is estimated to have significantly reduced nutritional profiles (vitamins and minerals) as compared to their ancient wild-grown counterparts, even those that are organically grown. As the name implies, mineral water is a major source of minerals, particularly calcium and magnesium, and we know from studies that people living near and using mountain stream water tend to live longer, healthier lives. So it behooves us to insure that the mineral water we are drinking is accompanied by high levels of these important minerals.

In the 21$^{st}$ century, one has to be creative and practical in order to fill in the missing ingredients and round out Nature's diet as best as possible. The following supplements help to do that, but please bear in mind that most food supplements are human-made or in some way tampered with so that they no longer have a counterpart in nature, no matter what the marketing folks would like you to believe. Therefore, these supplements have the potential of being toxic. One simple example is that virtually all capsule and tablet products use stearic acid or magnesium stearate as an added ingredient to speed up packaging. Theoretically, these ingredients can be sourced from seed oils, and perhaps even be hydrogenated. Fortunately, on the Wellness Diet, only a very few supplements are even suggested, and many of them are natural. As far as those folks on other diets such as the SAD diet, enormous amounts of supplements may be necessary just to keep them going.

As you recall from the dirt section of the diet, supplements to supply fulvic/humic acids as well as spore-forming bacteria were discussed. Because I consider them an intimate part of the diet itself, they are not repeated here.

## Vitamins

I have found that, until a certain amount of detoxification has taken place, taking large doses of vitamins as supplements can be very counterproductive because they feed the bad guys. As an example, the yeast Candida loves many of the B-vitamins, and taking large doses can easily contribute to its overgrowth. Actually, some B vitamins are normally produced for us by the microflora in our intestines, such as vitamin B6 [119], but as will be discussed in the detox section, many of us have disturbed gut flora due to toxins, so supplements can be helpful. If we look to MA for guidance, we find that another major source of B-vitamins for PA would have been the liver of prey animals, probably eaten raw. Most liver lovers like to eat it fried, and the attendant high cooking temperatures may destroy much of the vitamin content. Another modern concern in eating liver is its potential toxicity.

Many people, including myself, have assumed that taking a B-vitamin supplement can provide us with the equivalent of what is missing from our food sources. It was not until I did some serious research into the nutritional advantages of liver that I discovered many animal studies that showed this is not necessarily true. Dating back to the 1950's, Benjamin Ershoff, a medical researcher, ran dozens of experiments with rats to determine the effects of various nutritive substances on the health of the animals when they are subjected to various toxins and other stressors. In several of these experiments he tested the use of B- vitamin supplements versus small amounts of raw desiccated (dried) liver added to the diets of the rats, who were then subjected to various stressors such as swimming, x-ray radiation, thyroid hormone disrupters and the like [120, 121]. In each instance, he found that the rats fed liver outperformed and out-survived those fed synthetic B- vitamins. His conclusion was there is something in liver that we are unaware of that provides benefits beyond just B-vitamin supplementation. I don't know of any studies directed to finding out what these substances might be. We do know that the liver is the major detoxification organ, and perhaps some of these detox agents remain in raw liver and provide a protective effect.

Armed with this information, I set about looking at the various raw liver supplements on the market to see if any would be a suitable addition to the diet. My criteria were that it had to be derived from organic grass-fed animals in a protected environment to avoid toxins, and it had to be processed using low-temperatures to avoid damaging the tissue components. A final criterion was that the supplement should include both the water-soluble and fat-soluble portions of the liver, because Ershoff found that the combination was an important factor in its efficacy. Several desiccated beef liver supplements are available that are made from protected Argentinean free-range grass fed beef, and they use low temperature processing. However, I could only find one that was not defatted. It is supplied by Now Foods as a powder or a tablet [122], and is the product I use as a basic B- vitamin supplement. (The appropriateness of additional B- vitamin supplementation is discussed below in the various detox sections.) I happen to like the taste of liver, so I chew five tablets at each meal, or put one teaspoon of the powder in my fruit tea. For those who do not like the taste, swallowing the tablets is the way to go. Because this supplement is really a food, you can munch on it during the day for an energy boost. There is a long history of bodybuilders downing fistfuls of liver tablets for stamina.

Before leaving the subject of B- vitamins, I want to single out what I (and others) consider the queen of this group, and that is vitamin B6. It is responsible for more enzyme reactions in the body than any of the other vitamins, and its proper assimilation is easily interfered with by a variety of toxins, including candida overgrowth. We will visit this vitamin in more detail in the various detox sections, but I consider its supplementation to be important in conjunction with the modern implementation of the Wellness Diet for the following reason. There is some evidence that today's cultivated fruit is higher in sugars than the wild counterparts available to PA [56]. Studies have also shown that consumption of sugars has the effect of depleting vitamin B6 in the body [123] [124]. High levels of vitamin B6 are found in fruit as well as liver, important foods in the Wellness Diet. However, the importance of vitamin B6 to so many of the body's processes, coupled with a higher sugar intake from modern cultivated fruits leads me to add a daily vitamin B6 supplement to my regimen as a precautionary factor. It is usually found in supplement form as pyridoxine HCl, which must be converted in the body to the active form, pyridoxal–5'-phosphate (P5P). Because some toxins, including Candida overgrowth, can interfere with this conversion, I take P5P directly. Further, because P5P is easily damaged by stomach acid, I take it in the form of a sublingual tablet, placed under the tongue to dissolve and directly enter the bloodstream. The one I use, at four tablets per day, is Coenzymated B-6, made by Source Naturals [125].

Vitamin C is in the news almost daily as either being a panacea for major illnesses or being demonized for one thing or another. First, we need some definitions. Vitamin C is found in plant and animal products. In animals, it appears to be in the form of pure ascorbic acid, and this is the form usually called Vitamin C. In plants, primarily fruits and leaves, it is also found in the form of ascorbic acid, but it is virtually always found along with a group of compounds called bioflavonoids which I will call the "flavonoid complex". In the animal world, all mammals except for a small group including primates, humans, guinea pigs, the red-vented bulbul (a fruit-eating bird), a species of trout, and the Indian fruit bat can make their own vitamin C. This group apparently lost the ability to do so, supposedly because ample amounts were provided in their diet. Can we find some clues from MA as to what is going on?

Well, starting with fruit bats and the bulbul, they are major fruit eaters, eating the sweet stuff and spitting out the seeds as part of MA's plan to further plant germination. In the plant world, fruit, second only to some leaves, is the major source of vitamin C. Guinea pigs are not pigs, but rodents native to South America. There is precious little information available about their native diet because they have become so domesticated. There is even some discussion that they are now rarely found in the wild (they are a favorite food in many South American countries). Apparently, they like to eat grass, but so do many other rodents as well as rabbits, so I remain clueless as to why the guinea pig was singled out to lose the capacity to make vitamin C.

Primates eat a lot of fruit and leaves, so they should have a large intake of vitamin C. In one study, it was estimated that monkeys weighing about 15 pounds had an average daily intake of about 700 mg of vitamin C, while gorillas weighing 200-300 pounds had daily intakes in the 2-4 gram region [56]. I estimate a desirable human vitamin C intake in the range of 0.5-3 grams on the Wellness Diet. As you will see from the discussion below, Vitamin C needs can vary widely with stress level.

There is a lot more to the vitamin C puzzle than just my short analysis, and I have experimented with some enormous doses over the years, both orally and intravenously, while on the Wellness Diet. I can't say I received any particular beneficial or adverse effects (except diarrhea on high oral doses), even up to occasional 50 gram IV doses, but then again, I have not had a cold or even a sniffle while on the Wellness Diet. I do know that in general the human bowel tolerance for vitamin C changes drastically upward when the body is under stress. This takes us to another part of the puzzle: the observation that animals that produce their own vitamin C supply also have a built-in control system that increases the amount produced (sometimes up to several hundred grams) in response to stress, which we, of course, cannot mimic without taking supplements.

This animal behavior has led me to speculate as follows: let us say a band of PA hunters is in the chase to take down an African buffalo, and the buffalo knows it. Presumable, this is a high-stress situation for the buffalo, and consequently hundreds of grams of vitamin C are being produced and pumped throughout the animal's body. If so, when caught and eaten, perhaps PA was taking in from the meat somewhat massive amounts of vitamin C, information that I have not seen considered in past dietary studies. I don't have an answer, but we do know that PA favored glands and other organs from prey, and we also know that the adrenal glands usually contain the highest concentrations of vitamin C, so this is another source.

Since we and this small group of other mammals have lost not only the ability to make vitamin C, but also the ability to generate large amounts during stress, this leads me to another two-part theory as to why MA cut us off. First, we get enough from our diet, and second, we have evolved as low-stress animals (as compared to the rest of the mammal world), and hence not in need of the vitamin C stress-enhancement capability. I bring up this point again in the magnesium and chronic stress discussions below. I do not know of any studies in this area, but it would be a fun research project.

Regarding vitamin C (ascorbic acid) supplementation, many of the products on the market are derived from corn, most of which is GMO (Genetically Modified Organism). Some corn-free products that are available are derived from cassava root (also called tapioca), or sago palm, all of which appear to be synthetically derived. I use corn-free Vitamin C 500 mg by Nature's Plus. I take one ascorbic acid cap with each meal.

Regarding Vitamin E, the very term is ill defined. It generally refers to alpha-tocopherol, which is found in nature only as part of a complex of tocopherols and tocotrienols. I try to avoid supplements that contain alpha-tocopherol as an isolated nutrient, since it is not found in nature that way and there is now some evidence that it may prove toxic in its isolated form. A better choice is a vitamin E complex supplement that contains several E components, including both tocopherols and tocotrienols. There are several such E-complexes on the market, and the starting material for many is red palm oil (see for example U.S. Patent 5,157,132). This oil is extracted from the fruit of the oil palm, which, lo and behold, is a Wellness Diet food, having passed the ABC test. So instead of messing with the supplement products, one would ideally eat oil palm fruit, which is described as somewhat fibrous and oily. However, I am not aware of any readily available sources for the fruit. Instead, I suggest chugalugging some red palm oil (not palm kernel oil, which is derived from the nut), which is extracted from the fruit and which is readily available. Not only is it high in the E complex, it is also very high in the pro-vitamin A carotenoid complex, and in vitamin K.

Just as alpha-tocopherol is not found in nature as an isolate, beta-carotene is similarly not found that way, and I try to avoid any supplements that contain beta-carotene as an isolated ingredient. Some studies have shown that beta-carotene may be toxic in isolated form, particularly when Candida overgrowth may be present (see further discussion in fungal detox section). Red palm oil contains the carotenoid complex as found in nature, which includes alpha, beta, and other carotenoids yet to be defined. From my studies, red palm oil has the highest edible concentrations of Vitamin E and carotenoid complexes in the plant kingdom. Red palm oil is also high in vitamin K1, useful in controlling blood clotting, and as a raw material for enzyme processes in your body that helps keep calcium out of your arterial walls and bring it into your bones.

An interesting property of vitamins pro-A, E and K is that their absorption is increased significantly when consumed with fat, which is amply provided in the palm oil itself, as well as in the rest of the Wellness Diet. I take one to three teaspoons of the oil per day, right off the spoon. The kind I look for is Organic Virgin Palm Oil, which is red in color, originates in Africa, and is not refined, deodorized, or bleached. One source is Tropical Traditions [126]. Red palm oil has been demonized as unhealthy because it is high in saturated fat, a red herring for heart disease [127]. For those who want to forgo taking red palm oil directly, a trio of supplements would be needed just to replace the pro-A, E and K components. Some suggestions would be CarotenAll by Jarrow [128], and *Super K* and *Gamma E Tocopherol/Tocotrienols*, both from Life Extension Foundation [129].

Vitamin D is another critical nutrient, and acts both as a vitamin and as a prohormone. The ideal natural source is from the UVB spectrum of ultraviolet light impinging on unprotected skin, and I feel confident that PA had no shortage of sunlight in the tropics. I already commented above on my theory regarding skin cancer, and I go into more depth on this subject in the lifestyle section. Modernly, unless you happen to live in a tropical or semi-tropical environment, it is quite difficult for people in Western societies to get sufficient sunlight year round to produce adequate vitamin-D, which has been found to be necessary for bone strength and it is a potent anti-cancer compound [8]. Alternatives to getting natural sunlight include an artificial UVB source using a UV bulb (discussed in the lifestyle section); obtaining vitamin-D from the diet (liver is a source); and obtaining vitamin-D from supplements. Serious research into Vitamin-D is just beginning, and there is much that remains unknown, including all of the various forms that make up what will undoubtedly become the "Vitamin-D complex" some time in the future. Because we don't know yet what we are doing in this area, the best course of action is to follow MA, and get it from UV.

I personally prefer a UVB lamp, but supplements are an alternative. Before taking any, I suggest getting a Vitamin-D blood test. The test is called 25(OH)D, or 25-hydroxyvitamin D, and the latest consensus seems to be that an optimum level is above 30 and below 60 ng/ml. Excessively low or high levels can be harmful. If the level is low, Vitamin-D3 supplements are available (avoid Vitamin-D2 since it is poorly absorbed and interferes with magnesium absorption). One source I have used is Biotics Research Bio-D-Mulsion (available in 400 IU and 2000IU drops). Getting to the right dose (say between 1200 and 8000 IU per day) requires experimentation and monitoring using the 25(OH)D test [130].

As is the case in so many of the tests designed to measure levels of various compounds in the body, the vitamin D test results have generated confusion. A study was conducted where the 25(OH)D test was run on a group of people in Honolulu who habitually obtained a great amount of sun exposure. It was found that 51% of the tested group had a test level below the 30 ng/ml lower cutoff, indicating vitamin D deficiency [131]. This leaves for speculation whether the test is unreliable or a large subset of the population does not properly produce vitamin D, even with significant UVB exposure. Until this discrepancy can be sorted out, I continue to prefer UVB exposure as the natural way to obtain vitamin D, on the basis that at least MA knows what she is doing.

Regarding the relationship between UV and melanoma, the most deadly form of skin cancer, there are about as many studies showing incidence increase with excessive sun exposure as those that show the opposite [132] [133]. Something I find puzzling in these studies is that it did not strike the researchers that those people who sunburn easily might also be those with a compromised defense system, making them more susceptible to cancer, independent of sun exposure. At lease empirically, it is well- known that, for example, deranged fatty acid synthesis (typical of eating the SAD diet) can cause a person to be very susceptible to sunburning as opposed to tanning.

## Minerals - The Magnesium Factor

The title of this section is borrowed from a very important book of the same name, *The Magnesium Factor*, by Mildred Seelig, MD [33]. As you will see, magnesium, of all of the essential minerals, is not only the most overlooked and most deficient, but in my opinion, is also the most critical to our health. I will start with mineral supplementation in general, then move on to magnesium and finally to some of the support nutrients that work together to ensure an adequate supply of this critical nutrient.

Concerning minerals and the Wellness Diet, it would appear that PA derived certain of her/his minerals from two sources. The first is from food sources such as animal parts and fruit, and the second source is mineral water. Accordingly, I have divided mineral supplementation into two sections, one taken with food, and the other taken with water.

For food-based mineral supplementation, I take a multi-mineral to bolster what might be deficient in modern animal and fruit products. My preference is a supplement without copper (usually already elevated as a result of many toxins including Candida), and without iron (there is no shortage of iron in meat), and one where the minerals are bound to fruit acids. Examples of fruit-acid-derived compounds are citrates, fumarates, malates, and succinates. I also like a high magnesium/calcium ratio because of the importance of magnesium, discussed further below. There is no ideal mineral supplement, and they all contain human-made ingredients of one sort or another. I use *Citramin II* by Thorne Research [78], which is based on citric acid and is iron and copper free. I take three per day with meals.

For water-based mineral supplementation, the macrominerals calcium and magnesium appear in large quantities in natural mountain spring water. As you know from my discussion of water, I go to great lengths to ensure a high mineral content in drinking water. The water mineral content is dependent upon municipal water sources, which vary greatly, and the use of RO and distillation filters depletes water of these vital nutrients. One solution, mentioned above, is to supplement drinking water with small amounts of dolomite, which provide calcium and magnesium in the natural ratio of approximately 1.7 to 1. A protocol I have used is one dolomite tablet with water up to four times per day, for a maximum of four tablets. See the digestive rehabilitation section for more information regarding dolomite and stomach acid.

While we are on the subject of dolomite, as mentioned earlier, the minerals that are present in mineral water are in the form of bicarbonates, while the minerals in dolomite are in the form of carbonates. If we want to match exactly the bicarbonate form as a supplement, this can be done with some effort. Basically, mixing dolomite powder with carbonated water will do the trick. I have certainly experimented with this method, and have concluded that the carbonate form as found in dolomite not only has a long history of successful use, but works as well for me as the bicarbonate form. From a chemistry perspective, both the bicarbonate and carbonate mineral forms are expected to dissociate into chlorides in the body in the presence of stomach acid. However, I have found that orally taking chloride forms of these minerals does not produce the same positive results, so I intend to stick with dolomite.

Under "normal" circumstances, what I just described would appear to provide sufficient mineral supplementation, but we do not live under normal circumstances. Most of us live in a high chronic stress environment that has a major impact on depleting our body stores of magnesium, which I regard as the most important of all of the essential minerals. As you shall see from the following, I pay a great deal of attention to ensuring adequate levels of this mineral.

For this discussion of magnesium, I will be drawing upon the excellent research in Dr. Seelig's book [33], as well as the book *The Miracle of Magnesium* by Carolyn Dean, MD [34], and others. It is well recognized that those on the SAD diet have a deficient intake of magnesium from all of the processed foods being eaten. Further, as already mentioned, many of the seed- and nut-based foods in that diet contain natural mineral-binding toxins such as phytates and oxalates that block the uptake of magnesium as well as other minerals. On the Wellness Diet, we have eliminated the processed foods and the mineral-binders, and we get lots of magnesium from the water and fruit portions of the diet alone, so magnesium intake should not normally be a problem. In spite of this, we may end up with a magnesium deficiency because of our modern lifestyle. It turns out that *stress* depletes magnesium in great quantities from our bodies, so that amounts that were sufficient for PA are not sufficient for us with our chronically stressful modern lifestyles.

Readers may take exception to the conclusion that PA did not lead a chronically stressful life, but the studies of modern hunter-gatherers, such as those in Weston Price's research, show people who, for the most part, are happy, peaceful, and content with their lives. As previously mentioned, the fact that we do not make our own vitamin C tends toward the conclusion that, from an evolutionary perspective, our ancestor's lives were substantially less chronically stressful than our present lifestyle. I have no doubt that PA experienced times of acute (meaning short term) episodes of stress during hunting and predator evasion, but that is quite different from chronic stress that hangs around 24/7 in our modern environment.

Much has been written about the detrimental effects of chronic stress on our health, but there is little to pinpoint the relationship. Some believe that the increased levels of adrenaline and cortisol produced by the adrenal glands in response to stress contribute to illness, and then there is an entire "industry" devoted to the treatment of adrenal fatigue, which may well turn out to be the result of magnesium deficiency, usually in combination with a toxin overload. I can remember puzzling over the mind/body connection in relation to physical health for many years. How does stress make one sick? Well, Dr. Seelig maps it out very clearly. Everyday stressors that we take for granted, such as loud noises, reading the newspaper, listening to the news, politics, or even driving on the freeway cause our bodies to excrete large amounts of magnesium, which is needed for more than 300 critically important chemical reactions in our body. Physical stressors as simple as working in the heat or jogging use up or excrete large amounts of magnesium, as does exposure to toxins.

Magnesium deficiency can show up in many ways. Let's start with the one that first caught my attention: sudden death. I presume many of you can remember young, excellent athletes at the peak of health that suddenly drop dead when jogging. How about the patient that drops dead while on the treadmill in the doctor's office. Or the elderly gentleman who, in a fit of anger over some issue, grabs his chest and keels over. From my research, magnesium is the key to these disasters, and this is just the tip of the iceberg.

The above scenarios relate to the role of magnesium as a muscle relaxant, where it works in opposition to calcium, which causes muscles to contract. Some early signs of magnesium-related neuromuscular symptoms as a result of depletion include twitching, muscle cramps anywhere, including finger, toe, wrist, and back, heel and other bone pain, difficulty swallowing, headaches, tinnitus and hearing loss, spastic gut functions including reflux, and heart fibrillations. Further compounding the issue is the fact that magnesium interacts with other minerals, whereby a deficiency of magnesium can cause a deficiency of potassium [134], as well as zinc, and an over-abundance of calcium can interfere with magnesium absorption. Additionally, magnesium and vitamin B-6 assist each other in absorption, and the assimilation of this vitamin is, in turn, impaired by a variety of toxins.

A second major category of symptoms from magnesium depletion relates to its role in the production of energy. It is a critical factor in the production of ATP (adenosine triphosphate), which can be thought of as the body's batteries. Therefore, a deficiency of magnesium can result in serious fatigue and low exercise stamina. It is also thought by many to be a cause of Chronic Fatigue Syndrome. Now here is the Catch-22 with respect to fatigue. Many of the usual remedies to alleviate fatigue involve increasing the metabolism or energy state of the body, all of which require magnesium to do their job, further depleting the body's reserves and actually aggravating the fatigue.

Speaking of the body's reserves, much of the magnesium is found in the bones and muscles, so depletion can result in fragile bones and weak muscles. Depletion can also result in high cholesterol levels, and interference with essential fatty acid processing by the body. Magnesium deficiency is also implicated in kidney and gall stones, prostate problems, hyper-excitability, asthma, ulcers, depression, suicidal impulses, pituitary malfunction, and even body odor [62] [135] [136]. There are also studies that show magnesium supplementation halts the progression of polio if used early enough. By now, you probably get my drift that we are talking about a seriously important nutrient. A great deal of research on the effects of magnesium deficiency on the body can be found at several websites [59, 137]. Because it is involved in so many enzyme reactions in the body, the list of deficiency symptoms is very extensive.

I can personally tell you that if magnesium is depleted, many of the food supplements and detoxification remedies discussed here will not work and can produce adverse results. My analysis of this is that many of them require magnesium in particular to perform their functions, so they draw from an already depleted supply, thus increasing the depletion problem and leading to more symptoms. One example, discussed below in detail in the stress section, is the attempt to treat adrenal fatigue. It turns out that the typical remedies of hydrocortisone, DHEA, licorice, and thyroid hormone all deplete magnesium, and to some extent potassium, so it is quite important to achieve proper mineral levels before trying any of these remedies.

Magnesium replenishment is not so easy. The established approach for nutrient supplementation is to test for a deficiency and if there is one, to supplement to restore the level. For magnesium, there are challenges both to testing the body's level and to supplementation. For example, routine blood tests ordered by the majority of doctors do not test for magnesium. The standard chemistry panel only tests for three of the four body electrolytes (sodium, potassium, and calcium), leaving out magnesium, an incredibly important mineral. One reason is that a serum blood test for magnesium is virtually useless because magnesium is primarily stored in the cells. A more meaningful test would be a magnesium red blood cell test, which is a special lab order (meaning it costs more money), and even it is not extremely accurate [138]. A test that has been found to be more accurate in measuring all of the electrolytes is known as the EXATEST by Intracellular Diagnostics, Inc., and it may be covered by insurance [139]. This test uses cells scraped from the floor of the mouth to make the evaluation. Based on the test results, a supplementation program can begin.

Regarding magnesium supplementation, a problem with using oral supplements is a tendency toward creating diarrhea at the high doses that may be necessary to restore proper body levels. One method of finding the maximum tolerable oral dose is to increase it slowly until loose stools occur, then back off to a point where the stool is normal, referred to as the bowel tolerance point. Diarrhea should not be prolonged because it will flush most minerals out of the body, as well as cause dehydration.

Slow-release magnesium compounds have been developed in an effort to address the diarrhea problem, but the unknown with any timed-release or sustained–release product is how much is actually being absorbed in the gut. It is very much dependent upon the individual's gut environment, not exactly a controlled variable. One approach to oral magnesium supplementation is simply to ingest more magnesium carbonate, the form of magnesium found in dolomite. It is available as Magnesium Carbonate in 135 mg tablets from BodyBio [140].

There are many other choices for oral magnesium supplementation. Many of them combine the metal with either a fruit acid, such as citrates and malates, or an amino acid, such as glycine. A particularly serendipitous combination is magnesium and the amino acid taurine, which form magnesium taurate. Taurine actually exhibits some of the same properties as magnesium, and they complement each other in the body [141]. Further, as you will see in the detox section, taurine can be of great use in alleviating the symptoms of Candida overgrowth. One brand of Magnesium Taurate capsules is by Cardiovascular Research/Ecological Formulas, widely available with 125 mg of magnesium per capsule. Another brand is Magnesium Taurate tablets by Douglas Labs, with 200 mg of magnesium per tablet [142].

I use either the carbonate or the taurate form in conjunction with the dolomite protocol. Daily magnesium dosages required to sustain normal body levels can vary widely from, say, 400 mg to 2 grams, and may be a function of one's toxin level (including chronic stress), among other things. For example, if you have high levels of lead, which accumulates in the bones, it may take larger amounts of magnesium to displace and replace the lead in the bone matrix (more on this in the detox section).

Here are the oral magnesium supplement protocols that I have used in an effort to prevent diarrhea and assimilate large amounts of magnesium. I start with dolomite, and add additional magnesium as either magnesium carbonate or taurate or some of both. On an individual basis as part of the various detox protocols, and depending upon the toxin types and degree of toxicity being addressed, I would expect that daily doses of the various ingredients could typically range up to 4 dolomite tablets (containing 630 mg calcium and 350 mg magnesium) with 200-800 mg of additional magnesium. The dolomite tends toward constipation, and the magnesium has a laxative effect, so the objective is to balance the two to achieve normal stools and high magnesium intake. Taurine acts to stimulate the production of stomach acid, which assists in the assimilation of the dolomite.

Remarkably, even the above oral supplement protocol may not be sufficient to restore magnesium levels, or may take a long time to do so. One way to increase magnesium levels more quickly without causing diarrhea is to use a topical application. An established protocol is the use of magnesium sulphate crystals, known as Epsom salts, in bath water, which is quite soothing to some. Another protocol, and the one that I favor, is to wipe or spray on the skin a magnesium chloride solution - several such products are available. One that I use is Dr. Shealy's Biogenics Magnesium Lotion [143]. Apply an amount equivalent to about two teaspoons twice a day to random skin areas and either leave it on or wash it off after 20 minutes. You can also obtain from this same source magnesium chloride crystals for use in a foot or body bath. I believe the chloride portion of magnesium chloride will also assist in displacing toxic halides such as bromide from the body, which I discuss in more depth below.

I regard the topical application of magnesium as a very important adjunct protocol to aid in the restoration and maintenance of magnesium, and I plan to use it on a continuous basis. Dr. Shealy, a pioneer in the use of topically applied magnesium, estimates that it may take from 6 to 12 months to restore magnesium levels to normal using oral supplements [144]. For topical application, using the dosage listed above, he found that restoration occurred in 4 weeks. I apply the magnesium lotion twice daily, and I use a footbath several times per week with four ounces of the magnesium chloride crystals.

Still another approach to rapid magnesium replenishment is IV administration, as a slow drip of vitamins and minerals in what is known as a Myer's Cocktail [145], which usually includes magnesium sulphate. There are many variations of this cocktail, and the one I favor contains at least one gram of magnesium chloride. Ten drips may be sufficient to restore levels. Overdosing of magnesium is an unlikely occurrence unless a person has impaired kidney function, since excesses are readily excreted.

While all of the above magnesium replenishment protocols work well, I am experimenting with yet another one that I concocted and will discuss in the chronic stress portion of the detox section. It is specifically designed to deliver magnesium to the pituitary and hypothalamus glands to kick-start the endocrine system.

As it turns out, saturated fat in the diet interferes with the absorption of oral magnesium supplements. The theory is that magnesium binds with the fat in the gut to form insoluble salts, unusable by the body. Looking at PA's diet, where much of the magnesium was likely supplied by mineral-rich water, it is likely that a portion of his/her intake of magnesium occurred between meals, away from fat intake. So I take some of my magnesium and other mineral supplements with my water away from meals.

I am now going to go out on another limb (aren't trees handy) and speculate that this saturated fat/magnesium interaction may be a very important factor that has led to the incorrect demonizing of saturated fats. Let's begin with the proven fact that on the SAD diet in this modernly stressful world, most people are already marginally or very deficient in magnesium [33]. Even a slight increase in saturated fat in the diet could reduce the already deficient magnesium levels even further by binding up a portion of whatever magnesium is available, leading to a cascade of cardiovascular issues.

First, cholesterol levels may rise, leading to the incorrect conclusion that saturated fats are the cause of elevated cholesterol. Second, magnesium depletion is well known to lead to arterial plaque formation, hypertension, and virtually every other major sign of heart disease [33]. If my supposition is correct, this is yet another example of the medical community coming to the wrong conclusion regarding cause and effect relationships, analogous to the rat chow experiment, but with much bigger ramifications. My hypothesis seems to fit the fact pattern that some people can eat saturated fat and not have cardiovascular issues. It would be of great interest to measure their magnesium levels. I would bet that these folks have sufficient magnesium, while those that exhibit heart problems have a deficiency. It also explains why there is poor correlation between one's lipid profile and heart disease.

A lipid profile is actually an indirect reflection of body magnesium level, because there is not a consistent correlation between cholesterol level and magnesium level, just an inverse relationship. This is yet another example of measuring something indirectly that can be easily measured directly, assuming you know what to look for. What is needed is a study directly comparing magnesium level with CVD (Cardiovascular Disease), but there is no money in proving that magnesium supplementation is the correct treatment for CVD. What might really scare off statin-industry-paid researchers is that magnesium has the potential of reducing cholesterol in exactly the same way as do statin drugs, but without any side effects [36]. When you consider that virtually nobody in the medical field even bothers to measure body magnesium levels, you end up with the potential for a serious amount of faulty research being published. Because magnesium is *the* heart nutrient, at a minimum the magnesium levels of all participants in any cardiovascular study should be measured and published. This is not rocket science.

Now, let's look at some of the cofactor nutrients that work with magnesium. Our friend vitamin B6, previously discussed, is an important cofactor that aids in magnesium (and calcium) absorption in the body and is interfered with by many toxins, more reason to add it to the supplement list [146] [147].

Zinc is another mineral that appears to be depleted by many toxins, and it also requires sufficient body magnesium levels before it can be replenished. There is an interesting test, known as the Bryce-Smith zinc taste test (ZTT) [148], that is sometimes useful to gauge body zinc sufficiency, and here is how it works. You place about half a teaspoon of zinc sulphate solution in your mouth and swish it around for about 10 seconds. The objective is to experience a bitter taste somewhat immediately, indicating sufficient zinc, which is associated with the sense of taste. Delayed or no taste response is indicative of concomitantly lower zinc levels. Zinc sulphate solutions for use in this test are available from Biotics Research as Aqueous Zinc [104]. In the event of a deficiency, I have used zinc citrate and OptiZinc supplements (widely available).

The objective is to begin zinc supplementation and, about once per week, redo the taste test until the desired result is achieved; then reduce the supplementation to a maintenance dose. My personal experience has been that until magnesium levels are restored, it is impossible to pass this test, regardless of how much zinc is taken. I take 50 to 75 mg per day. Potassium supplementation is also usually required when magnesium levels have been depleted. My preference is to use potassium citrate (widely available), since it is also alkalizing. Dosing for potassium is discussed in the alkalinity section below, and is based on urine pH. Note that anyone with impaired kidney function or who is taking diuretics should consult their doctor before using potassium supplements. If more than 1000 mg is required to maintain alkalinity during detoxing, blood testing of potassium levels is suggested.

As you will see from my discussion in the lifestyle section below, I am not a fan of putting products on the skin that contain unnatural ingredients. However, there are some products with a low potential toxicity that can be used for a short period of time as an aid to restoring essential minerals and, for those, I make an exception. In the case of zinc, there are topical supplementation products available such as a zinc sulphate cream by Kirkman Labs [149].

While it would be great if we could normalize mineral levels before beginning detoxification, this may not be possible because of the effect of the toxins themselves. For example, mercury and other heavy metals along with Candida overgrowth can so derange mineral transport in the body that it is difficult to normalize magnesium, potassium, zinc and other essential minerals until the toxin load has been somewhat reduced. Therefore, the idea is to begin mineral repletion in parallel with detoxification.

## Salt

I already discussed the availability of large quantities of salt from animal blood. Drinking blood is not convenient for me, so I supplement my diet with an unrefined ancient seabed salt. I avoid all refined salts such as common table salt and most other salts, even those labeled as "sea salt." In the unrefined category, there are those salts that are harvested from the ocean, and those that are harvested from ancient seabeds that have been buried for millions of years. The latter are my preference simply because of the currently contaminated state of our oceans, and the fact that we have yet to identify all of these contaminants, let alone measure them. In theory, ancient seabeds have been protected from modern pollution, and the odds are higher that they have avoided modern contaminants. The one I use is *RealSalt* from Redmond Incorporated in Utah [150]. There are some ancient seabed salts advertised from various other parts of the world, but I am skeptical of the quality control and test methods used.

As you will see from a discussion in the detox section, salt has the ability to cause the removal of toxins from the body in ways that we do not understand. I love salt, use it to taste, and estimate I consume about 2 grams per day. Am I worried about high blood pressure? No. My resting blood pressure ranges from 90/50 to 110/60. As far as I am concerned, none of the research relating salt intake to high blood pressure is applicable to the Wellness Diet, where we use only unrefined salt, and eliminate all of the toxic foods. There simply are no studies for those conditions, except of course for the 99,000-generation one. An excellent book on the healthy aspects of salt, also showing that, for the most part, the increase in blood pressure from salt is a transient one, is *Salt: Your Way to Health* by David Brownstein [151].

## Glandulars

While we have already discussed liver, not a lot of folks like to eat the other organs of animals. Adrenals, thyroid, lung, and spleen, to mention a few, just do not sound appetizing. Therefore, unlike PA, we are thus missing some fatty acids, beneficial hormones, enzymes, and probably a whole lot more. We know there are benefits to be obtained because natural thyroid hormones from cow or pig are widely prescribed to people with low functioning thyroid glands.

To partially make up for my lack of raw organ/gland intake, I take a multi-glandular supplement, which is a freeze-dried version of the various glands from clean, naturally fed animals. There is scant evidence as to what survives processing in these products, but it is one way to hedge bets in this area. One I have used is Neonatal Multi-Gland by Biotics

Research [104], containing spleen, heart, pancreas, kidney, brain, liver, adrenal, thymus, intestine, eye, and pituitary. I take two per meal.

An interesting event happened in my house that buttressed my appreciation of glandulars. I previously mentioned our cats, raised on a raw food diet that includes as many glands and other organs as we can obtain, along with a glandular supplement. However, it is not a perfect rat. One day when I was in the kitchen preparing lunch I had put my supplements, including two glandular tablets, on the table and turned my attention to the oven for a couple of minutes. When I returned, all the vitamins were on the floor, but upon retrieving them, I noticed that only the glandulars were missing. It finally occurred to me that the cats, who were hanging around, had eaten them. As an experiment, I ground up a tablet and put it in front of the two cats. Whoosh - gone in a second! I repeated the experiment using the desiccated liver discussed above, with the same result. Usually, the cats are quite leisurely when they eat, but they gobbled up the glandulars, leading to the conclusion that they needed more than what was in their diet, so we have upped the amount.

As a result of toxins in the body, both adrenal and thyroid gland malfunction has become widespread, and a plethora of supplements are available, each claiming to support the gland in some manner. With respect to thyroid glandulars, the ones sold without prescription are required to have the hormone thyroxine (T4) removed. For a non-prescription natural thyroid extract, I have used GTA-Forte II from Biotics Research [104]. In the prescription category, there are synthetics and natural, usually extracts from pig glands. In keeping with the Wellness Diet, for thyroid hormone supplementation to treat a hypothyroid condition, the natural form would be preferable. The popular prescription natural brands are Armour® and Westhroid®, and there are several good websites describing the differences [152] [153]. There is a lot more discussion about the thyroid in the iodine and halogen portions of the detox section.

With respect to adrenal glandulars, for a non-prescription natural whole adrenal extract, I have used Cytozyme-AD from Biotics Research. It is a source of neonatal bovine whole adrenal gland. More information on adrenal fatigue will be found in the detox section.

## Gelatin

Gelatin is found in the skin and bones of animals, including mammals, fowl, and fish, and broth made from animal bones is a good source of gelatin. Contrary to popular belief, hoofs, horns, hair, feathers, or any keratin material is not a source of gelatin. For those not inclined to consume bone soup, a gelatin supplement is suggested. Most of us are familiar with gelatin in the form of desserts such as Jell-O®, but gelatin has many health benefits that make it an important part of the Wellness Diet. Gelatin is related to collagen, which may be thought of as the glue that hold our body together and is critical to bone, joint and skin health. The amino acids glycine and proline, found in abundance in gelatin, play an important role in building cartilage and preventing bone disorders [154]. Glycine is one of the amino acids necessary to form glutathione, an important peptide used to remove a variety of toxins from the body. Glycine also helps digestion by enhancing gastric acid secretion [155], an important factor in the protein digestion process, as discussed more fully in the digestive rehabilitation section below.

Gelatin, which mostly consists of protein, was given a bad name several years ago when it was discovered that it could not be used as a complete meal replacement because it was not a complete protein and was missing or weak in a few amino acids. Of course, gelatin was never meant to be eaten alone in the context of PA's diet. It was again given a bad name during the mad-cow scare, when it was thought that commercial gelatin could be contaminated. Many studies were conducted to show that gelatin rendered from animal skin and bones was not at risk, and the processing steps used to make gelatin further reduce any potential risks [156]. The majority of supplement capsules are made from gelatin.

The definitive references on the nutritional benefits of gelatin come from articles by Dr. Francis Pottenger, mentioned earlier in connection with his raw cat food studies, and the book *Gelatin in Nutrition and Medicine* by N. R. Gotthoffer [106], which includes much of the gelatin research conducted in the 19th century. The following are some of Gotthoffer's findings, which have also been reported by Kaayla Daniel in the article *Why Broth is Beautiful*, published in Wise Traditions by the Weston A. Price Foundation, Spring 2003, Volume 4, No. 1 [7].

Early in the 20th century, researchers showed that gelatin increases the utilization of the protein in wheat, oats, and barley, though not of corn; that the digestibility of beans is vastly improved with the addition of gelatin; and that gelatin helps the digestion of meat protein. The last appears to confirm the subjective reports of many people who say that meats found in soups and pot roasts--cooked with bones for a long time in a liquid to which a touch of vinegar has been added--are easier to digest than quickly cooked steaks and chops, and why gelatin-rich gravies are at the heart of many culinary traditions.

Gotthoffer reports the existence of more than 30 years of research studies showing that gelatin can improve the digestion of milk and milk products. Accordingly, nutrition textbook writers of the 1920s and 1930s recommended that gelatin be included in infant formulas to help bring cow's milk closer to human milk. Apparently, gelatin exerted a very important influence on the milk fat. It served not only to emulsify the fat but also, by stabilizing the casein, improved the digestibility and absorption of the fat, which otherwise would be carried down with casein in a lumpy mass. As a result, infants fed gelatin-enriched formulas showed reduced allergic symptoms, vomiting, colic, diarrhea, constipation, and respiratory ailments than those on straight cow's milk.

Gelatin's reputation as a health restorer includes its ability to soothe the GI tract and to dramatically improve rheumatoid arthritis as well as other degenerative joint conditions and inflammatory bowel diseases [157]. It has also been reported that gelatin will protect gastric mucosal integrity, at least in lab rats subjected to ethanol-induced mucosal damage [158]. Another study showed that collagen hydrolysate, an extract of gelatin, reduced pain in patients with osteoarthritis of the knee or hip and that gelatin held a significant treatment advantage over the placebo [159].

As you can see from the above, I think very highly of gelatin, which has been largely ignored by the mainstream medical community in favor of drugs. As a supplement, used in place of bone broth, I use Beef Gelatin made by Great Lakes Gelatin Company [160]. Gelatin is a tasteless and odorless powder that mixes well in hot water. One teaspoon (about 5 grams) per meal is a suitable starting dose. More uses for gelatin will be discussed throughout the sections of the book that follow.

## Essential Fatty Acids

According to the medical community, the essential fatty acids (EFAs) for humans are certain polyunsaturated fatty acids (PUFAs) in the omega-6 and omega-3 families, and they must be obtained from the diet. The body needs them for many foundational purposes, such as building healthy cell membranes, a properly functioning brain, and for a whole gamut of hormone-like substances that regulate, among other things, immune and inflammatory responses.

The alternative health community has bombarded us with a message stating the "importance" of getting enough omega-3 fatty acids in our (SAD) diet, by using supplements such as fish oils and flax seed oil. In the following discussion, you will see why omega-3 supplements are not only not required on the Wellness Diet, they should be avoided because they can promote illness by generating substantial amounts of toxins.

Let's see what these oils are supposed to nutritionally accomplish. There seems to be general agreement that the SAD diet has a preponderance of omega-6 fatty acids in it, as compared to omega-3s. Many studies, including some Paleo diet studies indicate that a healthy range of omega-6 to omega-3 is from about 1:1 to 4:1, but the SAD diet ratios are usually way over 10:1. A classic study of rats showed that the optimum ratio to maintain learning skills and resistance to pain was 4:1 [161]. The omega-6 overload in the SAD diet comes mostly from nut and seed oils, products consumed in great quantity in the modern diet, but are non-existent in the Wellness Diet, as is this whole issue of having to balance the two fatty acid groups. Many illnesses are being ascribed to this modern ratio imbalance, and we are told to increase dramatically our omega-3 intake to compensate for the omega-6 excess. As an astute reader, you may well ask why one would not just reduce the omega-6 dietary intake to solve the ratio problem, but to do that would gut the SAD diet of much of its devotees' favorite foods, and, gosh, it would start to look like the Wellness Diet.

On the Wellness Diet, including Tier One and Two food choices, PA would have obtained the EFAs primarily from animal sources. The omega-3s would have been obtained from grass-fed muscle meat and in larger amounts from eating the brains, liver and other organs of prey. It is my contention that the Wellness Diet provides all of the EFAs the body needs, and in the proper ratio.  No EFA supplements are needed, and it may be detrimental to add any of them.  I could (and should) stop right here and not waste any more time on this issue, but it has been so highly hyped in the media that I feel compelled to put in my two-cents worth. What follows is a summary of my research into the omega-3 supplement industry, followed by a discussion of how the Wellness Diet avoids all of the pitfalls I encountered.

I have found it very frustrating in dealing with the oil supplement industry – they seem to win the prize when it comes to hiding the ball. Let's start at the beginning.  There is general agreement that the essential fatty acids, particularly the omega-3s, are indeed fragile, and most oil products that contain them, such as the seed-based oils like flax seed and its blends, and the fish and fish liver (usually cod liver) oils, caution the consumer to "refrigerate after opening," to consume the refrigerated oil in a few weeks, and to not use it for cooking.  By fragile I mean they easily become oxidized or rancid.  Some brands boast of having the container back-filled with nitrogen to prevent oxidative damage from air.  Still others boast of being in a dark container (opaque plastic or brown glass) to protect against light damage.  The message to the consumer is loud and clear – these oils are easily damaged by exposure to heat, light and air.  If only the manufacturers would heed their own advice.  Flax seed and fish oils in their natural state have high omega-3 content, and virtually no omega-6 content.  Starting with flax (linseed) seeds, let's look at the processing of the oil.  There are various ways to get the oil out of the seed, including the use of chemical solvents such as hexane, and the use of mechanical presses to squeeze the oil out.

While solvents are still used for many vegetable oils, they are in disfavor in the health arena because they tend to combine with seed and oil compounds to produce toxic stuff, and sometimes require evaporation temperatures way above that of boiling water, not a smart thing to do with heat-sensitive oils.  Expeller pressing, sometimes called "cold pressing" is now the preferred method.  There is no definition in the U.S. for cold pressing, and in some cases "cold" is actually quite hot, above the temperature of boiling water.  Some oils are further refined, such as by being bleached, and deodorized.  Flaxseeds are not digestible in the shell (as Nature intended), but you could get the omega-3s directly from the flax seeds by grinding them yourself and eating the pulp. Unfortunately, the grinding operation might well heat the seeds significantly, so then you would be eating rancid seed pulp. In any case, you would be eating the natural toxins MA put in there to keep you from eating her seeds.

As you can see, seed oil processing is fraught with potential problems in which the oil may be subjected to the high temperatures consumers are cautioned against, and for good reason. The scientific community is still discovering the many ways in which heating and otherwise processing oils makes them toxic to humans. It started with hydrogenation, a true Frankenmethod of hardening vegetables oils, which led to the creation of trans-fats, which are now the bad fats du jour.

The lipid industry has made some valiant attempts to quantify the purity of food oils. As an example, efforts have been made to quantify the oxidation of fats and oils (the rancidity) by defining the Peroxide Index (PV). Well, they found this was not accurate enough to detect all forms of rancidity, so they added the Anisidine Value (AV), which alone is also not sufficient. Then they defined the Totox Value (TV), which is AV + 2PV. I am not a lipid chemist, but this numbers game makes me nervous. They have yet to make a dent in defining, measuring, or determining the other types of damage resulting from the processing of polyunsaturated oils and their effect on the human body, such as cyclic fatty acid derivatives, cross-linked fatty acid chains, dimers, polymers, cross-linked triglycerides, body-shifted molecules, and molecular fragments. The bottom line for me with respect to seed oils is this: in keeping with the precepts of the Wellness Diet, I do not want to mess with MA's seeds, and I do not need to on the Wellness Diet. A caveat is also in order here. For those on the Wellness Diet, which does not have an omega-6 overload, taking large amounts of a seed or seed oil like flax seed can be counterproductive, as it contains a lot of omega-3 but almost no omega-6, thus upsetting the diet ratio in the reverse direction (too much omega-3). See the book *Fats That Heal and Fats That Kill* by Udo Erasmus for a discussion of the dangers of this imbalance [162].

Onward to the fish-oil industry. Here we have plain fish oils extracted from the flesh, and liver oils extracted from the liver. Many of the same steps used in vegetable oil processing are also used here, including solvents and pressing. However, fish oils face an additional hurdle. As discussed above, virtually all fish are contaminated with heavy metals such as mercury and arsenic, as well as pesticides and organic contaminants such as PCBs. I have been told by industry representatives that the flesh contains most of the heavy metals, and the liver contains most of the pesticides and organic contaminants. Either way, there are basically two choices presented to the consumer: molecular distillation, a high temperature process used to remove contaminants; or un-distilled oil, which still contains the contaminants. In the flesh-derived fish oil business, the distillation process predominates, but the effect of heating the oil to high temperatures required for distillation may well result in damaged fatty acids, detrimental to health, and possibly leaving the consumer with clean but heat-damaged oil that, after the fact, one is now told to keep in the refrigerator!

There are non-distilled oils such as salmon oil that still contain contaminants, so that is the risk factor in this category. Other than various regulatory agencies such as WHO (World Health Organization) and the EPA (Environmental Protection Agency) and the FDA and the USDA ( U. S. Department of Agriculture) putting some numbers down on paper, we are clueless as to safe contaminant limits. The agencies, some supported by the fishing industry, are still bickering as to whose numbers are right. Another of these non-distilled oils is made from krill, small plankton that is reputed to have low levels of contaminants, and claims are made that high heat is not used for extraction. From what I could find in my research, the krill oil extraction process that appears to be used for some brands is that disclosed in U.S. Patent 6,800,299, involving a solvent-based system using ketones, which is probably an improvement over hexane. However, as stated in the literature, the issue with using solvent extraction is not only the solvent itself, but toxic compounds that can be formed between the solvent and the compounds in the oil [40].

Moving along to fish liver oil, in its natural form it could be ingested as a source of omega-3s in place of eating animal brain or liver. It has the advantage of not only containing the usual omega-3 fatty acids, but also the long chain varieties, such as DHA (Docosahexaenoic Acid), found in human and animal brains and to a lesser extent in their livers. Another nice feature of unprocessed fish liver is that it contains natural versions of vitamins A and D in a well-balanced ratio. Here again, as a supplement, the oil choices are molecularly distilled or un-distilled. Virtually all are distilled, which has the unfortunate effect of destroying most of the natural vitamins A and D, so these nutrients are added back in synthetic form, and in ratios that suit the whims of the manufacturer. At least one producer claims to remove the natural vitamins before distillation, and then return them afterward, using a proprietary process. The only process I could find for extracting vitamins from oil is to use solvents. Lastly, there is a recent market addition to the liver oil selection that uses fermentation to produce un-distilled oil, but the contaminant problem remains. An excellent article on the cod liver oil processing industry can be found on the Weston Price Foundation website [7].

I am not comfortable with any fish oil supplements currently on the market, and personally avoid them for the following reasons: while there is not a wealth of information on the subject, I feel quite strongly that putting damaged fatty acids into one's body is a very bad thing to do, particularly because of its impact on the cardiovascular system. Oxidized fatty acids are known to predispose one toward arterial plaque, and I doubt they have a favorable effect on the brain, which is mostly fat. I also do not have sufficient confidence in the lipid chemists that they know how to detect, measure, and evaluate the health consequences of damaged fats. It took them decades to figure out (or admit to) the problems inherent with hydrogenation and trans-fats. I also am not a fan of consuming environmentally contaminated fish products, and government agency "safe" levels on a piece of paper (frequently revised) also give me no comfort, as you will see in more detail in the detox section. Finally, the fact that the vitamins A and D in virtually all fish liver oils are actually the same synthetic stuff you can buy in a supplement bottle contributes to my lack of enthusiasm for commercially available fish oils.

Yet, there are many, many cases where people taking omega-3 supplements feel better. To see how it is possible that these oils are *healthy* (a comparative term) even if they may be damaged, we need to recall the rat chow experiment in conjunction with the latest thoughts on how the body processes damaged fats. The supposition is that when a person ingests a damaged fatty acid, say a trans-fat damaged version of an omega-6 fat, the body will put it in a site reserved for undamaged omega-6 fats, either because it cannot tell the difference, or because a damaged omega-6 is better than none at all. This characteristic can go one step further to translocation – if one does not take in enough omega-3 fats to satisfy the body's needs and instead takes in too many omega-6s, the body can start putting the omega-6s into the omega-3 sites.

So, now let's take the typical case of a person on the SAD diet, overloaded with omega-6s, most of which are damaged due to typical food processing (such as frying with unsaturated vegetable oils). We can presume the body has loaded all of the omega-6 and probably most of the omega-3 receptor sites with the ingested damaged omega-6s. Along comes some damaged omega-3 fish oil, and this person starts to take some. Well, the body can now put these damaged omega-3s into omega-3 sites in place of damaged omega-6s – quite an improvement, so the person feels better, and even the mostly meaningless blood tests show improvement. Voila, they are getting *healthy* (actually, less unhealthy). This is another example of how removing the bad stuff can make you somewhat less unhealthy as compared to your present state of health, even if you are replacing it with less than good stuff. This may be good enough for some people, in which case I encourage them to continue down this path.

The goal of The Wellness Project, however, is to put in the good stuff and take out the bad stuff. Sure, the body can process some amount of damaged fats eaten each day and get rid of them, but that takes defense system energy better reserved for more serious tasks such as eliminating cancer cells and fending off unwanted bacteria, viruses and yeasts. Why deliberately put in bad stuff if you don't have to? With this in mind, let's now take a look at the Wellness Diet and the need, if any, for essential fatty acid supplementation.

It would be nice to know the daily requirement for the essential fatty acids, but all of the efforts to estimate those are based on people who eat the SAD diet, and are thus not useful for our purpose. A major reason, discussed earlier, is that the large intake of damaged omega-6 from the SAD diet necessitates large offsetting amounts of omega-3. However, we can get some meaningful data from EFA studies of infant diets, where the total intake of fatty acids can be closely controlled. An EFA amount of as little as 0.1% of total calories appeared to be sufficient to prevent a variety of symptoms associated with EFA deficiency [163]. On a 2000-calorie daily food intake, this translates to a total of about 225 mg of EFAs. For purposes of discussion, let's use a 4:1 ratio and assign 225 mg to the omega-6 intake and 55 mg to the omega-3 intake as safe daily dietary levels to avoid deficiency.

In the Wellness Diet, research shows we obtain substantial amounts of omega-3 and -6 fatty acids in a proper ratio from our grass-fed meat [164]. If we ate clean liver, such as broiled calf's liver (not fried), this would be an added boost to both the -3 and -6 category, including the long chains. I understand the "Mad Cow" threat is a strong deterrent, but animal brain would yield even more omega-3s. Actually, in the Wellness Diet, grass-fed muscle meat alone produces ideal fatty acid ratios and more omega-3s than fish flesh. Beef and lamb liver are also excellent sources of omega-3s. A 1998 study of the fatty acid composition of grass fed beef and lamb liver found that 100 grams (about 3 ounces) contained 151 milligrams of EPA and 83 milligrams of DHA, and an omega6/3 ratio of 0.71[85]. For those who are not liver lovers, I already discussed a freeze-dried liver supplement that contains the fatty acids, and it may be a suitable EFA (Essential Fatty Acid) supplement.

If one wants to up the amount of essential fatty acids in the Wellness Diet, including the long-chain ones, a suggestion is already on the Wellness Diet list of supplementary foods: EGGS. In particular, I am referring to eggs from free-range hens fed a variety of natural foods that enhance their fatty acid profile in the right direction, producing healthy omega-6 to -3 ratios, and also yielding substantial DHA and EPA long-chain fatty acids. A suggested brand is labeled Christopher Eggs, and they are available at a wide range of markets [165]. I would avoid eating conventional grain-fed penned-hen eggs. Their fatty acid omega-6/omega-3 profile is close to 20:1, much like grain-fed beef. An interesting analogy can be made here. Remember the discussion above about how ruminants such as cows process toxic or indigestible plant matter, such as grass (their natural food), into something nontoxic that we are able to assimilate, like meat? Well, here we have chickens, whose natural food sources include seeds such as flax seed, which they are genetically designed to process, providing us with a food we can assimilate – eggs. Studies have been conducted on the fatty acid profile of egg yolks from chickens fed a high omega-3 seed diet, like flax seeds, and the results show omega-6/omega-3 ratios around 3:1, as well as high levels of DHA [166]. In fact, a single one of these egg yolks can provide more than enough

EFAs to meet the daily requirement on the Wellness Diet. I avoid omega-3 supplements such as fish and flax oils while on the Wellness Diet in order not to disturb the fatty acid ratio of the diet in the wrong direction of excess omega-3, leading to some very nasty symptoms.

From the above discussion, it is apparent that no EFA supplements are needed with the Wellness Diet. Further, there is evidence that increasing the PUFA intake above the small amounts necessary can be very detrimental one's health. As previously mentioned, PUFAs are very easily oxidized, and once oxidized in the body, they promote oxidative stress as a result of lipid peroxidation, which is another way of saying that they produce toxic substances in the body that significantly burden its defense system. It appears that the body will attempt to convert excess PUFAs into saturated fat, but inevitably dietary PUFAs still accumulate over time in cells and can increase the risk of cancer [167]. A multi-institutional prospective study in 2004 concluded that heart disease was directly correlated with PUFA intake, and inversely correlated with intake of saturated fat [168]. This study is sometimes referred to as the "American Paradox" because there are many other studies that appear to show the contrary. Antioxidants such as the vitamin E complex can sometimes slow the oxidative damage. Because of the inconsistent data on the effects of excessive PUFA intake, it would seem to make sense to minimize such intake. However, the thrust of the alternative health campaign is just devoted to balancing fatty acid ratios - add more omega-3 supplements to offset high omega-6 intake - while ignoring the absolute amounts of each being ingested. This may well backfire in the future if it eventually becomes apparent that the total amount of PUFAs consumed is as important as, or perhaps more important than the ratio, when it comes to the overall health of the person. Which brings me to a discussion of sesame seeds.

Researchers have found that eating sesame seeds can shut down the body's ability to make a crucial fatty acid that makes up about 50 % of our brain. A lignan (a phytoestrogen) called sesamin in sesame seeds interferes with an enzyme, delta 5 desaturase, which is part of the pathway that makes arachidonic acid (AA) from dietary intake of omega-6 linoleic acid. If that pathway is disrupted, there is a potential of shutting down at least a portion of AA production (the brain is about 50% AA). Doing so also upsets the amount of DHA that the body makes from omega-3 linolenic acid using that same enzyme, potentially increasing DHA production. The supplement community thinks this is great and actually puts sesamin in supplements for this very reason. You see, on the SAD diet, one gets too much AA and not enough DHA, so this is their way to fix it. Another way, of course, is to stop eating all of the seeds in the first place, since they are a major dietary cause of the problem, but that does not result in profits. Well, I can tell you that it could be bad news to eat sesame seeds on the Wellness Diet, which already has a natural fatty acid balance, because it could easily cause an AA deficiency [169] [170]. The point of this little excursion was to indicate how easily some of the foods in a SAD diet, like seeds, can mess with our fatty acid balance in unpredictable ways.

Speculating beyond sesame seeds, I wonder if some other plant food, (or maybe even sesame seeds) that we excluded from the Wellness Diet as naturally toxic, might result in *saturated* fat causing some detrimental effect on health in the SAD diet. Let us say, hypothetically, that we accept as correct the studies showing that people that eat a SAD diet and have high intake of saturated fat have a higher risk of heart disease. First, that is very different than saying saturated fat causes heart disease. Remember the rat chow experiment? They claimed that calorie restriction prolonged life, but what they had really proven was that rat chow is toxic. So, what may have been proven in these studies, if anything, is that if you eat a lot of saturated fat while also eating seeds, vegetables, dairy, processed oils, sugars, artificial sweeteners and tap water, it is unhealthy. I have already speculated above on the saturated fat/magnesium deficiency connection, and magnesium deficiency is rampant among SAD eaters. Those heart disease studies on saturated fats are not relevant to the Wellness Diet, where all of the toxic foods (like sesame seeds) have been eliminated, and magnesium is provided in adequate amounts.

It would be interesting to conduct studies to see which of the SAD diet components, if any, is the culprit in messing with saturated fat, just as they found that sesame seeds messed with polyunsaturated fats. My guess would be that it is also a seed-related compound, because the SAD diet is filled with foods from seeds. All grains are seeds (bread, pasta, cake, cookies, pizza, rice, etc.), and many are cooked using seed oils (canola, safflower, peanut). Well, if you eat MA's seeds (the reproductive agents of plants) in great quantity, this might be another way that it makes you sick so that you will cut it out.

My speculation regarding saturated fat and magnesium deficiency fits perfectly in the above model involving seeds. It works like this: seeds contain natural toxins that bind up minerals in the body, including magnesium, contributing to magnesium depletion. Saturated fat also binds with magnesium, aggravating depletion, which is a major culprit in heart disease. This is a fertile area for research, but it would have to be privately funded since it does not lead to the sale of any products other than magnesium supplements.

# Chapter 12 - Digestive Rehabilitation

This section is for people intrigued with the Wellness Diet, but who have had digestive problems in the past eating meat. The best way to make the transition from a SAD diet to the Wellness Diet is to do so slowly, introducing small amounts of easily digested meat, such as ground patties into the diet, while also starting to drop some of the SAD foods. This process can take many months, but is the most natural way to go. Remember that during the transition, a huge toxic load is being removed from the body in the form of MA's naturally occurring toxins. The body can actually go through a "die-off reaction," discussed in more detail in the detox section. The upshot of this is that one can feel lousy during the transition as the body adjusts to its natural diet. Further, some established parasitic toxins in the body, particularly Candida, get very unhappy when deprived of their favorite foods (which you will be giving up), and this can make one feel quite miserable until they are dealt with.

Many folks who have been, or are dealing with Candida overgrowth know that grains, sugars, and alcohol are the troubling foods. Having dealt with Candida issues for most of my life, I will spend a great deal of time discussing it in the next section. Fruit is sometimes identified as a problem Candida food. On the Wellness Diet, eating only limited amounts of carbs (typically less than 75 grams per day) in the form of whole fresh fruit (no dried fruit and no fruit juice), and taking the spore-forming bacteria seems to work quite well when combined with the fungal detoxification program outlined in Chapter 17.

Having said that, there are people who exhibit allergic reactions to certain fruit, including those that pass the ABC test. Examples are watermelon, figs, cherimoya and mango. Symptoms include itching, rashes, nasal congestion, and asthma-like reactions. Researchers have coined the term "latex-fruit syndrome" in an effort to explain this phenomenon [171]. They have found that many of those who exhibit this syndrome also have an allergic reaction to natural rubber latex, usually first detected upon exposure to latex gloves. Interestingly, several of the proteins believed responsible for the allergic reactions possess potent antifungal characteristics. Examples of such proteins are chitinases and glucanases, both capable of rupturing yeast cells.

As you will see in the detox section, yeast overgrowth in the body, particularly Candida, is a major obstacle to health, and rupture of those cells can produce all of the symptoms listed above for the latex-fruit syndrome. Personally, when I (unknowingly) had such a yeast overgrowth many years ago, I was allergic to certain fruits such as peaches and watermelon, and I used to get canker sores from eating citrus fruit. Now that the yeast is under control, all of those symptoms have disappeared, highlighting the importance of detoxification and its interaction with diet. Incidentally, all of my pollen allergies also disappeared, such as ragweed allergy and hay fever. So for those with fruit allergies, until you can implement some of the detox protocols of The Wellness Project, avoid or minimize eating those fruits known to produce symptoms. There is also some evidence that peeling the fruit, such as apples and peaches, before eating, can reduce or eliminate symptoms [172].

Beef allergy is considered to be very rare (pun intended), and I wonder how many of the few cases may be reacting to growth hormones or other adulterations found in conventional meat. I would venture that eating organic grass-fed free-range meat, along with detoxification, would eliminate even the few cases of meat allergy. As already mentioned, later introduced animal products such as chicken do have a record of allergy prevalence.

Some other roadblocks in the way of a smooth diet transition are a lack of hydrochloric (HCl) acid, a digestive secretion produced in the stomach; lack of digestive enzymes, mostly produced in the pancreas, and lack of bile, produced in the liver and stored in the gall bladder. Some of these shortages can be caused by many years on a SAD diet which did not required digestive support from these organs, and hence they have fallen into disuse (use it or lose it). In other instances, this digestive difficulty may be caused by various infections, such as H.pylori (Helicobacter Pylori) and Candida overgrowth, either of which could also be due to eating the SAD diet. Then there are all of the environmental and medical/dental-induced contaminants such as heavy metals and organic poisons that can wreak havoc with digestion. Those are discussed below. There is also some evidence that blood type has an influence, with type A generally having lower stomach acid levels than type O.

For individuals interested in making the diet switch, some digestive supplements might help pave the way during the transition, although I suggest that you use them only for a limited time. A caveat, however, is in order. Depending on the ultimate causes of digestive disturbances, these supplements may work fine, may not work at all, or may make digestive symptoms worse (this latter case is dealt with in the detox section). In other words, you should always be mindful of how your body is reacting to any type of supplementation and proceed conservatively.

## Bitters/Betaine HCL/Digestive Enzymes

Herbal bitters have been used for years as a remedy for digestive ailments, so let's look at these first. We know all about bitters from MA because of our fruit discussion, and we know we have separate taste buds just for bitter taste. Most digestive bitters are liquid preparations of the very parts of the plants that are avoided on the Wellness Diet because they are very likely to be toxic. From my point of view, this is why bitters seem to work to "wake up" the digestive system. This is a guess, of course, but consider that when the bitters are placed on our tongue and hit our bitter-taste buds, our bodies are programmed to expect that a load of toxic plant material is about to hit our stomach. In defense, the body starts cranking acid, pepsin, digestive enzymes and anything else it can throw at the stuff to try to detoxify it. On the one hand, this is a clever way to reawaken the digestive system using a natural process. On the other hand, we may be stressing the body unnecessarily to go on alert. Yet another concern is whether we are behavior conditioning our digestive system to awaken only when we consume something bitter. As a short-term solution, say only for a few months, perhaps this method could be used, for example, during the diet switchover period. There are many herbal bitter concoctions on the market for digestive relief, some of which are labeled Swedish bitters, and they are quite popular in Europe.

Instead of bitters, another approach is to approximate nature by directly replacing the missing elements in our digestive system. Let's start with HCl, which, when not sufficiently available, causes digestive upset and heartburn. Yet if you tell your doctor you have heartburn, he/she will probably give you an acid-suppressing drug or recommend antacids, which are a big business. Research, however, tells us that antacids don't really benefit you in the long run, and can lead to helicobacter pylori overgrowth (the cause of ulcers), pneumonia, and tuberculosis, just for starters. For a good discussion of the need for stomach acid see the book : *Why Stomach Acid Is Good For You* by Jonathan Wright [173].

Insufficient HCl is commonly blamed on aging and in some cases blood type (those with blood type A seems to have lower amounts than blood type O), but it could also be a result of accumulated toxins in the system, including those resulting from a poor diet. A supplement used for insufficient HCl is betaine HCl, a product widely available in health food stores, and it usually includes pepsin, a digestive enzyme also produced in the stomach. It should be taken with a meal, and the dosage is determined experimentally, varying from about 130 mg to several grams per meal. The goal is to simulate nature's wonderful system of secreting just the right amount for each meal, which varies with the meal size and content. At best, this is going to end up as a crude approximation, but fortunately, we are not after perfection. Anyone with a stomach ulcer should avoid this supplement until the ulcer is healed. One brand of Betaine HCL caps (with pepsin) is Twinlab [174].

There are a few tests available to determine stomach pH, and thus, indirectly, the need for HCl supplementation, but each has its drawbacks, so one can just start taking some small amounts of Betaine

HCl and see what effect it has on digestion. If a warm sensation in the gut is experienced while eating after taking the supplement, this may indicate an excessive amount of HCl, so the dose is reduced until the sensation is eliminated. A burning sensation is a sign to stop taking it temporarily, and instead take some supplements that may be helpful to heal an inflamed stomach, such as slippery elm, discussed below.

An HCl supplement with pepsin helps the body break down protein, among other things and, in theory, you will be able to tolerate animal products without discomfort, even if they haven't been eaten for a long period of time. This supplement can also help resolve a vicious digestive cycle. Here's the picture: with insufficient stomach acid, one cannot assimilate all of their food efficiently and, thus, they may not absorb certain nutritional elements, particularly minerals such as zinc, necessary for the production of stomach acid in the first place. For instance, the body needs chloride, which is from salt, and zinc and other minerals often deficient in today's refined diets. The HCl supplement jumpstarts the digestive processes and when the body's own levels come up, the digestive system should be able to resume the acid production operation on its own. In the above discussion of gelatin, it was mentioned that it could be used to correct stomach acid deficiencies. As an integral component of the Wellness Diet, I view gelatin as an important ingredient for the correction of HCl deficiency in the long-term.

A special note is in order here regarding dolomite, which contains minerals in their carbonate form, requiring HCl or some other acid for assimilation. As explained above, taking dolomite with magnesium taurate away from meals helps with acid production. If you know you are deficient in stomach acid, take the dolomite with one tablet of *HCL-Plus* by Biotics Research [104]. It supplies a small amount of HCl, insuring full assimilation.

Another way to improve digestion is with a digestive enzyme supplement. The body naturally produces digestive enzymes to break down food. Some are produced in the mouth while chewing food, and others are made in the gut and in the pancreas as food enters the stomach and small intestine. These enzymes have different roles. Some help to break down protein, still others break down fats, and others carbohydrates. Those who have followed a primarily vegetarian diet may be short on the enzymes that digest protein (proteases) and fat (lipases), and a deficiency can lead to indigestion, discomfort, and an inability to assimilate all of the food. People tend not to be deficient in the carbohydrate enzymes (amylases).

There is some controversy about whether enzyme supplements become habit-forming and prevent the body from gearing up its own. I haven't seen that happen, but I would only take them during the diet transition period. Further, some fruits in the Wellness Diet contain digestive enzymes, making it even less likely that the body will shut down its own ability to make enzymes from ingesting them in supplement form. In the animal world, the pancreas of an animal would be a source of digestive enzymes if, in fact, PA consumed the pancreas. From my point of view, it is much more likely that PA's supplementary digestive enzymes came from fruit. Tropical fruits such as papaya (papain) and pineapple (bromelain) are typically the source for plant-based protease enzyme supplements. Well, wouldn't you know it, these fruit enzyme profiles fit perfectly into the Wellness Diet.

For an enzyme supplement during the diet transition phase, I would eat papaya (but only if it is labeled as not genetically modified) and/or pineapple with meals, to help digest meat protein. A second choice is to get papain or bromelain in the form of supplements and take those with meals– there are many brands. Look for those where the only ingredient is papaya or pineapple. Usually, portions of the fruit that are not on the Wellness Diet are used, such as the leaf or a part of the unripe fruit. Since this supplement is for short-term use, I don't have a problem with this implementation. Because of the GMO issues with papaya, I prefer a bromelain supplement. One example is Bromelain by Now Foods, available in tablet or capsule form, and one per meal is a good starting dose [122]. If the enzymes work, one should experience better bowel movements as well as less bloat and discomfort after eating. For those with an inflamed gut, however, protein-digesting enzymes can aggravate the condition, requiring one to stop or severely cut back on dosage if gut pain or headaches are experienced. In such case, see the section below regarding gut repair.

It is interesting to note that there are two distinct ways in which digestive enzymes can be used. One is to help digest food, in which case, the enzymes are taken with food. The second usage is aimed at digesting certain proteins present in the bloodstream, some of which may have originated as remnants of undigested food, and which are involved in inflammation and allergic reactions. Some people target these proteins in an effort to help reduce inflammation, pain, and allergies, simply by taking the enzyme supplements between meals. The goal, of course, is only to use the supplements during your transition to the Wellness Diet. After a time, the combination of eating the right types of fruits and one's own pancreas waking up should make you digestively self-reliant.

## Bile salts

Another digestive area that may need supplementing is the gall bladder, which could have either gone to sleep and/or been congested by being misused on the SAD diet. Unfortunately, many people have already had it removed because of gallstones and/or a strange notion within the medical community that people don't really need it, but they do. The liver makes bile, which is then stored and concentrated in the gall bladder between meals. The bile is then secreted into the small intestine to emulsify fats and get them into a form that the body can assimilate and utilize. This function is particularly important when eating animal fats. Some indications of insufficiency are pale stools, perhaps gray in color (bile gives our stool its characteristic brown color), and/or floating stools, which are full of undigested fat. As you will see in the detox section, bile is an important pathway for the excretion of toxins, hence an insufficiency of bile can impair the ability to detoxify.

For those with a gall bladder, bile salt tablets may be useful as a supplement to ease the transition to animal fats. The protocol recommended by the supplement manufacturers is to cycle doses to avoid dependence upon the salts. They suggest starting with one tablet with meals the first day, two tablets with meals the second day, three on the third, and then back to one tablet the next day. Going up and down like this apparently prevents a dependence on the bile salts during the diet transition period, after which the gall bladder should be functioning normally. For those without a gall bladder, they suggest that one to two tablets with each meal is generally effective and can be used for life. Examples of bile salt supplements are Beta Plus by Biotics Research [104], and Cholacol by Standard Process [175]. Checking stool characteristics and tracking gastric symptoms would be a good way to monitor progress.

## Probiotics

In the mucous lining of your intestinal tract is a teeming world of bacteria, fungi and other microorganisms. It is estimated that hundreds of species are present, some detrimental, some beneficial, and others than can become either, depending on the circumstances. These creatures number in the countless billions, more in fact, than the total number of cells in the body. If all of them were piled together, they would tip the scales at several pounds.

As of the writing of this book, we still have not identified the majority of the microbes in our gut, but a government-funded initiative has been officially announced that is planning to do just that. It is known as the NIH (National Institutes of Health) Human Microbiome Project, and their objectives include determining whether individuals share a core human microbiome, and trying to understand whether changes in the human microbiome can be correlated with changes in human health. Recently, there has been a renewed interest in gut microflora and its role in illness and inflammation [176], and I predict they will find it to be an important link in the riddles of illness.

The gut microorganisms that are carried around 24/7 in the body (but actually outside of it because the intestines from the mouth to the anus are actually outside the body, separated by the intestinal wall) are pivotal to quality of life and it's the balance among them that is vital to your existence in ways you never imagined. They can include bacteria, viruses, fungi, and a variety of parasites including worms, amoeba, and protozoa. In reality, all of these could be considered as parasites because many live off us, the host. Healthy bodies supposedly harbor huge colonies of so-called friendly bacteria, otherwise known as beneficial intestinal flora. The most famous of these bacterial "good guys" is the lactobacillus genus, among them the acidophilus strain, which is active in the lower portion of the small intestine. Bifidobacteria, another genus of bacteria, is primarily active in the colon. In addition are the spore-formers, which should be a part of the mix but are usually missing. Estimates are that 80% or more of the body's defense system is in the gut, so the gut flora is intimately involved with overall health. A big part of

The Wellness Project is devoted to tending to this teeming mass, for unless it is performing properly, illness is likely.

In the alternative health world, there is a great deal of emphasis placed on the use of conventional probiotics, which are supposedly bacterial clones of the "friendly" bacteria that should be in your gut. Taking them in quantity (from 1 billion to 1 trillion) each day will theoretically squeeze out the bad guys, and reestablish a healthy colony. For the purpose of our diet makeover, some may find it helpful to take a probiotic, since gut microbes are intimately involved in the digestive process, and many previously living on the SAD diet are likely to have a mess in their gut. Before we can answer the question of which probiotic to take, if any, we need to step back and look at the big picture.

Based on my research, here is my take on what might be going on in our gut. When we are born our gut is sterile, and we are designed by MA to colonize it from the bacteria in our mother's birth canal on the way out. Well, that moves us to the hospital room, and brings up the following questions: Have the well-meaning staff swabbed the birth canal with anything that might disturb the natural flora? What about the anesthesia or other stuff dripped or injected into the mother – does that affect the natural flora? What about a caesarian section [177]? In the latter instance, we can forget about the birth canal, and assume the baby will colonize his/her gut from a passing nurse, lab technician, or orderly. Not a fun prospect, but wait.

An observation from all of this concerns the general belief that a child can genetically inherit food and other allergies, skin problems, and gastric upsets from their mother. Well, if the gut colonization process works as designed, the baby "inherits" at least some of these characteristics from the birth canal bacteria, which reflects the health (or illnesses) of the mother as reflected by her lifestyle, and is not genetic at all, but it is passed on. So, if you were a C-section baby (possibly itself indicating a less than healthy mother), and the nurse that held you, cleaned you, played with you, and breathed on you was a healthy specimen, you might be way ahead of the game! I can think of a fun animal research project (perhaps it has already been tried) where just before birth, a portion of the mother's birth canal is cleaned of the bacteria in it. It is then replaced with what are hopefully the ideal mix of friendly bacteria to give the offspring a good head start in life, particularly if it is known that the mother has pre-existing health issues.

There is also ample evidence that breast milk is a second source of probiotics from the mother, particularly bifidobacteria for colon colonization, increasing the importance of breast feeding [178]. Along these same lines, we know from anthropological studies that MA's method for human females to give birth is by squatting. I wonder what differences there would be in birth canal probiotic colonization of the child as a result of this position versus the conventional supine position. Certainly, the birth canal would be at a very different angle when squatting, perhaps enhancing colonization.

So, here we are today with a gut full of stuff that has changed over time as a function of just about everything we put into (or even on) our bodies, as well as everything the medical/dental communities put in us. My personal opinion is that if we were to have available to us the gut microbial contents of PA and compare it to anyone now living, there would be few similarities. I would expect to see in the guts of modern humans not only new critters, but also mutated old critters, and this is one reason why I do not think the medical research community will be able to define even a substantial part of our gut contents any time soon, if ever. So far, they have only identified a handful of the hundreds of mutating critters, and by the time they get to the end of that list, hundreds more new ones will have evolved. If my analysis is correct, we actually no longer have a specimen of a healthy gut, so it becomes a guessing game.

In the probiotic industry, they have identified what they believe to be the healthy strains, some of which may be human or animal based, and these are grown using a variety of media (food), including dairy and such esoteric plant products as garbanzo beans. Some require refrigeration and others do not. If the A excludes B theory of new bacteria replacing old were the only thing going on in the gut, perhaps probiotics would always be a good idea, but I do not think it is that simple. I see no reason why Darwin would not be at work in our guts, where survival of the fittest reigns among competing strains and even species. A simple assumption is that they all feed off our bodies, which I am sure many do, but I also would expect to see what are called epiparasites, which are those that feed off other parasites – critter eating critter.

If my assumptions are correct, let's see what might happen if we willy-nilly start taking multi-strain probiotics in large quantities. Depending on what is waiting at the other end of our esophagus, we may well be sending down food to feed many of the bad guy epiparasites that live off some of these strains, strengthening them and making us sicker. Or, the strains used in the probiotic, for some reason or other, do not match any in our gut, but are close enough so that they can somehow combine with similar strains to create yet a new mutated friend or foe. Please remember that the gut critters we are talking about are not just bacteria, but include the whole gamut of fungi, viruses and various parasites, and it is wishful thinking to assume they do not interact with each other.

I will cover this in more depth in the detox section, but suffice to say that it has been my experience that you can make yourself sicker (or healthier) with probiotics, and it is somewhat of a dice roll [179]. The issues become more complicated for those probiotic supplements that include prebiotics, a food source designed ostensibly to provide nourishment to enhance only the growth of the good guys. Basically, the bad guys may get to it first, and you end up nourishing them. In fact, a recent study of the use of the popular prebiotic known as FOS (fructo-oligosaccharides) in rats found that it actually increased gut permeability (leaky gut), and caused salmonella bacteria to spread outside of the intestines, both of which can contribute to illness [180].

Yet another problem is Small Intestine Bacterial Overgrowth (SIBO). Normally, the stomach and upper portion of the small intestine should be devoid of large colonies of bacteria, but due to improper diet and toxins, the small intestine, in particular, can become host to a variety of bacteria, leading to malabsorption and a host of other symptoms, including IBS (Irritable Bowel Syndrome). There is a simple breath test to determine the presence of SIBO, and the usual treatment is with an antibiotic such as rifaximin [181]. From my research, it appears possible that the bacterial strains normally found in probiotics may end up colonizing in areas where they don't belong [182], another reason not to begin high dose probiotics until diet and detox protocols are in place. Here is my protocol.

It appears that L. acidophilus is a required bacteria strain in the gut, so it should be represented in the product. In addition, B. bifidum and B. longum appear to be somewhat universal, so I limit my intake to those three, and I prefer a human-derived strain, if available, grown on a dairy-free medium. The one I use is Kyo-Dophilus by Wakunaga [183], and I take from one to three per day, with meals. Look for improvement in gut function, such as elimination of gas, diarrhea, and/or constipation, and you may also find some fruit allergies are alleviated [184]. There may be an adjustment period of a few weeks during which some symptoms may be aggravated. Once detoxification has taken place, particularly in the area of parasite cleansing, multi-strain and higher dose protocols might be employed. I believe it is very important also to be taking spore-forming bacteria to complement conventional probiotics. These have been already been discussed in the diet section, and will be discussed further in the detox sections.

At this point, I am going to speculate and peer into the future as to the potential impact of the gut microflora on our diet. If you recall from the evolution and environment section of the book, I singled out gut microflora as a unique bridge between our heritage and our environment. It is a part of our heritage because it is naturally intended to be inherited from our mother at birth. It becomes a part of our environment when it proliferates in our gut, which is outside the body. Finally, it plays a major role in the digestive process. This raises the issue of whether in the future our gut bacteria could be tailored in such a manner that we would be able to digest foods other than those in the Wellness Diet without ill effect. In other words, perhaps we could bypass the geneticists and accomplish some amount of additional alignment between our heritage and today's environment by fiddling with gut bacteria. Let's see if MA can shed any light on this proposition.

From the discussion of natural toxins in plants, tannins surfaced as a prevalent toxin. A large intake of tannins may cause bowel irritation, kidney irritation, liver damage, irritation of the stomach, and gastrointestinal pain. A correlation has also been made between esophageal cancer in humans and regular consumption of certain foods with high tannin concentrations [185]. Ruminant animals also have difficulty digesting and deriving nutrition from plants with high tannin levels, and hence avoid them unless foods that are more nutritious are not readably available.  A research study was conducted in Ethiopia on East African ruminants, including sheep, goats and antelope, where these animals had been found to be eating small amounts of plants with high tannin content, such as the leaves of Acacia trees [186].   Upon examination of the gut bacteria from these animals, they found previously unknown strains, which had the unique property of being able to digest tannins and derive nutrition from them.  It is not known how these strains were derived – did they come from long-term ingestion of the Acacia leaves themselves, or did these animals inherit the strains as a biological fluke?  In another study, researchers found that they could transplant tannin-digesting bacteria from one mammal (a Hawaiian goat) to another mammal (an Australian goat), who then acquired the ability to safely eat some tannin-containing foods [187].

The upshot from the above studies is the intriguing possibility that similar cultivation and transplanting of gut bacteria in humans may be a way in the not-too-distant future of accelerating the alignment of our evolutionary heritage with today's environment, at least in the area of food digestion.  For example, could the transplantation of gut flora from a healthy pie-and-soda-eating winner to an *other* convey those same health "benefits" useful in our modern environment?

## Gut Repair

Many people have inflamed, angry, and dysfunctional intestines, a likely result of the way they have eaten, the medications they have taken, and their burden of toxicity.  This condition is sometimes referred to as chronic gastritis.   Each factor undermines the balance of beneficial bacterial flora colonies in the gut lining.  If this has taken place, betaine HCl or digestive enzymes might cause some negative reactions such as local pain and headaches.   Important elements in gut repair are the fulvic/humic acids and spore-forming bacteria from the diet, which displace some of the bad guys and repopulate with good guys, thus speeding the healing process.

There are several approaches to healing an inflamed (and possibly porous or leaky) gut.  One approach uses plant extracts for short-term relief, and the other uses animal products for ultimately healing the lining of the gut.  I will discuss the plant extracts first.

Slippery elm bark is a soothing and healing herb for an irritated gut, and can be taken as a tea, powder, or capsule. Large amounts of slippery elm can be taken often, and over time it can help to patch up the gut. Once intestines have healed, HCl and digestive enzymes are more likely to be tolerated. There are many brands on the market, and one can take many grams per day during the healing process, which could take months. Marshmallow root, also widely available, may be used as an alternative to slippery elm bark.

For at least several thousand years, people in the Mediterranean region have used resin from a particular shrub belonging to the Pistachio family for gastrointestinal ailments. The resin is called mastic gum, and it is produced commercially on the Greek island of Chios. Some reports have shown that it has the ability to eliminate the H.pylori bacteria that causes stomach and intestinal ulcers, and it also has anti-fungal properties. Other studies, backed by the pharmaceutical industry, have concluded that it does not reduce H.pylori concentrations, so this is somewhat of a personal trial-and-error process. Like slippery elm, many brands are available and one can take several grams per day.

Notice that the healing supplements in this section use portions of plants that we have eliminated from the Wellness Diet, like bark, root, and a resin extracted from the bark. This is in keeping with reserving these plant parts for short-term medicinal use, not as nourishment. Depending on one's level of toxicity, none of the above remedies may work. For example, large amounts of mercury can keep the gut in a state of inflammation until sufficient amounts have been removed through detoxification.

Now, let's turn to animal-based gut healing, in the form of gelatin. It was already mentioned in the above discussion of gelatin that it has soothing properties. Like slippery elm and marshmallow root, gelatin also forms a hydrophilic colloid, meaning a water absorbing gel, which coats the intestines and leads to healing. Because gelatin is an integral part of the Wellness Diet, its long-term use will maintain the integrity of the gut wall.

Last, but by no means least, is clay. Because it is discussed at length in the next section, I will only briefly mention its use here. Clay is known to adsorb or otherwise render harmless the natural toxins found in foods that you have probably been eating most of your life, and will continue to eat during the diet changeover period. During this diet transition time, sucking on clay tablets between meals during the day may be helpful. One source of clay tablets that I have used is the Terramin brand by California Earth Minerals [188]. I suck on one at a time until it has "dissolved." Swishing the clay around in the mouth is a very good idea (I happen to love the taste of clay). I find that it triggers the thirst response, which may have been long dormant, so I drink lots of water with the clay and avoid taking it with food supplements because it may adsorb them. Many annoying digestive issues may disappear with clay, including food cravings.

## Chapter 13 - The Portable Diet

This section is devoted to the busy person who may be on the move a great deal of the time and would like to have a portable version of the Wellness Diet, so here it is. For animal fat and protein in portable form that requires no refrigeration and will not deteriorate for many months, it is hard to beat pemmican, so I would take along several bars. My favorite is the one from US Wellness meats [27]. Liver tablets are also a good source of protein and easy to transport. For fruit, I take along fresh fruit. For eggs, I take along hard-boiled eggs. The food supplements are easy to tote except for the red palm oil, which can get somewhat messy. I have been looking for a source of the oil in gelcaps, but have not yet found one. Individual pro-A, vitamin E and vitamin K supplements can be substituted. I do get many stares on the airplane, but a discussion of the Wellness Diet is sure to break the ice in any conversation!

What happens if I am away from home for some time and cannot get the Wellness Diet raw materials? Well, my analogy to that is times when, due to environmental disruptions such as long-term drought, PA could not get his/her diet raw materials. To avoid starvation, PA needed to eat items that he/she would normally consider unacceptable. Visit the clay section in the detox section below and you will see that PA was able to manage on a short-term basis by consuming clay with the food, which adsorbed enough of the toxins to enable survival. (Note that adsorption means to form a bond on the surface, as opposed to absorption, which means to diffuse together to form a solution.) So, I add to the portable diet a good supply of clay – don't leave home without it! There are no formal guidelines for this, but taking 1-4 capsules of clay with a "toxic" meal should help matters.

# Chapter 14 - Questions Relating to the Diet

I have tried to put on the hat of a reader, and pose questions likely to be asked after reading the diet section.

Isn't the Wellness Diet like the Atkins diet? The Atkins diet is a low carb diet that allows for: grain-fed as well as commercially-processed meat such as bacon, fried foods, vegetables, dairy, nuts, seeds, artificial sweeteners, fish, fowl, processed oils, and beans such as soy, and does not control the types of liquids. The Wellness Diet is much more restrictive, disallowing all of the above.

Isn't the Wellness Diet like the gluten-free/dairy-free diet? The GF/DF diet, as it is known, restricts dairy and gluten-containing grains, but allows other grains, vegetables, juices, nuts, seeds, fish, fowl, grain fed meat, and processed oils, and does not control the types of liquids. The Wellness Diet is much more restrictive, and perhaps we should call it the SF/DF/VF/SF/NF/RF/OF diet! Did I leave something out?

Isn't the Wellness Diet like the Paleo diet? There are many so-called Paleo diets out there, but most of them are centered on the late Paleo period after the introduction of cooking, fishing, and bird catching, ignoring the previous 2.4 million years of our heritage. Therefore, they presume that toxic vegetables, nuts, seeds, fish, and fowl were acceptable ancient foods. They also presume that a diet low in saturated fat and salt were standard fare. The result is a diet very different from the Wellness Diet.

Can't I have a bagel with cream cheese just once a week? Nobody is perfect, so if you "cheat," take some clay with the meal. Closely monitor how you feel afterward to see if you can detect any negative effects.

I am healthy, so why should I consider the Wellness Diet? Perhaps you shouldn't consider it. Here is one plan that you might follow. If you believe you are in a good state of health, there may be no reason to modify any of your food choices at all. If you are the self-experimenting type and/or are interested in illness prevention, you could try various combinations of the Tier One, Two, and Three food choices, knowing the relative toxin issues relating to each. If you are suffering from health issues, you might want to gravitate to the Tier One Wellness Diet, beginning as slowly as you wish, to see if you notice improvements.

If I follow the Wellness Diet, will my [insert symptom or illness] go away? The only way I know to answer this question would be to try the diet, along with the rest of The Wellness Project. Please remember that to achieve overall health, detox may be just as important as, or more important than diet. Because everyone's health history is different, I do not believe it is possible to predict the degree of success that can be achieved. The diet itself is the essence of simplicity and, while some of the detox protocols are a bit complicated, overall, participating in The Wellness Project is not rocket science!

What do you think of [insert name of supplement or treatment]? As a researcher, I am very open to reviewing what others are doing in the health field, and I have been doing so for decades. The Wellness Project is a distillation of this research, and contains what I currently believe to be the essentials for health. I am no longer a supplement junkie, and try to minimize using anything that was not available to PA. I fully intent to continue my research and to discuss any updated findings at www.projectforwellness.com . Because we have become accustomed to the take-a-pill-feel-better approach of big pharma, I have seen many people pick and choose among supplements in an effort to get a quick fix (I used to do it, too). The Wellness Project does not work that way, and piecemeal supplementation may provide unpredictable or no positive effects.

The Wellness Diet and all the supplements are expensive, so what should I do if I can't afford it? It is certainly true that organic grass-fed meat and organically grown fruit are more expensive than macaroni and cheese, and some of the supplements I suggest are pricey. Illness is also expensive, in terms of treatment, loss of work, and the impact on one's lifestyle. Each person must make a choice regarding the use of his or her financial resources. It would be great if, instead of subsidizing "health" care (it is really *illness* care), the government offered to subsidize illness prevention, but it is doubtful that we will see such a shift in our lifetime.

What do *you* eat on a typical day?  First, bear in mind that I eat the purist, Tier One, version of the diet, primarily because I feel better when I do, and I like to self-experiment.  Of course, I cheat occasionally, keeping my clay nearby.  I do not expect many others to follow Tier One as closely as I, unless they are motivated to do so by some health issues. For breakfast, I might have a baked organic-grass-fed free-range rib-eye steak with a half-grapefruit and some hot fruit tea made with mineral-rich water.  I use plenty of salt on the steak and grapefruit.  If I want a morning snack, it might be one or two lightly boiled high omega-3 egg yolks and a green apple, perhaps with some desiccated liver.   I drink a glass of mineral-rich water between meals.  For lunch, a baked ground-buffalo burger, salted, with a bowl of blueberries, and some hot water or fruit tea. If I want an afternoon snack, pemmican and a slice of melon are good choices.  I drink another glass of mineral-rich water between meals.  For dinner, I might have a couple of baked organic-grass-fed loin lamb chops, or perhaps baby-back pork ribs, salted, with some pineapple, and bone-stock soup.  I avoid eating after dinner, but drink more mineral-rich water.  All of the animal foods are cooked in glass dishes in a convection oven.   I take the food supplements mentioned in the diet section, including liver, glandulars, and red palm oil.  As a reminder, Appendix B is a chart summarizing the diet, including supplements.  Appendix C is a list of resources for obtaining the various foods and supplements used in the diet.

# Section Three - Detoxification

*We need a Bill of Rights against the poisoners of the human race.*
– Supreme Court Justice William O. Douglas

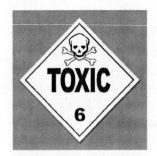 The purpose of this section is to discuss methods of getting the bad stuff out of the body, and it is with a great deal of frustration that I finally have written it. While this section is filled with some important clues from MA, it is also filled with a litany of technical blunders that have subjected many of us to needless toxins that read like a bad science fiction movie. The result is that, in many instances, the toxic load on our bodies has far surpassed what nature has evolved us to handle, and hence even her clues are not always adequate for the job.

At first blush, it might seem puzzling that there is not a major effort by modern medicine to research and develop detoxification products and protocols. If, as studies have shown, everyone on the planet, including polar bears, is loaded with toxins, from an economic point of view (if altruism isn't enough motivation) there would seem to be an enormous market, and hence profit potential, in this area. However, as an experienced lawyer, I have some insights into how exploiting this commercial opportunity within the health industry would have some serious financial drawbacks. Let's say a pharmaceutical company asked one of my fellow lawyers for a legal opinion on getting into the market of developing products to remove mercury from the body. Assuming the lawyer was astute, he might advise the company as follows. Since the company might make or have made certain drugs and various consumer products containing mercury (such as common vaccines), it could be setting itself up for one of the largest class action lawsuits of all time, as well as providing the general public with strong evidence of the company's culpability. In the field of tort law known as products liability, under certain circumstances, the doctrine of "subsequent repair" can be brought into the picture. This doctrine states that if a manufacturer of an allegedly defective product subsequently performs "repairs" in connection with the defect, this can be admissible evidence that indeed the product was defective.

There is a lot of tension regarding this doctrine because of its chilling effect on a company making repairs or coming up with remedies, which are usually in the best interests of the public, so sometimes this evidence is excluded. Because of the political clout of the pharmaceutical companies, I would not be surprised if they were able to successfully lobby for a special law excluding them from liability under this doctrine, and in fact they have been somewhat successful in doing so for the production of vaccines. From my perspective, the bottom line is that we are not likely to see any meaningful research in the field of detoxification in the near future, unless it is privately funded, and one of the goals of writing this book is to get like-mined individuals interested in pursuing such a worthy cause.

By adopting at least portions of the Wellness Diet and putting the good stuff in the body, one can take a giant step to stop ingesting natural toxins at every meal, thus relieving a burden on those portions of the defense system used by the body to detoxify. One reason detoxification is part of The Wellness Project is because, even if we eat the perfect diet, the accumulated toxic load of a lifetime can prevent us from assimilating nutrients, and also block and disrupt critical processes throughout our body, causing a great deal of illness. Fortunately, eating the proper diet enhances the entire detoxification process. Put another way, eating the wrong foods not only repeatedly toxifies us, but also interferes with our ability to get rid of both natural and human-made toxins already stored in our body.

As discussed in the first section, to go from cause to effect, we need to examine the nature of each cause in detail. In the case of The Wellness Project, both diet and detoxification are each necessary to achieve health, but neither is sufficient in itself. It takes both to reach the goal. A body loaded with toxins cannot achieve full benefit from the Wellness Diet, and such a person might find that supplements and even healthy foods act in a paradoxical fashion, either not achieving the desired result, or causing an opposing result.

What I will be concentrating on here is in understanding and finding ways to clear from the body a lifetime of toxins that one has accumulated from environmental sources and from the medical and dental communities. The term toxin as used in this section refers to any substance that causes illness, whether organic or inorganic, and whether originating from outside the body or from inside. I refer to detoxification (sometimes shortened to "detox") as a broad term covering the processes used to render toxins harmless. These processes can include removing the toxin from the body, destroying the toxin and removing the residue from the body, changing the structure of the toxin so it is no longer harmful, reducing the amount of toxin to a level no longer harmful, moving the toxin to an area of the body where it no longer causes harm, and binding or encapsulating the toxin in a manner that it is no longer harmful even if it remains in the body.

In this section, we are going to look at major categories of toxins, some of which have been with us since Ancient times and others that are of an origin that is more recent. We will then look at various detox strategies, beginning with natural ones and moving on to artificial ones developed to cope with modern toxicity issues. Had we not lost our operating instructions from MA, we would have known that detoxification should be an almost daily ritual, as it is in the animal kingdom, to avoid toxin buildup. For those readers interested in the myriad ways in which animals self-heal and detoxify, I highly suggest the book *Wild Health* by Cindy Engel [9].

Because most of us have lacked information on the subject of toxin removal, we are now faced with a toxic burden that has accumulated over the years, and is now distributed throughout our body. The result is that, in some cases, the processes of removal can be quite daunting. My plan is to visit the various categories of toxins we are likely to harbor, and discuss natural and synthetic methods for removing them. Following the discussion of physical detoxification protocols is a section on emotional detoxification. Therapeutic protocols are presented that have a record of accomplishment for clearing emotional toxicities, which in turn enhance physical detoxification.

First off, it is important for readers to understand some basics surrounding detoxification. Often, it can be a slow and somewhat frustrating process, which largely is a result of the accumulated toxic burden we are carrying. Reading the side box labeled Detox and The Die-off Reaction will give you a feel for some side effects that are most assuredly going to occur. Second, keep in mind that patience is not only a virtue, but is mandatory in detoxification. Many of the toxins we will be discussing involve metals with very long half-lives in the body, some in excess of 30 years (the time it takes for the body to remove one-half the burden if no intentional detoxification is used).

## Detox and the Die-off Reaction

A sustained detoxification program dislodges the body's entrenched toxins at variable and unpredictable speeds. Toxins are not only being eliminated from the system but also being redistributed as well. This movement from one place to another has the potential to trigger a variety of discomforting symptoms—different in different people with different levels of toxic burden—known as a "die-off reaction," or as a Herxheimer "herx" reaction. In some detox programs, living toxins are being killed, and during the process, they can release potent toxins, causing great discomfort. Discomfort could be slight, moderate, or extremely intense. Symptoms can mimic the original symptoms caused by the toxins, or present as a completely new set of symptoms. The classical ones are headaches, rashes, and pain.

There are support groups to help people through the process, and a few health professionals and spas specialize in detoxification. One tricky issue is to distinguish symptoms that are a result of the detox itself from those caused by an allergic or other reaction to the detoxifying agent.

From my own personal experience, I have found that slower is better in any kind of detoxification process, and one should certainly be prepared to feel worse at times, on the way to feeling better. There is no way to know total level of toxicity and how quickly the body can excrete these toxins, so trying to push the cleansing can wind up making one feel ill.

Couple this difficulty of removal with the body's limited capacity for safe rates of toxin excretion, and the timeline for some of the detox protocols can be very long. One informal estimate based on the collective experience of several who have detoxed is to take the number of years over which toxins may have been accumulating in your body, and divide by ten – the result could be the detoxification time needed to reduce the levels to those that no longer produce symptoms. Yes, we can be talking years – some lucky folks can achieve some success in months, but it is not possible to predict. Once the process is begun, many of the programs should continue for a lifetime to avoid a recurrence of buildup. Detoxification should become a normal part of one's life, because exposure to toxins surely is. As we go through this section, various detox supplements will be discussed, some natural, some not, and some require a prescription.

Now that I may have scared many of you, you might ask why do it at all? Well, it depends on your current state of health, and your future expectations. In my opinion, the ultimate level of health achievable by any person will be limited by their toxin load. Unfortunately, there are no completely reliable tests to determine the overall body burden of most toxins in the body, increasing the suspense. On the other side of the coin, people who have gone through detox programs have finally achieved relief from life-long symptoms that the conventional medical community has been unable to address.

How might you know if you have been exposed to any toxins (aside from food), and what are the symptoms? If you have ever been vaccinated (mercury, aluminum, viruses); have or have had in the past any amalgam fillings (mercury); had root canals or extractions (bacterial toxins); bathed, showered or drank city water (chlorine, fluorine); eaten bread (bromine); used a hot tub (chlorine, bromine); live with commercial carpeting (bromine, formaldehyde); eaten fish (mercury, PCBs); eaten at a restaurant (parasites); been alive when fuel contained lead (lead); taken antibiotics (Candida); played on a golf course or in a city park (pesticides); used a cell phone or lived under power lines (EMF); drank water from a plastic bottle (antimony, BPA); worked around products enclosed in plastics (bromine), worked in a building without natural circulation (mold); used artificial sweeteners (formaldehyde, chlorine); or taken prescription drugs (the drug itself), there is a good chance you are harboring some toxins. The list could have been much longer, but many toxins and their sources have not yet been defined. The symptom list could go on for pages, and is expanding daily. The problem here is establishing a cause-effect relationship when we know so little about how the toxins affect us. I will try to identify some of the major symptom clusters in the sections below. Note that Appendix B is a chart summarizing the detox protocols, some of which can become quite involved. Appendix C is a list of resources for obtaining the various supplements and other products used in detoxing.

Now, let's begin our journey into detoxification where, as a starting point, I have presumed that at least some portions of the Wellness Diet and food supplements are already in place so that the body has a head start in relieving the toxin burden. In this regard, perhaps certain days of the month can be devoted to detox and, on those days, the Wellness Diet is followed more closely. Appendix B includes some detox schedule suggestions.

The body removes wastes and toxins through several familiar pathways:

- the kidneys through urination

- the bowel through defecation

- the lungs through breathing

- the skin through sweating

In the case of acute poisoning, the mouth also becomes a pathway through regurgitation, and tears, nasal secretions, nails, and hair are also minor pathways, but we will concentrate on the big four listed above, as they play a major role for conditions of chronic toxicity.

# Chapter 15 - Natural Toxin Excretion Pathways

## Urination

Generating and passing urine through the kidneys is a major pathway for toxin excretion. In order for the system to work properly, sufficient liquids and a correct mineral balance are required. Water intake is easily under our control, and an amount that maintains a pale urine color is usually deemed sufficient. Unfortunately, some toxins can so mess with the body that one's urine is always pale, regardless of water intake. These toxins can also mess with our thirst sensors so that we no longer know when to drink. Yet other toxins can cause frequent and excessive urination by causing hormonal imbalances. In many cases, it may be necessary to endure some discomfort until detoxification provides relief. A general rule of thumb during detox is to drink one-half your body weight in ounces daily, which is useful as a starting point.

Excess water intake can be quite harmful, since it can cause dilution and excretion of essential minerals. Some fruits have a diuretic effect we have yet to understand, and that can be cleansing. Watermelon is an example of a beneficial diuretic fruit. Because it is not natural to drink when there is no thirst sensation, one must keep track of water consumed, and make a conscious effort to drink a sufficient amount. During detox, sufficient water is important to the process, and dehydration is common, due in part to mineral derangements. One approach is to drink a glass of water after each urination. Sipping commercial bottled water, especially RO water, from a plastic container as a detox strategy is self-defeating, because the toxins from the plastic may completely offset any gain from drinking the water, which means you will be continuously increasing your toxic load with every sip.

There is an old treatment that has been used somewhat successfully for generations where people intentionally drink (or even inject) their own urine to treat illnesses and allergies. Considering that urine is designed to carry waste products and toxins out of the body, I would caution against using these treatments in today's highly toxic environment, as it may well have the undesirable effect of reintroducing toxins into the body.

For some people, eating certain foods such as asparagus results in a very strong urine odor, not very desirable when it comes to avoiding predators. So, I regard this as yet another whisper of wisdom from MA to stop eating her leaves and stems as food. By the way, this may also be a sign of magnesium deficiency.

Lastly, it has been found that the pH of urine has an effect on the excretion of toxins by the kidneys, whereby an alkaline pH increases excretion of some heavy metals [189] and may have other benefits. As you will see, in several of my detox protocols urine alkalinity turns out to be an important element.

## Defecation

Generating and passing fecal matter through the colon is another major pathway for toxin excretion. In order for this system to work properly, you need the colon to work as designed, removing water and some minerals from the fecal mass, and consolidating it into stool. We do not fully understand how this works, but it definitely requires the cooperation of the large biomass of bacteria and fungi and possibly some other parasites in the colon to make it happen. In fact, the bulk of the stool is made up of gut bacteria. The muscle system controlling the gut must also be operating correctly to generate the peristaltic action necessary to move the digested food along in the gut. Some toxins can seriously mess with normal defecation. For this reason, my belief is that in the future we will discover that illnesses with names such as irritable bowel syndrome (IBS), irritable bowel disease (IBD), and Crohn's disease are all various manifestations of toxin disturbances of the gut.

For those readers who are squeamish, I am about to launch into a somewhat graphic description of bowel movements (BMs), and I hope you will not shy away from it. As in the case of any chemical factory like the human body, it is very important to analyze not only what you put into the body, but also what comes out of it. Paying attention to the condition of one's bowel is a simple way of detecting intestinal problems at an early stage, yet even mentioning such a subject is shunned as culturally and socially unacceptable. The goal of this analysis is to try to determine what comprises the perfect bowel movement, in terms of frequency, consistency, odor, and color. Sort of like a Wellness BM! If we can do that, then for those who have a disturbed gut, we can use *stool as a tool* to measure our detoxification progress.

It is rather amazing how little research has been done in the area of defecation, considering its importance as a diagnostic tool. There is a funny analogy here. Much like asking ten nutritionists what to eat and getting ten different answers, if you ask a group of gastroenterologists to describe a healthy bowel movement, you are also likely to get little agreement. Just the simple question of how often one should have a movement elicits widely varying answers, with the so-called normal range being from once a week to several times a day. There is no doubt that what you eat, as well as your toxin load, can have a major effect on your bowel movement frequency. We don't know exactly how many bowel movements PA experienced on the Wellness Diet, and most modern indigenous groups do not follow that diet, but we can take a look at the animal community for some clues. Chimps are known to have multiple movements each day, but their diet is loaded with fibrous foods we could not possibly digest, and they spend most of their time eating.

When on a natural diet, cats, which are obligate carnivores, have one movement per meal, and dogs, which are mostly carnivores, when on a natural diet also have one movement per meal. From my experience, one BM for every meal is ideal, with a minimum of once per day. I would view more than once per meal or less than one per day as potentially a gastric abnormality. On the other hand, bowel movements of normal frequency are no guarantee of bowel normalcy.

What should "normal" stool look like? Would you believe that it took the medical community until *1990* before someone first addressed this question in a formal matter? In that year, some enterprising researchers at the University of Bristol in the United Kingdom came up with what is now referred to as the Bristol Stool Form Scale to categorize various stool forms. They devised a seven-point scale in which stools were scored according to cohesion and surface cracking as follows: 1, separate hard lumps like nuts; 2, sausage shaped but lumpy; 3, like a sausage or snake but with cracks on its surface; 4, like a sausage or snake, smooth and soft; 5, soft blobs with clear cut edges; 6, fluffy pieces with ragged edges, a mushy stool; and 7, watery, no solid pieces. Some of the tests they performed were on patients with irritable bowel syndrome, where they were able to inverse correlate the stool scale number with actual whole gut transit time, where the lower the number the longer the transit time [190]. This data is difficult to interpret because of the varied diets of the participants, none of which match the Wellness Diet. Further studies have inverse related gut transit time with dietary fiber, which on the Wellness Diet is controlled by fruit consumption.

Ah, but we do have more clues from MA. There is no toilet paper in the animal kingdom! Yes, chimps have been known to use leaves for occasional anal wiping (usually a sign of toxicity), and some species are famous for doing that for each other. However, by and large, there is no need for anal wiping because the form and consistency of their stool is such that there is no significant residue. Enter toilet paper.

Apparently, toilet paper was used in China as early as 900 A.D., but that's like a minute ago on the human timeline. Even more recently, in step with the nineteenth century advent of the toilet, flat sheet paper, and then roll paper, came of age. Before that, people used newsprint or mail order catalogues, and before that they used their hand (left or right depending on culture), and some still do. This to me serves as a clue as to how our stool should shape up. We should not need toilet paper, which is probably one of the first things we would grab in case of an evacuation. The fact that we need toilet paper to wipe away residue is testimony to our dietary detour and the resultant ill health of our gut. Referring back to the Bristol Scale, categories 1-4 qualify for leaving no or minimal residue. Category 1, however, is clearly a case of constipation and is usually accompanied with straining, eventually leading to hemorrhoids, hardly part of MA's plan.

So, from my analysis, a normal stool should be sausage shaped, varying from a rough to a smooth exterior, eliminated without straining and occurring at least once a day. As you may remember, toilet paper was on my list of Faulty Human Trials in Table 1. It seems to me that the mere fact that it is in such widespread use is clear evidence that our bowel movements are unnatural. Further, the use of toilet paper has conditioned us to accept this state of affairs, and to pay little or no attention to what is in the toilet bowl, allowing gut problems to go unnoticed for years, if not a lifetime.

Next on the stool list is the age-old question of floaters versus sinkers. As discussed earlier in the section on bile salts, floating stools can be a sign of excessive fat content, symptoms of maldigestion that may be related to the gall bladder. A second reason for floating stools is excessive trapped gas, also a sign of maldigestion. So, the winners are the sinkers.

Moving on to color, the foods we eat can have a dramatic effect on stool color. In the Wellness Diet, the types of fruits eaten may affect stool color, particularly those with high carotenoid (orange) content. Typically, stool color is a dark brown. Green or yellow (bile color) may indicate excessive bile in the stool, usually from very fast transit time, not allowing for bile recycling in the small intestine. Normally, only about 5% of the circulating bile is excreted. Pale stool color, such as grey or whitish, may well be a sign of insufficient bile, and the use of bile salt supplements might be a good idea. If you find during detoxification that your stool tends toward numbers 5-7 on the Bristol scale, your colon may not be removing and recycling sufficient water, leading toward dehydration. One idea is to drink a large glass of water after every bowel movement.

Finally, strong stool odor is a sure sign of maldigestion, whereby undigested food is being excreted, and strong odors would not have been amenable to survival in PA's environment. Rodale found that taking dolomite could reduce stool odor, indicating that it has a strong effect on normalizing digestion [62]. This completes the description of stool, and here is a concise summary: the goal is soft, sinking, sienna, stinkless sausages. Now, onward to clues from MA on how to defecate.

From studies of indigenous societies and animals, we know that the natural way to defecate is to squat—not to sit—and in much of the undeveloped world, squatting is still very much the norm. It was less than 150 years ago, in the latter part of the nineteenth century that the toilet arrived on the scene and slowly changed the style of how most of us learned to defecate. What has the toilet revolution wrought? Some studies show that the colon actually lines up more effectively in a squatting position, and that, in theory, you get a more relaxed and thorough bowel movement. The long-term benefits may include less stress and strain on the intestinal and urinary tracts, more complete elimination, and other benefits yet to be determined. Some keen-eyed medical observers over the years have noted that many different bowel, bladder, and pelvic conditions, previously rare or unknown, suddenly became commonplace in the Western world in the last half of the nineteenth century. Their observations suggest that by returning to squatting, as MA intended, we may eliminate problems such as hemorrhoids.

If you are interested in experimenting with the concept of squatting to line up your colon naturally, the least expensive method is to elevate your feet, say, about eight to ten inches from the floor using books or bricks, while sitting on the toilet. A more elegant solution is to purchase one of the many devices for this purpose, which I affectionately call "stool stools" [191]. These devices put you in a squatting position as you lean forward, and it doesn't take long before you feel very comfortable and natural with it, so much so that when you're traveling and you don't have it, you feel like something's wrong. This issue may seem somewhat humorous because we have all grown up on the toilet, so to speak. However, it's really just another example of how we have deviated from what MA intended with unknown consequences simply because of our arrogance in thinking we know what we're doing. Children are potty trained, but it may well be that adults need to be potty retrained.

It has been my experience that deviations from the ideal in the realm of defecation result from diet and detox issues, and a goal of The Wellness Project is to restore order to the gut. This accomplishes two purposes: first, it will improve nutrient absorption, and second, it will maximize the use of the defecation pathway for toxin removal. The dirt components of the diet, such as spore-forming bacteria, can be instrumental in restoring bowel movements to normal by providing the right mix of bowel flora.

I want to make it clear that I am not saying everyone has to meet The Wellness Project BM criteria to be healthy. I have no doubt that there are people out there who can have two messy BMs per month and lead a very long and healthy life. Probably these same folks can thrive on cake and soda, and are the *winners* for the moment. I doubt they are reading this book.

## Breathing

Breathing gets rid of toxic chemicals through gas exchange in our lungs, where we take in oxygen and expel gaseous wastes. While we can promote that process with breathing techniques that can be learned as part of some yoga and meditation practices, there are additional ways to enhance this detox pathway. Deep breathing requires unrestricted movement of the belly, ribcage, and diaphragm. Enter tight clothing.

I'm not going to suggest you walk around with a loincloth but there are some lessons to be learned from Flintstone® fashions. One would assume that hunter-gatherers figured out how to clothe themselves using the skins of animals. Whatever they wore would have been minimal and it would have been loose, whereas today (except for baggy-panted juveniles) we tend toward the tight in order to show off buns, boobs, and biceps.

What's the difference between loose and tight? Studies have shown that tight clothing does affect both the anatomy and physiology in ways that may be detrimental to health. One example is brassieres.

Indigenous women did not wear them, but throughout recent history, women have used a variety of garments and devices to cover, restrain, or elevate their breasts. From the sixteenth century onwards, the corset hoisted the breasts of wealthier women. Then, in the latter part of the nineteenth century, clothing designers began experimenting with alternatives that by the early twentieth century had morphed into what we now recognize as contemporary bras and a multi-billion-dollar industry. The emphasis has pretty much shifted from functionality to fashion, with an underlying assumption throughout this evolutionary process that no harm is being done.

However, at least one set of studies I am aware of has investigated the possibility that brassieres may contribute to the incidence of breast cancer. These studies were featured in a widely publicized 1995 book entitled *Dressed to Kill* [192]. The authors collected striking evidence directly correlating the number of hours per day a woman wears a bra with the risk of breast cancer. Women who wear tight-fitting bras 24 hours a day are 125 times more likely to have breast cancer than women who do not wear bras at all. One theory behind this correlation is that bras may be constricting the flow of lymph from the breast area, and restricting the flow of lymph into the axillary lymph nodes under each arm. As I mentioned earlier, the lymph system is poorly understood, but it is a major system within the body for transporting toxins and getting them into the blood stream for evacuation. To the extent that process is interfered with, it may contribute to toxin accumulation in the breast. See the side box entitled HealthBra™ for a short description of my efforts in this area.

For those female readers wanting to experiment, not wearing brassieres is clearly what MA intended. Other than that, it would seem prudent to wear them as loose as possible, for the shortest time possible, and as unstructured as possible (perhaps without an underwire, which usually can be removed with a scissor). If you can see indentions in your skin upon removal, this may be a clue that your bra is indeed causing restriction of some sort, such as lymph or blood flow or the ability to take full deep breaths, none of which is a good idea. Some companies have produced bras designed to include lymph massage as a feature [193].

As tight bras are to women, tight briefs may be to men. Researchers have found that they hold a man's testicles close to the body and raise the temperature of the sperm. This decreases its lifespan and could affect fertility. In some problem infertility cases, men have been asked to switch to loose-fitting boxers. Guys, take this as a clue from MA – loosen up. Is there a difference between wearing a belt or suspenders? It seems logical that constricting the abdomen with a tight belt for many hours a day could adversely affect abdominal blood flow and the digestive system, as well as the ability to take deep breaths. Avoiding tight belts and pants are among the lifestyle changes suggested by some doctors to overweight patients with heartburn issues.

---

# HealthBra™

A disturbing incidence of breast cancer in prior generations in my family inspired me to suggest to my wife and daughters that they abandon their brassieres. The suggestion was not well received, so I set out to design bras that would minimize the restriction of lymph flow. I eventually created a variety of designs with the help of some product designers, and patented them (US Patents Nos. 6,086,450 and 6,361,397). In my conversations with the authors of *Dressed to Kill*, they predicted there would be little interest from the undergarment industry to produce products of this kind, and the authors themselves had been threatened with a lawsuit when they were about to publish their book. In the introduction to this section, I mentioned the "subsequent repair" legal doctrine. One could imagine the difficulty of a brassiere manufacturer producing a bra that is designed to overcome what might be negative health effects of their previous designs. I remain optimistic that this area will ultimately get the attention it deserves.

---

Bad breath may be another sign from MA that you are excreting bad stuff through your lungs. Faulty diet, and/or toxins from bad dentition and gum problems, or from gut backup or throat infections, can all cause it. Below, I will discuss the use of clay to absorb a lot of this junk during the detox process, and the use of spore-formers to get rid of putrid gut bacteria. The breath should be sweet day and night in a healthy body.

## Sweating

Sweating has proven to be a major detoxification pathway for a variety of reasons. First, the large surface area of the skin enables significant amounts of sweat to push or carry toxins to the surface along short, direct pathways from virtually any part of the body. Second, unlike urination and defecation, we have some control over when and how much we sweat, leading to a detoxification program that can be scheduled. Third, it bypasses the digestive system, which in many cases is not functioning properly because of the toxic load. That is not to say, however, that toxins do not interfere with the ability to sweat, which I can attest to personally. As an example, magnesium deficiency, caused by many toxins, can suppress normal sweating.

The easiest way to promote sweating is to heat the body. One way is through the natural fever we develop when ill, which is certainly a clue from MA and should never be suppressed unless necessary to prevent brain damage. A more pleasant way to sweat naturally (at least for some) is through exercise, and in fact, I consider sweating as a major health benefit of exercise. Yet another way is artificially to heat the body with an external source, such as a sauna. I will be going into this topic in some depth in the next section, as external heat is an extremely important detoxification tool.

This brings me to the subject of antiperspirants. Using antiperspirants is really fooling with MA on several counts. First, it is suppressing the very mechanism we so heavily depend upon to excrete toxins. There are large sweat and lymph glands under the arms—major detoxification pathways and outlets near the heart and lungs critical to keeping the body clean. Antiperspirants interfere with their natural function. Second, the chemicals used to create these products are themselves toxic and usually include aluminum and possibly zirconium. Applying aluminum under the arms (and with women, it's often freshly shaved underarms) is really not a good idea since it can be absorbed in large amounts, further toxifying the body. Aluminum is believed to be a neurotoxin and has been implicated as a possible cause in Alzheimer's disease, so daily use of an antiperspirant could contribute to a dreaded disease [194]. To absorb sweat, consider pads of some sort. I will also discuss below the use of clay and magnesium as other alternatives.

Regarding deodorants, if you have extreme body odor, that is likely an indication of improper diet and/or significant toxins. Remember that a strong body odor is not conducive to survival in the wild, as it attracts predators, another clue from MA. Because sweating is a natural detoxification pathway, food odors passed through the skin may well be a sign that you are eating the wrong stuff. We can all remember being around others reeking of garlic and onions (plant bulbs not on the Wellness Diet), and this may actually be a smelly clue from MA to leave her bulbs alone. So, if you smell like dinner, you probably ate the wrong food, and your body is trying to get rid of it. Many in the medical field dismiss body odor as simply a normal bacterial decay process, but they have nothing with which to compare it. The word *normal* has no real meaning unless you can compare it to some *baseline*, which is, of course, a major Wellness Project goal.

Having said all that about odors, I feel compelled to tell you about a natural body deodorizer – magnesium! Buried in the archives of early magnesium research are some fascinating experiments and observations showing that taking sufficient magnesium supplementation (actually, dolomite was used in the studies) completely eliminated underarm, body, urine, stool, and foot odor [62]. I am not aware of any studies to determine why magnesium acts in this manner, but it surely points to a detox effect of some sort. As readers know by now, I am not shy about speculating, so here is something to ponder. Many of us have heard the expression "the smell of fear," which is loosely defined as an odor emanating from an animal or person in a highly fearful situation. Well, magnesium is quickly excreted when we are under stress, so could the origin of this expression be the depletion of magnesium (resulting in body odor) as a result of extreme stress (fear)?

# Chapter 16 - Natural Detoxification Agents

This section is a discussion of some of the more important detoxifying agents that would have been easily accessible to PA, with the exception of a sauna, which is a modern day substitute for PA running around in the tropical sun with few clothes on.

## Sauna

Sauna is a Finnish word for a small room or house in which one can experience dry or wet heat sessions. Indigenous tribes have used sweat lodges for a very long time as a ritual means of cleansing through sweating. The wet sauna uses various methods to produce steam, resulting in a humid environment with air temperatures in the range of 175-200 degrees F. Unless purified water is used to produce the steam, it is possible to inhale and absorb toxins such as chlorine or fluoride, much like the shower situation, and fungus growth is another possible issue. The closest analogy I can think of to a wet sauna in nature would be hot mineral springs, which can be quite healing.

The modern dry sauna is called the FIR (far infrared) sauna, and is one of my favorite detoxification tools. It is well known that the human body radiates infrared (IR) energy at a wavelength of about 10 microns, well within the warming portion of the spectrum of sunlight. The idea behind FIR sauna is to generate IR energy in a range of wavelengths near this value in a sauna environment. There is much anecdotal information on the detoxification benefits of FIR vs. wet sauna, mixed in with a lot of marketing hype. I and others with whom I have consulted have found saunas to be of great benefit in promoting the excretion of a variety of toxins, from heavy metals to pesticides to prescription and recreational drugs. Some excellent books on the subject are *Sauna Therapy* by Lawrence Wilson, and *The Holistic Handbook of Sauna Therapy* by Nenah Sylver [195] [196]. How do we know it works? Well, personally, I can see it in my skin, which for most of my life has been my visual indicator of toxicity. My observations, in conjunction with the pioneering work of Paul Dantzig into the cutaneous signs of mercury poisoning, provided me with a handy way of evaluating progress in my own mercury detoxification program, and I could track it as a function of sauna use [19, 197-200] [201]. I also feel better than usual when I use the sauna regularly. Since the mantra of the dermatology community is "name it, we tame it," I will take this opportunity to hereby name the constellation of undiagnosed skin manifestations due to mercury toxicity as *Mercuroderma*!

Although quite controversial because of its ties to a religious organization, the Narconon program of drug rehabilitation has apparently been successful in using sauna treatment to sweat out drugs. More recently, a similar program was used to treat New York City firefighters exposed to a wide range of toxins in the 9/11 debacle, with reported successes. There are anecdotal stories of past drug users reliving "highs" during sessions, and still others report seeing and smelling various substances in their sweat that they remember taking decades ago. The bottom line for me is that I intend to use my sauna regularly for life in an effort to keep up with the unavoidable toxic load in today's world. With some caveats, the concept seems to fit well within the natural experience of being exposed to the warming rays of sunlight, and it actually feels that way. Unlike the wet variety, the FIR sauna has a lower air temperature, in the 90-120 degree F range, so it is much more comfortable, and the lack of use of water eliminates problems such as chlorine and fungal contamination.

It is helpful to put the FIR sauna experience in perspective with respect to nature. The FIR frequency spectrum is within that of normal sunlight, and the air temperatures are within the range one might find in the summer in some desert resorts such as Palm Springs and Scottsdale, or tropical locales. Actually, if you live in or have access to these locations, you could start a detox program simply by sitting outside wearing minimal clothing in an area receiving sunlight energy, directly or indirectly. If not, here are some suggestions in purchasing an FIR sauna.

There are many FIR sauna manufacturers, some reputable and some not. My preference is one built of wood, using a species (at least on the inside) such as poplar or alder that has minimal outgassing of volatile compounds. Many on the market have an interior made of cedar, which outgases terpines that may be irritating to some people. The sauna should have a large complement of ceramic FIR emitters, and a temperature control. One brand that has a good reputation is Thermal Life made by High Tech Health [202].

Less expensive models, called cabinets, wrap around the body, leaving the head exposed, and for some people, this is more comfortable.

It may also have an advantage if there are medical or dental problems requiring avoidance of heating the head (the issue of dental amalgams is discussed in a later section). One concern I have about some of the cabinets is their use of plastic for the enclosure, since the elevated temperatures of the unit may well cause these plastics to outgas toxins that are absorbed or inhaled by the user. For another option, you can inexpensively build your own sauna in an area as small as a closet, as described in the Wilson book cited above [195]. Here are some sauna protocols.

Sauna therapy, like any other form of detoxification, can cause a die-off reaction as described above, and may be harmful to those with specific medical conditions or implants. For this reason, begin by using the sauna in a very slow, low dose manner. There is actually some controversy as to the harmful effects of sauna, and there are rare reports of cases of toxic individuals who seem to get worse, but this is no different from possible responses to most of the other detox protocols. I encourage anyone with a serious medical condition or taking a lot of medications who would like to begin sauna therapy to read Larry Wilson's book on the subject, and perhaps consult with him [203] or others with experience in the field. Two that come to mind are Dr. Dietrich Klinghardt [204], and Dr. Hans Gruenn [205], both of whom use sauna therapy in their detox practices. In any event, at the beginning, it might be prudent to have a buddy along to monitor you during sessions.

I would also suggest reading the section below on alkalinity, since I believe it can enhance all detox protocols, including sauna. Finally and most important, note that body stores of magnesium (and other minerals) are depleted as a result of elevated body temperature and sweating. Therefore, I encourage sauna beginners to first test their magnesium levels and begin a supplement program if needed. Interestingly, there is some anecdotal evidence that magnesium supports sweating, so perhaps an inability to sweat is a marker for magnesium deficiency.

Along my journey in the world of sauna therapy, I was fortunate to have Dr. Wilson as a coach to coax me along as I got started. Knowing I was mercury toxic, with the usual attendant hypo-metabolic issues, including the inability to sweat very much, I began very cautiously, and I would encourage others to do the same. I used the low temperature setting (about 90 degrees F), and started with only a five-minute session time once every other day. After a month, I went to daily sessions and began to notice an increase in sweating (I was also supplementing with magnesium). I slowly raised the temperature and increased the session time to 20 minutes, and now (several years later) I enjoy the 120 degree F setting and sweat quite profusely. It is important to replenish water and minerals (particularly magnesium and potassium) after each session, using the protocols described above. Doing so insufficiently is very likely to be quite unpleasant, particularly if you experience muscle cramping. After each session, I suggest quickly showering in warm water to wash off the toxins, and not reusing (or sharing) towels until they have been washed.

While we are on the topic of washing clothes, how about a soap derived from fruit? The fruit from the Chinese Soapberry tree (Sapindus Mukorossi), referred to as a soap nut, is not a sweet fruit that would qualify for the Wellness Diet, but it is very high in saponins, a natural detergent, and makes a soap for washing clothing and other items. It is supplied in its natural nut form [43], in powder form [206], and as a liquid [207]. It is hypoallergenic and biodegradable, with many uses.

In an FIR sauna, you are surrounded by electrical wiring, which can subject the body to a substantial electrical field. This can easily be measured using a digital AC millivoltmeter connected between an electrical ground terminal and your body. I have measured voltages as high as 8 volts AC on my body in the sauna, and although I do not know what effect this may have on the detox process, this electrical field induced charge is quite easy and inexpensive to eliminate. In the section below entitled the EMF (Electromagnetic Field) Problem I go into some depth regarding the potential advantages of keeping our bodies in electrical contact with the earth. It is there that I will show examples of how to do so, even in the sauna. Because I have adopted sauna therapy as a part of my lifestyle, I built my house to include a room devoted to detoxification, including the sauna, a system for connecting myself to earth ground, a connection to the house music system, and both a filtered mineral water spout and shower just outside the sauna. I feel it is important to make taking a sauna a fun experience that you can look forward to, either alone or with others.

Before leaving the sauna discussion, I want to mention some products that are also based on the use of FIR energy, and that have proved quite useful in treating chronic detox symptoms and pain in general. They are FIR heating pads that can be used locally to deliver FIR energy to specific parts of the body. The purpose of these devices is not to cause sweating, but to create healing effects which result either through the heat itself or the particular wavelength, or from reasons we have yet to discover. The brand I use is *Thermotex*, and the pads come in a variety of sizes [208]. Their successful use with horses and other animals prompted my wife and me to acquire one designed as a pet bed, and our cats love it. My personal theory is that, for indoor pets, it recreates the natural experience of lying on warm earth heated by sunlight. If you use an FIR pad, I have found it helpful to be aware of the possibility of referred pain while detoxing, where your neck pain may be due, for example, to toxins accumulating in the gut. So, experiment with the pad to see what areas of the body work best. It may be that using the pad on the abdomen will alleviate neck pain. In other words, do not assume that the origin of the pain is the part that is hurting.

## Alkalinity

Those readers familiar with detoxification may be puzzled by the inclusion of alkalinity as a detox protocol, but from my research, it is an important factor, without which many conventional detox protocols will not work, or will work poorly. As many of you know, acidity and alkalinity are conveniently measured using a pH scale, where values from 0-7 are considered acidic, and from 7-14 are considered alkaline (the value 7 is considered neutral).

My research on this subject actually took shape when investigating how heavy metals such as mercury, lead, and cadmium are dealt with by MA in the outside world. The results were somewhat astonishing, and had to do with dirt and pH. It is well known that humic and fulvic acids in the soil can act as heavy metal scavengers, adsorbing and transporting them. Adsorption occurs when a substance, such as a heavy metal, forms one or more of several types of bonds with the surface of an adsorbing material such as the soil acid matrix. This is as opposed to absorption, where two substances diffuse into each other to form a solution.

It is also known that the soil acids have the capability of desorbing the metals, or dropping them from the fulvic/humic acid matrix [209]. Much research has been performed on these issues, because heavy metal sequestration is an important issue in toxic site remediation [210]. Several factors enter into the desorption phenomenon, but the one that caught my attention was that an increase in pH vastly increased the strength of attachment between the soil acid matrix and the metals. Conversely, at low (acidic) pH values, the soil acid matrix lets go of the metals. The same scenario takes place when clay, fulvic/humic acids, and heavy metals were mixed together [210].

The reason that pH caught my eye is that it had come to my attention before in my research into spore-forming bacteria. Remarkably, spore-formers also have the ability to bond with heavy metals via adsorption, and they too can release the metals under certain conditions, including low pH (an acidic environment) [211] [212] [213]. So, now we have three elements of soil that I consider important to health (humic/fulvic acids, spore-forming bacteria, and clay), all capable of binding with heavy (and other) metals, where the pH of the mix is a determinant as to the strength of the soil-metal bond, and hence whether the soil will hold onto the metals or release them. This adsorption/desorption characteristic is actually used by environmental scientists for toxic cleanup. For example, soil bacteria, also called biomass, can be used to grab toxic metals at a high pH level, and then made to let go of them at an appropriate reclamation site by lowering the pH. Thus, the metals get to be recycled into industry, and the biomass can be reused again for toxic cleanup by re-alkalization.

You may ask what all of this has to do with human detoxification. I am conducting a personal detoxification study, which I call the Dirt Detox protocol™, detailed more thoroughly in the next section on dirt, in which the pH of urine plays a critical role. For this section, I will concentrate on ways in which one can measure and adjust urine pH. There are no end of books and supplements devoted to body alkaline/acid balance, many of which seem to contradict each other, but there is general agreement among authors that diet has an impact, with fruits and some vegetables (not seeds) having an alkalizing effect. In the Wellness Diet, fruit, mineral water, and dolomite act as natural alkaline balancers.

During detoxification of heavy metals, particularly in the case of mercury detox, I and others have found it difficult to keep urine pH in balance (it tends to be too acid) without some supplement help. This is important because it has been shown that alkaline urine promotes the excretion of mercury [189]. The first step is to get some pH paper to measure your urine. I use pHydrion brand pH sticks with a pH range of 5.0 to 9.0, or their pH paper in roll form with a range of 5.5 to 8.0 [214]. The objective is to measure urine pH a few times per day, with the goal of keeping it neutral or higher, say between 7 and 8.

In addition to the natural alkalizing agents of fruit, mineral water, and dolomite (calcium and magnesium carbonates), there are two supplement categories that have been used to alkalize urine pH. The first are mineral citrates such as potassium citrate, which may be taken with or without meals. I experiment with the dose until I find the minimum that keeps urine pH above 7 for most of the day when detoxifying heavy metals [215] [216]. Those taking drugs or those who have kidney issues need to monitor potassium levels (preferably red blood cell levels) while taking potassium supplements.

Another alkalizing approach is to use bicarbonates such as potassium and/or sodium bicarbonate (baking soda). There are many alkalizing bicarbonates on the market, and they should not be taken with meals because they tend to neutralize stomach acid, interfering with proper digestion. My preference is to use additional mineral citrates to achieve daytime alkaline urine when detoxing heavy metals. Alka-Seltzer® Gold is one example of a commercial product that provides sodium and potassium citrates. On the days when not detoxing heavy metals, I do not take supplements to alkalize urine, and let my body establish its own acid/alkaline balance. The subject of alkalinity will be further discussed in the experimental Dirt Detox Protocol™ below.

# Dirt

In this section, I am going to revisit the four soil components discussed above in the diet section, with an emphasis on their use in various detox procedures, culminating in the Dirt Detox Protocol that I have developed, which can play a role in some detox procedures.

## Clay

Would you walk miles through the jungle to get to a particular type of dirt that you then proceed to eat in great quantity? Well, many animals (including humans) do so, for reasons that are still unfolding. The dirt types they are seeking are generally referred to as clays, one of MA's secret weapons in the game of survival and, remarkably, one that takes us full circle in the quest for a toxin-free diet. It is not fully understood how clay-eating interacts with animals, but several theories have been put forward. The six explanations most discussed among zoologists, anthropologists, and doctors are to assuage hunger, to provide grit for grinding food in the stomach, to buffer stomach contents, to cure diarrhea, to serve as a mineral supplement, and to adsorb toxins [217].

We are going to discuss the last explanation first – toxin adsorption. As you recall from our diet discussion regarding excluded plant foods, the main reason for avoiding them was the load of natural toxins they contain. While we in the Western world are fortunate that we have available to us year round the animal and fruit products used in the Wellness Diet, our Paleo ancestors were not so fortunate. It is easy to image how, for a variety of environmental reasons, a shortage in animal food periodically could have occurred in the Paleo era. In such a case, PA might have had to resort to plant sources of protein such as seeds, tubers, and roots, along with their attendant toxins, as a survival strategy. Enter clay.

Humans ate clay to protect themselves against these plant toxins. For example, modernly, some South American Indians regularly dine on bitter, toxic wild potatoes containing a nasty alkaloid that by itself would cause stomach pains and vomiting. However, the Indians have learned to make the potatoes safe and palatable by eating them with an alkaloid-binding clay. California Indians and natives of Sardinia used to make a bread from nutritious acorns whose sole drawback was that they contained bitter, astringent, and toxic tannic acid. Both the Indians and the Sardinians mixed the acorn flour with a clay that reduced tannic acid by up to 77 percent. These peoples did not understand alkaloid chemistry or adsorption, but they did discover empirically that eating clay made these foods edible and thus avoided starvation. Wild animals and birds worldwide do the same thing, and are able to consume plants with potent toxins such as strychnine [6]. I am certainly not advocating eating non-Wellness Diet foods on a *regular* basis, relying on clay to clean up the toxins. Not enough is known about the types and amounts of clay to be used for a given toxic food. Further, whenever available, animals eat their native foods and only deviate when necessary. I intend to follow that example.

Returning to some of the other explanations for eating clay, some clays are believed to act as mineral supplements as well as immune system boosters in ways we do not fully understand. Pregnant and lactating women in indigenous regions are known to crave soil, consuming more than an ounce per day. Clay in the form of kaolin was used for many years in the preparation Kaopectate® to ameliorate diarrhea, and supposedly was removed from the product because of some form of contamination. We will cover the clay contamination issue below. Regarding assuaging hunger, the Ottomac Indians of South America made soil balls six inches in diameter and ate more than one pound per day during the flood season when it was difficult to find food, and clay eating has also been reported in Western Europe during famines. In this detox section, we are going to make use of several of these clay characteristics. Unfortunately, as in many of the other fields we have traversed, little research has been done in the area of clay as it relates to human health (there is no money in it), while there are a wealth of studies on its use in water treatment and other toxic abatement applications.

Beginning with the adsorption of toxins, anecdotal evidence abounds in the curative properties of clay with respect to toxin removal [218] [219] [220, 221] [222], and a website dedicated to the healing applications of clay, created by Jason Eaton, has a wealth of information on the subject [223]. Because the Wellness Diet removes virtually all natural toxins, this enables clay to be used as necessary in detox protocols to remove modern toxins such as heavy metals, pesticides, parasites, and bacteria. Here are a few caveats. Since we don't know for sure what is adsorbed and what is not, it is prudent to make sure we take clay an hour or more before or after taking food or detox supplements or medications.

Second, it is imperative that the clay material we start with is clean (devoid of toxins), to prevent unintentionally toxifying ourselves with "dirty clay." Regarding toxins in clay, they naturally contain aluminum hydroxide and iron, but eons of use have demonstrated that neither produces an excess of aluminum or iron in the body. Third, clay only works if it is hydrated, that is, mixed with water. So taking clay if you are dehydrated is unproductive and could be dangerous by allowing the formation of a blockage in the gut. Clay should always be taken with water, or dissolved in saliva before swallowing.

Here are my suggestions for ingesting clay as a detox agent. I plan to use clay as part of a lifetime detoxification regimen on the basis that we are continuously exposed to environmental toxins. The widespread use of clay for millennia in the animal world is a good enough "clinical trial" for me. I have used and evaluated three U.S. sources of clay. Two are considered to be calcium-bentonite types (also referred to as Montmorillonite), and the third is a sodium-bentonite type. These three are all from the smectite family of clays that have been found overall to have the most favorable healing characteristics. There are hundreds of other types from various parts of the world, all with their unique following. The first source is called Pascalite clay [224], and is available as a powder or in capsules for ingestion. The second source is called Terramin [188], and is available as powder and tablets for ingestion. The third, Redmond clay, which is the sodium-bentonite clay, is only available in powder form [225]. All of the companies referenced have an excellent reputation and have been supplying clean clay for many years. As far as which brand is best for you personally to use, I know of no other way to determine this except by experiment.

How you ingest the clay depends on several factors, the first of which is whether you like the taste of clay (I do). If you do not, the choices are to take it as capsules or tablets. For a short term detox dosing schedule of five days every two weeks, I take two capsules or tablets or a half-teaspoon of the powder upon arising and at bedtime. I am sure to drink at least 8 ounces of water with them. As reported in the literature, you may see a wide range of symptom relief from eating clay, including digestive, skin, pain, and mental clarity areas, all pointing to a reduction in toxic load.

Some people are distressed by the prospect of eating clay, and for them we have the art of pelotherapy, the topical use of dirt, covering everything from mudpacks to medical poultices to clay baths. Both Pascalite and Terramin brands also sell topical preparations for use in various applications, some pre-prepared. The references cited above will provide a lot of information on the topical use of clays, some of which seem to border on the miraculous, including curing somewhat incurable skin ulcers and flesh eating infections [223].

Among the various topical uses of clay, for general detoxification I prefer clay baths which, while somewhat messy, are well worth the effort. Large amounts of clay are needed for baths, and the clay I use is designated as Microfine Volclay HPM-20 by American Colloid Company [226]. It is a fine-mesh high purity sodium bentonite clay which I purchase in 50 pound bags from Laguna Clay, a nationwide distributor [227]. To prepare the bath, while it is filling, hand distribute the clay on the surface almost as if you were sowing seeds, to avoid clumping as much as possible (some of which will happen anyhow). The more clay the better from a detox point of view, and the typical range is from 2 to 20 pounds at one time. The bath setting I use is a water temperature around 100 degrees F, and I stay in it for 20-30 minutes. The wet clay becomes very slippery, so care is required getting in and out of the tub. Draining the bathwater is straightforward, and only minimal cleanup is required. Municipal sewer systems apparently have no problem with the hydrated clay, but there is some concern that septic systems may eventually become clogged. I again refer you to Jason Eaton's site for some of the healing effects of clay baths, including Jason's personal story [223]. The frequency of clay bathing is a personal choice ranging from once per month to several times a week.

While I have mentioned the adsorption characteristics of clay with respect to natural toxins in potential sources of foods, I do not believe it is of much benefit when it comes to eating foods that we are intolerant of because of their particular protein content. Examples have already been discussed, such as casein and whey in dairy products, gluten in some grains, etc. In general, those foods should be avoided, but when that is not possible, as discussed above, gelatin can be employed to encapsulate and assist in the digestion of these proteins, providing some short-term relief.

## Humic/Fulvic Acids

In the diet section, I discussed dirt as an ingredient of PA's diet, and in particular, the group of soil compounds called humic/fulvic acids. These acids are known to bind with mercury and also to methylate it, potentially making it more toxic. However, regarding methylation, there is also evidence that the normal bacteria in our gut methylates mercury, so I do not regard this as a sufficiently important risk to disregard the use of these useful compounds [228] [229] [230]. A Hungarian company, Humet, has extracted a humic/fulvic acid compound they call HumiFulvate® from a peat bog in Hungary and have studied it as a heavy metal detoxifier [231]. The product is available in the U.S. as Metal Magnet™ by PhytoPharmica [232]. From my research on humic and fulvic acids, they appear to act as bioaccumulators, able to bind with heavy metals, and to let go of them easily, which is where the alkalinity protocol will come into play. One to two capsules per day during short-term detoxification is an average dose.

## Spore-Forming Bacteria

Next, we come to the important topic of spore-formers, discussed above in the dirt section of the diet. Their ability to stimulate the immune system, to generate unique antimicrobials that disseminate system wide, and to competitively exclude pathogens from taking up residence in the gut make them ideal agents to be used in a variety of detox protocols. Of the two spore-former species I discussed above, bacillus laterosporus has a history of controlling Candida overgrowth in even the most difficult of cases, and the developer of this spore-forming strain, Boyd O'Donnell, has obtained a patent covering its use as an antifungal (US Patent No. 5,455,028). Spore-formers adsorb minerals, so it is very important to use the mineral repletion protocols already described. I stay on a maintenance dose of one per day to ensure I keep the gut flora under control. Undoubtedly, spore-formers also act as a fungicide and do kill off some Candida, but I have found the side effects to be minimal, such as occasional diarrhea.

## Dolomite

Last on the list is dolomite. Dolomite is widely used in pollution control systems to adsorb heavy metals from flue gasses, polluted stream water and even lakes [233] [234]. In the case of lakes, an experiment has been proposed where large quantities of dolomite are added to increase the water pH in an attempt to reduce the methylation of mercury in the water. I do not know of any research on the use of dolomite in humans to remove or render harmless heavy metals, but it is quite persuasive from the wide scale use in industry that it has such an effect.

## The Dirt Detox Protocol

For this protocol, for which a patent application has been filed, I have combined several natural substances. The goal is to determine if there is a synergistic detox effect in the combination that may make it more effective than the individual components. Perhaps it may be even more effective than the conventional detox protocols that are presently in use, particularly for removal of heavy metals.

The basic concept for this protocol is to combine clay, fulvic/humic acids, and spore-forming bacteria with alkalizing agents (including dolomite) that ensure the urine pH is neutral or alkaline. The rationale for this protocol is that each of the soil components individually is known to bind with metals in soil, and the strength of the soil-metal bond in each case is increased in an alkaline environment. What I am counting on is that the pH factor as applied in the human body will be the answer to the long-standing question for many detox protocols as to how to ensure that the detox agent does not let go of the toxic metal before it is excreted from the body.

The alkalizing agents can take the form of more fruit in the diet, dolomite, and/or supplements such as magnesium and potassium citrate. Here is an example of how I combine the individual components for detox purposes. Twice a day, upon arising and at bedtime, I take each of the following, all of which have been previously described: Pascalite clay (2 capsules), Immune Boost 77 (1 capsule), and Flora-Balance (1 capsule). In addition, during the day I take dolomite with water, as well as potassium citrate in sufficient quantity to ensure neutral to alkaline urine. Terramin clay tablets can be substituted for some or all of the Pascalite, Metal

Magnet can be substituted for one of the Immune Boost 77, and Lactobacillus Sporogenes can be substituted for one of the Flora-Balance. Sodium citrate or bicarbonate can also be used as alkalizing agents. Because the soil components are known to adsorb essential minerals as well as toxic ones, it is important to replenish minerals, some of which is accomplished by the dolomite. For a dosing schedule, I use this protocol for five days every two weeks, which allows for essential mineral replenishment during the off time.

## Charcoal

Most people are familiar with the use of charcoal in emergency rooms for poison control, and in that regard, it works in a somewhat similar fashion as clay in that it adsorbs toxins from the body. Charcoal powder is somewhat messy to use because of its black sooty consistency, but it is widely available in capsule form under many brands. If clay is not available or not to your liking, activated charcoal caps, usually about 250 mg each, can be used instead, or they can be mixed together in powder form, which makes the charcoal somewhat less sooty. Like clay, charcoal has a long history of animal use. For example, after a lightning-caused forest fire, returning animals are known to chew on charred branches to get at the charcoal. The activation process used to make modern charcoal acts to increase the available surface sites for adsorption. Charcoal does not appear to have the high mineral content of clay, which might make it somewhat less attractive for use, and it will turn your stool black, quite harmlessly. Otherwise, it is an excellent detoxifying agent. There are several good sources for products and information [235].

## Minerals

I single out two essential minerals in particular that have demonstrated detoxification potential by what appears to be displacement and replacement. It seems that these minerals, iodine and magnesium, have the capability to dislodge some toxic elements and then move into the now unoccupied locations.

## Iodine

There is a very exciting story to be told about iodine, one of the body's essential minerals, and for me it illustrates how difficult it can be at times to tell whether a reaction to a compound is an allergic one or a die-off reaction resulting from some detoxification process. The conventional wisdom regarding iodine has been that its primary function is in the production of thyroid hormones, and with insufficient intake, goiter (an enlargement of the thyroid gland that resembles a swollen neck) will result. The RDA for iodine, an essential element, is 150 micrograms, which was chosen as the dose necessary to prevent goiter.

Iodine is one of the halogen family of minerals, including chlorine, fluorine, bromine, and astatine (which is a radioactive element). Doses of iodine that exceed the RDA have been thought to be toxic because of the symptoms that arise. These symptoms can include unstable thyroid activity, seemingly creating hypo- or hyperthyroid conditions, a variety of skin problems known as iododerma, and a cluster of other symptoms called iodism, including excess salivation, fever, acute runny nose, swelling and tenderness of the salivary glands and tear ducts, and canker sores. Some years ago, in experimenting with supplements naturally high in iodine, such as kelp, I experienced virtually all of these symptoms, declared myself allergic to iodine, and stayed away from it. That is, until I met up with those MDs whom I refer to as the three musketeers of iodine research: Guy Abraham [236], David Brownstein [237], and Jorge Flechas [238]. Over the last three years or so, they have joined together in an Iodine Project [239] devoted to researching the health aspects of iodine and how it really interacts with the body, the results of which have been startling. I will discuss some of this research in more detail in the section below entitled "The Halogen Problem." A lot of this research is still quite new, and much of the medical community is either unaware of it, or in their usual fashion, dismissing it.

At this point of the iodine discussion, I will highlight some of their findings, while referring the reader to an excellent book on the subject by Dr. Brownstein: *Iodine, Why You Need It, Why You Can't Live Without It* [240]. In the realm of detoxification, Abraham, Brownstein, and Flechas discovered that iodine acts to displace the other halogens (which are toxic in all but the smallest amounts) from iodine receptor sites in the body, restoring health.    During this displacement activity, symptoms appeared that were believed to be allergic reactions to iodine, but actually were signs of toxic-halogen detoxification.    In the realm of general health, they found that the thyroid gland was just one "user" of iodine in the body, and that in the female, the breasts and ovaries are also large users.

They developed a simple urine test to evaluate the body iodine status, and I suggest that everyone take this test, which can also be ordered from the Flechas website [241].    Out of their research also came an iodine supplement in the form of a tablet called Iodoral, and it is a convenient way to supplement if the test establishes a need.    Both Iodoral and the test kit can be ordered from Vitamin Research Products [242].    They also discovered, based on both research and common sense, that the iodine RDA is set too low by a factor of somewhere between 100 and 300. Healthy Japanese routinely consume about 100 times our RDA, or about 15 milligrams of iodine per day.

As explained in Dr. Brownstein's book, the urine test will evaluate your present level of iodine sufficiency.    Once a supplement regimen is in place, periodic tests can monitor your improvement. Virtually everyone tested so far (thousands of people) have shown iodine deficiency.    Besides being a detoxification agent with respect to other halogens, iodine is also a powerful antibiotic and antiviral, and is probably the most popular choice of doctors and hospitals worldwide for wound disinfection in the form of povidone iodine products like Betadine®.    Last, but certainly not least, iodine in the elevated doses mentioned above has been shown to eliminate cysts of all kinds, including breast fibro cysts and ovarian cysts.    To me, anyone with a cyst problem anywhere on their body could benefit from iodine supplementation.    In addition, ongoing research into iodine insufficiency and its impact on thyroid illnesses and cancers of all kinds is producing very positive results.

The type of iodine used for supplementation is extremely important.    Human-made organic iodine compounds are, in general, highly toxic and should not be used.    Also, avoid the drugstore tincture disinfectants, as many are toxic for internal use because they contain wood alcohol.    For the last 100 years or so, doctors routinely used an inorganic solution called Lugol's solution, a liquid with one drop containing 6.25 mg of elemental iodine, comprising 5% iodine and 10% iodide as the potassium salt. The suggested daily intake for iodine supplementation was about 12.5-37.5 mg of elemental iodine (2-6 drops). Lugol's was widely available at this potency until very recently, when the DEA stepped in and decreased the potency of the OTC (Over The Counter) product sold in any quantity over one ounce, to less than half the original. There are several sources of Lugol's solution [243]. As I indicated earlier, it is best to be tested before using either Iodoral tablets or Lugol's solution as a supplement, and then use the dosages described in the Brownstein book.

For experimenters, while waiting for test results, you might have an interest in the topical iodine test. It involves painting some Lugol's on clean skin in, say, a 2-inch circle or square. It will stain the skin a typical orange color (it also stains clothes until it dries). Note the time of application, and peek at the spot every few hours. The objective is to see how long the stain remains visible. The rule of thumb is that if the stain disappears in less than 24 hours, you are iodine deficient. Repeated daily applications on different areas of the body has been known to extend the stain time, so it seems likely that transdermal absorption of some sort is taking place, with the body decreasing its rate of absorption as its iodine stores are replenished.

This is a very crude test because there are so many variables such as the evaporation rate of the liquid from the skin, and the absorption characteristics at different parts of the body, so don't expect highly consistent results. Once the stain stays for, say, 24 hours, the idea is to cut back the application, and just use the test occasionally, say once per week, to monitor level. Women who have applied the solution to the breast area have reported significant decreases in breast cysts. Various oral iodine dosing schedules can be found below for different applications. As a general precaution for anyone taking thyroid (or possibly other) hormone therapy, taking iodine supplements may require an adjustment of the dose of one or more of these hormones. Others and I have also found that large doses can radically affect thyroid test results until the thyroid reaches a normalized state, which may take some time. As an example, the thyroid hormone TSH may be elevated for as long as six months on this protocol. Note that for highly toxic people, even the skin test can provoke symptoms of a die-off reaction.

A question to ponder is where would PA get a large dietary supply of iodine? Of course, fish and sea algae have quite high levels, but for about 2.4 million years, PA had not yet learned to fish, and, of course, not all of our ancestors lived near the sea. Modernly, iodine deficiency disorder (IDD) is occurring in epidemic proportions in tropical populations, causing untold hardship. In the Wellness Diet, a calculation of the iodine content in the blood of a typical bull or cow is about 100 milligrams [244], and there is about another 100 milligrams in a bull or cow thyroid gland [245]. Additional amounts are found in other organs, so the animal portion of the Wellness Diet has a high potential yield of iodine, with smaller amounts being contributed by mountain spring water. In general, the iodine content of plant foods is low and extremely variable, being dependent on soil conditions [246].

Other than for detoxification purposes, iodine is a great antiseptic, especially for topical applications. However, one annoying side effect of the topical use of iodine, other than for the skin test above, is that it *does* stain the skin, which, for some people, has limited its antiseptic applications because of cosmetic issues. To overcome this objection, I came up with a combination of iodine and clay (see side box entitled Clayodine™), which enables topical iodine to be used without staining. Moreover, the antibiotic, antifungal, and antiviral properties of iodine are now combined with the toxin adsorption characteristics of clay.

---

## Clayodine™

I ran several experiments in an effort to remove the skin-staining effects of iodine without compromising its antiseptic properties. The result was a combination of two of my favorite detox compounds, iodine and clay. Some of the applications are poultices, bandages, toothpaste, mouthwash, gargle, soap, shampoo, a cosmetic base for troubled skin, and, of course, internal consumption. Here is how it works. For topical applications, first mix clay (e.g. Pascalite, Terramin, or Redmond) and water to form a mixture whose consistency fits the application (e.g. thick for a poultice, thin for a shampoo). Then mix the iodine (typically Lugol's Solution) with the hydrated clay to a maximum concentration, which is arrived at by experiment. The objective is to find the limit of iodine at which the combination does not stain the skin when used topically. This amount may be different for different clay compositions. For non-topical applications (see the lifestyle section for toothpaste), the iodine can be added to dry clay up to a maximum concentration where the iodine remains adsorbed in the clay. A patent application is pending.

Note that this application is different from the de-colorized iodine preparations on the market, which are typically potassium iodide, not iodine, and they lack many of the antiseptic qualities of iodine itself. The Clayodine preparation is intended for antiseptic use, not detoxification use, where the preferred products are Iodoral tablets and Lugol's solution.

## Magnesium

In previous sections, I have said much about magnesium as an essential mineral. Here, I want to review its role as a detoxifier. In particular, magnesium has been found to displace and replace lead from the bone matrix, and is also known to increase the excretion of aluminum and cadmium [247]. Magnesium may well prove to be an alternative to EDTA (ethylene diamine tetra-acetic acid), a lead chelator, in the removal of lead from the body [248]. (A chelator is a compound capable of forming an ionic bond with a metal.) There is also evidence that magnesium can be used prophylactically to inhibit lead and cadmium from depositing in the body [249] [250]. While there is not much in the way of research into the role of magnesium in detoxification, I believe it will be shown in the future to be enormously effective in dealing with many areas of toxin accumulation other than that of heavy metals. Of course, its ability to eliminate body odors of all sorts is another indication of its detox potential. Its uses in specific detox protocols will be discussed below.

## Salt

Salt was discussed in the previous section as a part of the Wellness Diet, but it has also been found that when it is used in large doses (several grams) it has detoxification properties that are not well understood. Its uses in specific detox protocols will be discussed below.

## Herbs

In addition to looking for clay, animals with gut problems also go searching for particular plants to cure themselves. Generally, these are bitter to the taste and contain what would normally be toxic compounds, not eaten for food, and are from the parts of the plant that are considered unacceptable as food items on the Wellness Diet. One objective is to use the plant toxins to kill or at least dislodge parasites from the gut, which is a major and recurring problem in the animal world. As you will see in the parasite discussion below, it is also a major but usually ignored problem for humans.

## Fiber

Fruit supplies natural fiber in the Wellness Diet, which has been shown to have a detoxifying effect in at least some applications where the toxin binds with bile. Because the body recycles most of the bile during the normal digestive process, these toxins can remain in the body for a long time. Fiber can act as a bile-sequestering agent, binding up some of the bile, which is then excreted, as opposed to being recycled in the normal manner.

For detoxification purposes, particularly when the target is mold, it may be advantageous to increase the amount of fiber in the Wellness Diet by using a supplement. The easiest way to do that is to add fruit pectin, such as apple pectin [251]. There are many pectin supplements on the market, but many are made with the rind and other parts of the fruit that are not acceptable. One example of a product I have used is *Apple Pectin USP* by TwinLab at two capsules per meal [174]. The most popular fiber supplements on the market today are made from psyllium, a seed, and are usually used to regulate bowel movements. In keeping with the principles of the diet, I avoid them. Large amounts of fiber can also interfere with essential mineral absorption, so I see no reason to go overboard on quantity.

# Chapter 17 - Specific Detox Problem Areas

In this section, it is my intention to discuss specific physical toxin problem areas prevalent in today's environment, along with some targeted detox protocols others and I have used with some success. In the following section, I will discuss emotional detoxification protocols.

## The Chronic Stress Problem

You might wonder why stress is listed as a toxin problem area, but its effect on the body and on detoxification in general is so pervasive, it deserves star billing before discussing the other toxin protocols. In the magnesium factor section of the diet, I outlined the relationship between stress and magnesium depletion, and much of what I cover in this section is an extension of that relationship.

When I refer to chronic stress I mean any activity or event that stimulates the fight-or-flight impulse in the body for long periods of time. The range of precipitating events can be everything from loud noise to a life-threatening experience. Under stress, the adrenal glands in particular are responsible for generating large quantities of certain hormones including forms of adrenaline and cortisol. All of these activities act to deplete the body stores of magnesium, B-vitamins, and vitamin C. The amount of such depletion is affected by genetic heritage, acclimation to stress, and stress reduction activities. There are endless activities that have been featured as stress reducing, such as yoga, tai chi, meditation, prayer, and the like, and I will not go into details regarding these, other than to say that any activity that reduces stress is certainly advisable.

Regarding the depletion of B-vitamins and vitamin C, I already discussed typical supplements that I use that seem adequate for my lifestyle. However, anyone leading a high stress lifestyle may want to consider even larger doses of the B-vitamin group as well as vitamin C, and this is quite easy to accomplish, with the caveat that high doses of B vitamins may interfere with certain other detox protocols, as discussed below. One B-vitamin exception that bears mentioning is vitamin B-5 (pantothenic acid), and a biologically active form of it called pantethine. Neither appears to feed the bad guys in the gut, and instead support the growth of friendly bacteria. Pantethine, in particular, supports the production of cortisone and other hormones by the adrenal glands, improves lipid profiles, and is an important addition to several detox protocols. They are discussed in more detail below. Vitamin B6 is also depleted by stress, increasing its importance as a supplement [252].

On the subject of adrenal glands, one of the more serious effects on the body of chronic stress is what is referred to as "adrenal fatigue," where the ability of the adrenal glands to continue pouring out the elevated hormones necessary to support the high stress level eventually becomes compromised. The result is general fatigue as well as a compromised defense system. Many protocols have been developed in an attempt to correct these hormonal deficiencies, and I will review some of them in this section.

There are several tests for measuring the hormone output level of the adrenal gland, particularly the hormones cortisol and DHEA. A saliva test is quite popular, and a typical fatigue profile shows low levels of both hormones [88]. There are dozens of programs out there offering support protocols with a variety of glandular and other products that go on for pages. I already referenced a natural adrenal extract in the glandular section above that may be helpful for those that test with an adrenal hypofunction. Another protocol using a prescription drug that works for some people is known as the Jefferies protocol [253], where small physiological doses of hydrocortisone are taken orally during the day to supplement the amount produced by the adrenals. If the total daily dose is kept below the level produced by a normally functioning gland (about 30 mg per day), none of the nasty side effects of pharmacological doses of cortisone occur. When it works, it seems to restore levels somewhat to normal, and the person feels much better and apparently can stay on it for years, if necessary, without adverse effects. Then there are the prednisone tapers, which are proposed to combat fatigue, but they require close monitoring, are adrenal suppressive, and can be quite dangerous.

I first experimented with the Jefferies protocol years ago, with negative results. While my adrenal tests indicated low cortisol and DHEA levels, taking the small support doses of cortisone aggravated all of the adrenal fatigue symptoms. Consulting with several MDs using the Jefferies protocol, they confirmed that a significant fraction of those who have tried it do very poorly for unknown reasons. After some careful experimentation, I realized that increasing the levels of stress hormones requires the support of magnesium, and if there is a deficit, the replacement therapy will not work, and the initial symptoms will get worse. Bringing magnesium levels (and iodine levels) up to normal, along with heavy metal and toxic-halogen detoxing, may completely obviate the need for adrenal or thyroid hormone replacement therapy. Remarkably, Dr. Shealy has found that restoring body magnesium levels also restores DHEA levels [144], leading to the intriguing possibility of hormone replacement therapy being a natural function of magnesium replacement therapy. Since magnesium is so intimately involved with hormone activity, I wonder what the effect of magnesium normalization might have on hormone issues related to menopause.

One of my theories as to why many anti-fatigue remedies do not work properly is due to the depletion of magnesium, along with vitamins B-6 and B-5. A unique form of vitamin B-5, pantethine, has been found to support the production of cortisol by the adrenal glands, making this an important supplement for stress related issues. A more thorough discussion of pantethine, outlining its other benefits, appears in the fungal detox section below. As part of my detox protocol, I take a 300 mg softgel of pantethine with each meal, available from Jarrow Formulas and others [128]. I also complement it with the conventional form of vitamin B-5, pantothenic acid (widely available), which I take with every meal at a dose of 500 mg. Neither of these supplements appears to interfere with any of the detox protocols. Virtually any supplement that increases the metabolic activity of the body will require magnesium, and those people with toxins such as heavy metals or candidiasis are generally deficient. Therefore, I also view the protocols described previously for topical magnesium and sublingual P5P replacement as an important part of any adrenal fatigue treatment protocol.

On the basis that magnesium deficiency may be a precipitating factor in fatigue in general, and thyroid and adrenal deficiency in particular as the result of excess chronic stress, I propose the following experiment. Both the adrenal and thyroid glands are controlled by the pituitary gland, located at the base of the brain at about the middle of the head. There is research showing that magnesium is necessary for proper function of the pituitary [62], leading to the speculation that providing magnesium somewhat directly to the pituitary might have a positive impact on fatigue. When surgery is to be performed on the pituitary, they usually operate by going through the nose, as a short path to the gland. My approach was to create a magnesium nasal spray that could be safely used, in the hope that the magnesium could be sufficiently absorbed through tissue to find its way to the pituitary gland somewhat directly. See the side box labeled Magnesium Nasal Spray for the formula.

Another major concern for those under chronic stress is the development of cardiovascular disease (CVD), and that concern itself can act as a stressor! There is little doubt that magnesium depletion as a result of chronic stress can lead to CVD by causing calcium deposits in the arteries as well as causing arterial and heart muscle spasms. Interestingly, Dr. Seelig has shown that magnesium acts to regulate cholesterol levels in much the same way as statin drugs, by acting on a coenzyme known as HMG-CoA, but with none of the drug side effects [36]. So for those concerned about cholesterol levels, be aware that normalizing magnesium levels may result in improvement in all portions of the lipid profile.

---

### Magnesium Nasal Spray

The source of the magnesium is a solution of magnesium chloride such as Cardiovascular Research's Magnesium Solution 18%, widely available. For a container, I empty out and clean a commercially available bottle of nasal spray with a removable top, and fill it with filtered mineral water (free of chlorine and fluoride). I add 10 to 20 drops of the magnesium solution per ounce of water, and shake well. For those who want to add a preservative, add one drop of either Lugol's solution or grapefruit seed extract. Spray each nostril several times per day. If a burning sensation arises in the nostril, dilute the spray mixture. While salt-water nasal sprays, using sodium chloride, have enjoyed widespread use, in this experiment, magnesium chloride (and some magnesium acetate) is being substituted for the sodium chloride. I have been using the spray for a short time without any difficulties, and I do notice an energy boost.

---

## The Heavy Metal Problem

The term *heavy metal* has many definitions in the field of health, so for the purpose of this chapter, I am going to narrow it down to a discussion of two particularly nasty and prevalent toxic metals in our environment and in our bodies: mercury and lead. Many other heavy metals are also no fun to have around in excess. They include cadmium, antimony, arsenic, aluminum, nickel, palladium, tin, platinum, bismuth, and others.

I will begin the discussion with mercury and wish to advise the reader that from my research and personal experiences, mercury toxicity is intimately bound with Candida overgrowth, covered in depth in the following section on fungal problems. Therefore, I suggest these two sections be read together so that the entire spectrum of this toxic combination can be fully appreciated.

Mercury is considered the most potent non-radioactive neurotoxin found in Nature. A neurotoxin is a compound that acts on nerve cells in a detrimental manner, either disabling or killing neurons and other portions of the nervous system. Examples of other natural neurotoxins are the venom of bees, spiders, scorpions, and snakes. Human-made neurotoxins are chemical in nature, and include nerve agents used in chemical warfare, which, ironically, were developed from research into insecticides, most of which are also neurotoxins. Neurotoxins have many harmful effects on the body, from simple tremors to loss of body functions to death, and virtually everything in-between.

What do you do when a caring dentist places a compound in your body a few inches from your brain, one half of which is the most potent neurotoxin in Nature, in an amount that will slowly leak out as a vapor to all parts of your body over your entire lifetime? Well, I used to say thank you, pay the bill, and make an appointment to have more installed later. What do you do when a caring pediatrician injects into the body of your child (or perhaps you in the form of a flu shot) a compound including this same neurotoxin? Well, I used to say thank you, pay the bill, and make an appointment to have more injected later.

These dental and medical practices eventually may be recorded in the annals of history as possibly some of the most tragic technology errors in the fields of dentistry and medicine (closely followed by root canals and fluoridation, but more on those later). To add to this story, except for the financial issues involved, none of this would have taken place. In the case of mercury amalgam fillings (no, they are not silver fillings), they were developed over a hundred years ago as a cheap replacement for gold alloy fillings that do not contain mercury. In the case of adding thimerosal, a mercury-containing preservative, to vaccines, the motivation was to make more cost-effective vaccine dispensing systems where multiple persons could be vaccinated from the same vial. If individual dose glass vials are used, no thimerosal is required.

I do not believe either of these practices has taken place with evil intent or in any manner intended to cause harm. The reason I say that is because those connected with the development and implementation of these blunders have also personally been the recipients of these same blunders. I have many friends in the medical and dental field, and the majority have mercury amalgam fillings in their own mouths, as well as in the mouths of their family members. They have all been vaccinated with thimerosal, as have their family members. With this as a prelude, I do not believe it is productive to belabor the mistakes of the past in any more detail. I strongly support all the grass-roots efforts around the country to promote legislation to stop the damage, but until then, there will be endless arguments and denials, fueled by conscience and the threat of lawsuits.

Our real work ahead as individuals is to find ways of removing mercury from our bodies, and seeing to it that no more is intentionally added. The major sources are amalgam fillings, vaccinations, and seafoods. As I mentioned above, there are many adults and children that can withstand large amounts of mercury without ill effects, and then there are the *others*. At least among vaccinated children, it is looking like the *others* are approaching 1 in 150, which is the current autism rate.

Before beginning any mercury detox program, it is important to support the body with additional nutrients that mercury either depletes or interferes with. The list of such support agents could (and does) fill a book [254], but I will highlight some that I have found to be particularly useful. Several more are discussed in the fungal section below. Because mercury interferes with the transport of minerals throughout the body, the additional mineral support previously described, particularly magnesium and zinc, is important, and I suggest the testing of mineral levels before detoxing.

Liver and high omega-3 eggs are good essential fatty acid support foods during detox. Regarding vitamins, for some, the gut is so deranged from heavy metals that oral vitamins are not well absorbed. One alternative is a sublingual (dissolved under the tongue) coenzymated B-complex, available from Source Naturals [125]. Note that this supplement comes in orange and peppermint flavors. According to the company, the peppermint flavor is free of wheat, gluten, and soy, while the orange flavor contains trace amounts of these in the flavoring. One per day should be enough. Remember that we want to minimize feeding the bad guys. Another approach to non-oral vitamin and mineral support is the IV administration of vitamins in a Myer's Cocktail [145], which is a favorite IV mix of vitamins and minerals mentioned earlier. I try to have a set of five of these twice a year, particularly to boost magnesium levels.

Many other support supplements have been suggested during heavy metal chelation to make the process more comfortable, particularly in the realm of fatigue. The HPA/T (hypothalamus, pituitary, and adrenal/thyroid) axis of the body is particularly vulnerable to heavy metals. The thyroid will receive a lot more attention in the halogen section below. Adrenal exhaustion is the usual suspect for fatigue as mentioned above, but I have found that this is not always the case. The HPA/T axis involves a variety of what are known as closed-loop control systems, an area in which I have had extensive experience in connection with spacecraft design. I do not know if the study of endocrinology includes courses in control system theory, but it certainly should. The bottom line is this: what appear, via test results, to be adrenal or thyroid problems may just as easily be hypothalamus or pituitary problems. However, since endocrinologists do not know how to control those glands, the adrenals, which can sometimes be supported with small doses of hydrocortisone [253], and the thyroid, which can sometimes be supported with thyroid hormone, get all the attention. Enter magnesium, again.

There is some evidence that magnesium is a key factor in the proper functioning of the pituitary gland [62], and I have personally found that restoring magnesium levels can have a positive effect on restoring hormone activity. For example, a long-term program of oral, topical and IV magnesium supplementation restored my low body temperature to normal, where adrenal and thyroid hormone replacement alone failed to do so. Where possible, my preference is to support the glands with the Wellness Diet and the supplements previously mentioned, and wait for the detox regimens to restore the glands to health. I will have more to say about the use of cortisone supplements in the fungal section below.

There is controversy over the use of vitamin B12 supplements, based on the concern that this substance might act to convert some mercury compounds to methylmercury, a particularly toxic mercury compound. There is some scattered research on the subject indicating that such conversion is possible [255], but I do not believe B12 supplementation would normally be required on the Wellness Diet because of its naturally high concentration in animal food. There is also evidence that humic and fulvic acids can methylate mercury. However, they are so important in correcting gut issues - insuring healthy bowel elimination, a major detox pathway - that I have no concerns about using these soil elements, particularly in conjunction with the alkalinity protocol. Remember that the bulk of stool is gut bacteria, so having the right kind in the colon can improve bowel excretion of toxins.

Regarding amalgams, from the work of Weston Price discussed above, and from Paleo skeletal evidence, if we did not live a life disconnected from our heritage there would be no need, barring accidents, to ever visit a dentist, much less have cavities filled. It is my hope that those who adopt at least portions of the Wellness Diet and the rest of The Wellness Project early enough in life will be spared the necessity for any restorative dental care.

Dental restoration amalgams are typically a combination of mercury, silver, copper, tin, and zinc, and a threshold question is whether you have or have had them. Many folks believe they can merely look in their mouths for metal color to make a determination, but that is not so. In many cases, tooth colored crowns have been placed directly over amalgam fillings, and the only way to know if that is the case is either to consult detailed and correct records from your dentist as to what work was performed, or to have the crowns pulled to look underneath. X-rays cannot tell because the metal crown material hides what is underneath. By the way, gold crowns are really alloys of many materials including gold, and porcelain crowns are usually porcelain fused to gold or another metal alloy. Nickel and other alloys are also used for dental materials. One problem with having many different metals in the mouth is that they set up galvanic reactions, forming miniature batteries, with saliva as the electrolyte. Perhaps you remember making a battery by putting a copper penny in one end of a lemon, and a zinc nickel in the other end. That is what happens in the mouth, causing currents and voltages that can disrupt the entire nervous system and lead to all kinds of symptoms, which just add to the already long list of mercury caused symptoms [256, 257]. So, for a definitive reading on your amalgams, you need either dental records, or possibly crown removal, not a fun prospect.

Before we temporarily leave a discussion of amalgams, there is an indirect way in which you could have been exposed to large amounts of mercury (and other toxins) from the dental industry even without having amalgams installed. The source of that exposure can be a friend or family member who works in a dental office or in a dental lab, and you spend a lot of time around that person. Unless they practice some sort of decontamination, it is quite likely that they will bring home clothing, shoes, and other personal materials loaded with mercury. A particular problem is mercury or other toxins on shoes, which are then brought into a home containing carpeting. The carpeting becomes contaminated, and babies and young children playing on the floor acquire the toxins.

Moving on to vaccinations, if you have recently had a flu shot, it most likely contained thimerosal, the mercury preservative. Going back in time to childhood shots or those needed for travel, the only way to tell if they contained thimerosal is by doctor's records, if they exist, which should have recorded lot numbers for each vaccine. These lot numbers permit tracing by the manufacturer to see if it was a mercury-dosed lot. There are online sources to check the history of various vaccines and their ingredients that may be useful [13]. Thimerosal-containing vaccinations have come under great scrutiny as a potential cause of autism, which has now reached epidemic proportions. It is not rocket science to image the damaging effects of injecting large amounts of mercury into a child, and I strongly support all of the organizations attempting finally to get mercury and other toxins out of vaccines. If you find it necessary to be vaccinated, perhaps it would be wise to insist on single dose vials, and even then, to ask to see the ingredient list.

Next, we move to seafoods. You have already read my love affair/horror story with fish, but sea algae such as seaweed, kelp and the like are also contaminated. After all, the way fish accumulate mercury is from direct or indirect ingestion of sea algae, which have the unique ability to bioaccumulate toxins, including mercury. Fortunately, in the Wellness Diet, seafoods are unnecessary, as they have been for most of our heritage.

From the above, you can get an idea of your lifetime exposure to mercury. Does everyone exhibit symptoms of toxicity from mercury exposure? No, once again there are those who, through past mutations and/or evolutionary luck, possess the ability to be exposed to large amounts of mercury without ill effect. One guess as to why is that they have the natural ability to mobilize and excrete large amounts of mercury before it can cause damage. Are you one of them? One approach to answering this question is to see if you have any of the symptoms. However, the symptom list goes on for pages, and is undoubtedly not complete. I would have a tough time categorically ruling out mercury, at least as a contributor to the worsening of any symptom I could think of, so that is really no help.

Next is testing, but unfortunately there is no test for one's body burden of mercury, short of an autopsy! Blood tests for chronic mercury exposure are mostly useless because the mercury is swept from the bloodstream into cells everywhere shortly after exposure. However, there is a specialized blood test to detect if you are hypersensitive to mercury. It is called the Melisa® test, and it can check for hypersensitivities to a number of toxic metals, including such seemingly innocent ones as titanium and nickel [258]. It is very worthwhile if you have or are planning to have metal implants for whatever reason. If you test positive to mercury hypersensitivity, and your history includes mercury exposure, it ups the odds that it is ruining your day.

A urine mercury test without a provoking agent (a compound to push mercury out of the body via the kidneys) is also not very useful because without a shove, mercury is quite content to stay in your body for, say, 30 to 50 years. The downside of a urine challenge test with a provoking agent (a large single quantity of DMPS or DMSA, described below) is that it can cause the redistribution of large quantities of mercury throughout the body. Another type of urine test is starting to gain popularity, one that indirectly measures the effect that mercury has on porphyrins, organic compounds normally found in the body [259]. It is called the Urine Porphyrin Profile Analysis (UPPA), and several labs offer the test. Derangement of porphyrins has been correlated with mercury toxicity, and the tests have been particularly helpful in diagnosing autistic children poisoned by thimerosal [260].

A hair-minerals test may be useful, and certainly was for me. Unfortunately, many folks carrying a large burden of mercury are not very good at excreting it in their hair, and so get a false negative. Many autistic children fall into this category. Another indirect way to use a hair test for mercury is to measure the essential and other non-toxic elements in the hair, because mercury is well known to cause deranged essential mineral transport. You can order a test which measures both toxic and non-toxic minerals through Direct Labs [261], which has an arrangement with Doctors Data, a well-respected medical laboratory [262]. Andrew Cutler, a chemist and past mercury toxicity victim, has devised methods of interpreting hair essential mineral test results in an effort to determine if mercury toxicity is an issue, and has written a book on the subject [263].

While the neurotoxic properties of mercury can wreak havoc with one's personality (e.g. the Mad Hatter syndrome and Mozart's madness) [264], there are some other clues that can point to a mercury problem, not the least of which is persistent Candida overgrowth. As you will see from a discussion in the fungal section, it is very difficult to eradicate Candida when mercury is present, and in many instances, it is counterproductive to try to do so. Another clue to mercury or other heavy metal toxicity is that supplements and other remedies don't work the way they are supposed to, and may even aggravate the condition they are supposed to alleviate. Yet another clue is dry skin with or without bizarre skin outbreaks. A final but significant clue is a gut that just will not behave, switching from diarrhea to constipation and everything in between, at a moment's notice. Spore-forming bacteria and magnesium play a major role in alleviating some of these problems while mercury detox is underway.

My personal opinion is that, if a person has amalgams in their mouth and also has health problems, there is a likelihood they would not achieve optimum health without proper removal. This should be followed by a detoxification program to begin to eliminate the lifetime of mercury that has collected throughout their body, including in the brain.

The mercury detox problem is somewhat more complicated because having amalgams in place limits the detoxification protocols that can be safely undertaken. If you wish to keep your amalgams, and yet are interested in some detox protocols, here are the issues. Because you have a large reservoir of mercury from your teeth continuously leaking into your body, attempting major detoxification can quickly overload the body's ability to handle the potentially large amounts. One result is that mercury can end up redistributed throughout the body, making you much sicker and potentially making it much harder to remove the now scattered mercury, not a good idea at all.

There are a few things others have tried to minimize mercury release from amalgams, one of which is to avoid chewing gum, since tooth pressure increases mercury excretion. Minimizing the drinking of hot beverages may also be useful to decrease excretion. The only detox protocols I can think of using with amalgams in place are the natural ones such as sauna, fiber, clay, spore-formers, and fulvic/humic acids. The alkalinity technique is designed to work with these protocols to reduce the amount of redistributed mercury, but I am not aware of any testing to support my theory. In any case, the mineral supplementation protocols, particularly transdermal magnesium along with sublingual P5P, are very worthwhile to support the body.

If you decide you want to get your amalgams removed (I did), here are some suggestions. The first step is to find a dentist trained in amalgam removal, which begs the question of "trained by who"? There are many removal protocols out there, and frankly there is no perfect way to remove mercury. The best you can do is to minimize the amount of mercury inhaled and ingested during removal. Of course, the next issue is what to put in its place. Ironically, most of the replacement materials are also toxic, containing various plastic materials including the ubiquitous bisphenol-A (BPA) of bottled water fame. Trading one toxin for another is not a fun prospect, but the reality is any foreign material put in the body will generate some toxic reaction.

Your dentist needs to be fully trained in replacement materials, which hopefully are not other metals! There are materials compatibility tests that can be run for both crown materials and bonding agents [265], but they are not foolproof. After much research and a few false starts, I decided on dentists trained by a pioneer in safe amalgam removal. His name is Hal Huggins, and he is a dentist who has personally suffered from mercury toxicity. As a typical pioneer, he ended up with arrows in his back and license revocation for daring to question the mainstream dental community. He offers a dentist referral service on his website [266], which is a good starting point. My dentist, David Villarreal, in Woodland Hills, California, was trained by Huggins and did excellent work for my wife and me. Another organization listing dentists claiming to be trained in amalgam removal as a specialty is IAOMT, International Academy of Oral Medicine and Toxicology [256], and they have a referral service. For thoroughness, I would further check out the potential candidates by running them through a grass roots organization called DAMS, Dental Amalgam Mercury Solutions [267], which collects data from patients reporting their experiences with various dentists.

Going hand-in-hand with amalgam removal are the issues of permanently damaged teeth, raising the prospects of root canals, implants, and bridges. I am not a fan of implants because that is reintroducing metal back into the mouth, permanently altering the jawbone, and possibly leading to infections and cavitations. If you still wish to follow this route, a Melisa test would be of use to see if you have an intolerance of materials such as titanium. I discuss the folly of root canals in the section below on bacterial problems, and I consider this procedure another major technology blunder that can lead to potentially serious health problems for some people. In my case, I had a tooth nerve-damaged during amalgam removal, and rather than risk a root canal, I had the tooth extracted, using a Huggins extraction protocol, and a permanent zirconia bridge put in its place.

Let's say you have decided on a dentist for amalgam removal, and have chosen a replacement material (I chose zirconium oxide). Before beginning the procedure, it would be a good idea to find a practitioner skilled in detoxification therapy so that after amalgam removal you are fully prepared to begin removal of the mercury stored in the rest of your body. Such a practitioner can also advise you on preparation for the amalgam removal procedure. Unfortunately, finding detoxification support is not so simple, as most dentists are not qualified in this area and there are as many mercury detox protocols as there are detox supplements on the market. I have studied many of them, and my findings are listed below. In this discussion, I am presuming the reader is already following the Wellness Diet or something similar, because anecdotal evidence has shown that animal fat and protein are important to support detoxification. After the discussion of the conventional detox protocols, I will bring in the Dirt Detox Protocol as a supplementary or possibly even alternative approach to dealing with the heavy metal problem.

The first category of conventional protocols I will be discussing concerns those compounds that can be truly described as chelating agents. While there is a wide range of chelating agents in nature, for purposes of this book, we will use the strict definition in which the toxic metal ion is bound to two or more atoms of the chelating agent. For mercury, a class of compounds known as dithiols meets this criterion, but they all leave a lot to be desired. I would like to reiterate at this point that it can be problematic to use these agents if you still have amalgams in your mouth, because of the redistribution problem.

DMPS (2,3-Dimercapto-1-propanesulfonic acid), also known as Dimaval, is a pharmaceutical agent developed in the Soviet Union fifty years ago and is widely used in Europe as a treatment for mercury intoxication. It is not approved by the FDA for such use, but it can be obtained from U.S. compounding pharmacies with a doctor's prescription. It binds to mercury, lead, cadmium and arsenic [251]. It also binds to some essential minerals including zinc, copper, and chromium, which can be replaced through supplementation. There is wide disagreement as to how DMPS should be administered – whether administering it by IV, oral, or transdermal means is best. Drs. Klinghardt and Gruenn, mentioned earlier, both have wide experience in this area. My personal chelation preference, described in the Cutler and other references [254, 263], and one that I have pursued for some time, is low-dose oral administration, taken every 8 hours for three days every two weeks, and then repeated. The dosing period is designed around the half-life of the chelator (also true for other chelators) in an attempt to keep an even amount in the body, minimizing the redistribution of un-excreted toxins. Starting doses can be as low as 5 milligrams, and increased slowly while monitoring detox reactions. I personally do not go above 30 milligrams per dose for any of the chelators. The idea is to stay comfortable during the process. I would suggest consulting with DAMS

Intl. for referrals to practitioners in your area who are skilled in these protocols [267]. I also believe in keeping the urine alkaline while taking DMPS in the anticipation that alkalinity will greatly enhance its efficacy, and may also reduce adverse reactions.

Another chemical chelating agent is DMSA (Dimercaptosuccinic acid), also known as Captomer. It is available over the counter as an oral chelating agent, and my preference would be to take it about every 3 hours for three days every two weeks, and then it would be repeated. A safe starting dose would be 5 milligrams, which is not easy to achieve because the available potencies start at about 25 milligrams, so you must manually split doses. Others and I find DMSA produces more gut related symptoms than DMPS, particularly with respect to Candida overgrowth, and this is discussed further in the fungal section below. My comments regarding urine alkalinity also apply here.

The third chelating agent is ALA (alpha-lipoic acid), a compound appearing naturally in the body in small amounts, and found in organ meats. It is widely available as an antioxidant supplement, but, unlike DMPS and DMSA, it has the ability to cross the blood-brain barrier and theoretically chelate mercury out of the brain. My preference for ALA is to follow the same protocol as for DMSA, taking doses every 3 hours. It, too, is only available in large doses, and needs to be manually split up for a safe starting dose. If tolerated, it can be taken along with DMPS or DMSA. There are some studies that show ALA may interfere with the production of thyroid hormones [268] and aggravate hypoglycemia [269] and, and for some people it can only be tolerated after a significant amount of mercury has already been chelated from the body. My comments regarding urine alkalinity also apply here. Dr. Broda Barnes, one of the early pioneers in the use of natural thyroid hormone, identified hypothyroidism (as well as hypoadrenal and hypopituitary issues) as a major cause of hypoglycemia in his book *Hope for Hypoglycemia* [270]. So, it should come as no surprise that ALA's interference with thyroid hormone production would also raise issues of hypoglycemia. Personally, I have found that many of the adverse symptoms associated with the use of ALA as a mercury chelator can be avoided if thyroid and adrenal issues are addresses prior to use.

Another chelator, EDTA, bears mentioning, and historically has been used for lead chelation, although both DMPS and DMSA also chelate lead [271], but more slowly. EDTA has also been used both orally and in IV formulations to open partially blocked arteries in patients with cardiovascular problems. The way in which this is accomplished is not well understood, but EDTA has antifungal properties (so does aspirin) and this may be a factor [272]. There have also been some studies that show EDTA can combine with mercury in the body in a manner that increases toxicity [273]. It may have some uses for those who are mercury-free and have arterial occlusions. As mentioned above, magnesium may well be an alternative to EDTA in the removal of lead from the body and in the transport of calcium from the arteries to the bones, where it belongs.

There are many issues surrounding the above chelating agents, with little agreement in the detox community as to the way they should be used and the outcomes expected [251]. A major problem is that while the chelators may initially bond well to toxic metals, the bonds are not strong enough to prevent un-bonding of some of it on the way out of the body, thus redistributing the toxins in a sort of "musical chairs" scenario. It is quite common to have a worsening of symptoms while using these agents, and cycles of symptoms that disappear and reappear quite randomly. That is why I suggest having a coach available who is skilled in supporting you if you wish to go this route. What would be a breakthrough is a chelating agent where the bond strength is sufficient to lock up the toxin all the way out of the body. Until that agent becomes available, we are stuck with the above protocols. Having said that, and as part of an ongoing experiment, I am pursuing the approach that alkalinity may be one answer to redistribution. For those interested in keeping track of new developments in this area, DAMS is usually an excellent source of information.

I will refer to the next category of heavy metal detoxifying agents as bioaccumulators for want of a better term. This category includes certain algae from the sea. If we back up and look at the fish/mercury problem, it becomes apparent that the chain of events begins with small fish eating sea plankton and algae, which accumulate toxic metals as well as organic toxins such as pesticides. The big fish eat the small fish, and the accumulation cycle concludes with humans eating the toxic big fish. For this reason, I avoid naturally occurring sea algae such as seaweed, kelp and spirulina, as they may already be contaminated. However, some enterprising supplement makers have devised ways to grow algae, particularly chlorella, in a clean environment so you can buy it uncontaminated. The thought is that by eating algae, it will accumulate the toxins in your body and escort them out. Well, maybe.

Anecdotally, there are mixed reviews on the use of chlorella for mercury detoxification, and I can think of at least one reason why. Clearly, when fish eat contaminated sea algae, they become contaminated. Well, it is not rocket science to conclude that contaminated algae is quite willing to give up its toxins to its host, so one inference is that the algae-toxin bond is quite weak. This leads back to the problem of how much mercury-loaded chlorella in your body will get excreted as opposed to being redistributed. For those interested in trying it, a well-respected brand of chlorella is Yaeyama, sold under various labels. My gut won't tolerate it, so my body has made the choice for me. There is some anecdotal evidence that a lactating mother with a mouth full of amalgams can keep mercury out of her breast milk by taking chlorella supplements, which is a very good thing for the baby. What is unknown is where the mercury ultimately ends up in the mother's body.

I will refer to the next category of detox agents as mobilizers, which actually covers all detox agents to some extent. In this case, I am limiting the list to those agents that simply mobilize, but do not bond with or excrete toxins. The presumption is that they dislodge toxins from their present location, begging the question of what happens next. For example, cilantro, from the leaf and stem of the coriander plant, has been attributed with some detox characteristics, probably as a mobilizer [274], and there are many products on the market that contain chlorella and cilantro in various formulations. Cilantro (coriander) has antifungal properties, which may contribute to its effect in mobilizing mercury, as described in the fungal section. In the case of mobilizers, the questions are what takes the place of the dislocated toxin, which was presumably sitting on a receptor site normally reserved for some good guy, and where does the mobilized toxin end up? This is really a rhetorical question, because I really don't expect anyone to have the answers.

The minerals iodine and magnesium fall into the mobilizer category, but they are unique because they act as displacers and replacers. In other words, when they push a toxin out of its location, they (iodine and magnesium) are the ideal elements to replace that toxin in that location.

The last category includes adsorbers which, in the natural detox agent category, includes clay, charcoal, fulvic/humic acids, and spore-forming bacteria, as discussed above. There are also products on the market that use modified zeolites (chalks), and some sellers make outrageous claims for these products. From my vantage point, it is hard to beat the natural agents. It is generally believed that none of the adsorbers are systemic in action, being limited to operating in the gut. However, users of adsorbers for detoxification report symptom relief that would appear to require systemic detoxification. Therefore, I think it is premature to make any statements limiting their action, even if they themselves are physically limited to the gut.

While the above discussion has concentrated on the removal of mercury, the same protocols may be used for lead and cadmium. In particular, magnesium has been found to displace and replace lead from the bone matrix, and is known to also increase the excretion of cadmium and aluminum, so maintaining body stores of magnesium, as discussed above, is definitely part of the heavy metal detox protocol.

As you will see from the discussion of fungal problems below, it is my belief that mercury toxicity and Candida overgrowth are intimately related, and hence the protocols in that section are very relevant for use in conjunction with those presented here to deal with the combined problem.

In summary, to simplify this section of the book for the reader, here is what I suggest. Given what I know now, after years of experimenting and researching in this area, daily sauna is my number one choice for heavy metal detoxification, followed by daily magnesium supplementation. Next, on a schedule of five days every two weeks, are alkaline urine, clay, and the other soil elements of humic/fulvic acids and spore-formers, which form the Dirt Detox Protocol. I know of no studies that would contraindicate the use of these items for people that still have amalgam fillings in place, because none of these items are chelators that might pull mercury from fillings.

For those that want to take heavy metal detox to another level, an UPPA or hair mineral test is next on the list if you wish to quantify your level of toxification. Depending on test results and dental records, amalgam removal would be next, followed by oral chelation therapy on a schedule of three days every two weeks, where these three days are not the same days as used for the Dirt Detox protocol. Chelation would include DMPS in small doses, using the protocols I discussed above, and ALA, also in very small doses. I find that if I take ALA with DMPS, I can use the eight-hour dosing schedule for both. I presume DMPS acts to clean up any un-excreted mercury mobilized by the ALA. Appendix B summarizes these protocols in chart form.

Let's take a closer look at the Dirt Detox Protocol as it is applied to the removal of heavy metals such as mercury, lead and cadmium. As stated above, it is known that fulvic and humic acids adsorb heavy metals, particularly mercury, and the product Metal Magic is a commercial example of this type of detoxifying agent. From the previously cited references, it is also known that spore-forming bacteria (biomass) adsorb metals, including mercury, cadmium and lead, and clay also has a history of metal adsorption. A concern in the past with adsorbers has been the weak bond, raising the issue of whether the detox agents will let go of the metal on the way out, redistributing it.

My approach is to use alkalinity as the "glue" to hold the metals to the soil elements. As a way of testing the efficacy of this protocol, I am planning a program of self-experimentation, paying attention to redistribution as evidenced by the reappearance of previously resolved symptoms. Further, I will set up a schedule of urine-challenge testing, where, similar to the DMPS or DMSA challenge test, I collect urine after administering the protocol, to see if and to what extent heavy metals are being excreted in the urine. Humet, the company that makes the active ingredient in Metal Magic, has observed some excellent results for mercury excretion in urine testing, using just the humic/fulvic compound alone. The results have been reported by Doctor's Data lab, and they can be found in the research section of the Humet website [231]. I am hopeful that the combination of ingredients in the Dirt Detox protocol will show even better results, and that this method may end up as a replacement for some of the conventional detox methods.

I want to emphasize the use of activated charcoal to quickly deal with acute detox symptoms, should they be experienced with any of the protocols. Charcoal's huge surface area makes it the idea choice when you are suddenly hit with the typical detox symptoms of head, neck and shoulder pain. After much experimentation, I have found that, in my case, this is referred pain from the gut, and charcoal caps (10-15 at one time) can mop it up fast. Remember that doses of charcoal for routine poison control can range from 20-100 grams (equivalent to about 80-400 capsules!) Another fast-acting remedy for some detox symptoms is to add alkaline foods and supplements, as discussed above.

There are a few online support groups that discuss some of the various heavy metal detox protocols covered here, other than the Dirt Detox method. Look for Yahoo groups with the word *chelation* in the title. You will see as we discuss other toxin issues (even including the subject of indoor lighting) that mercury will continue to rear its ugly head. Which bring us to the fungal problem.

## The Fungal Problem

A discussion of body fungal problems will usually center around Candida. Earlier in this book, I described the work of Drs. Truss, Crook, and Trowbridge in uncovering the role that overgrowth of Candida and related yeasts (candidiasis) in the gut and elsewhere can play in causing illness. It is well established that taking large and/or frequent doses of antibiotics can predispose one to this condition, and often probiotics are prescribed in an attempt to prevent the problem. The theory is that the antibiotics reduce the bacterial population in the gut, allowing for fungal overgrowth. Well, that may be the start of the fungal problem, but it certainly is not the entire picture for many people.

There are many natural treatments for Candida overgrowth, and since I have had a very long relationship with this issue, I have probably experimented with most of them. They included oregano in all forms, olive leaf extract, grapefruit seed extract, digestive enzymes, pre- and probiotics, caprylic acid, undecenoic acid, tea tree oil, fiber, garlic, pau d'arco, artemesia, silver, other yeast products, EFAs, vitamin C, B vitamins, and others I can no longer remember. In the prescription category, I have experimented with nystatin, ketoconazole, itraconazole, fluconazole, amphotericin B, terbinafine, and clotrimazole, among others. Of course, I followed the various anti-Candida diets very closely over the years, as reported earlier. They all worked in their own way to alleviate symptoms, which were mostly gut and skin problems for me. However, for some reason, I could never really get rid of it completely. Re-enter mercury.

Candida is a genus of yeasts, and the *albicans* variety appears to be the most significant. It is found in our gut, skin, and mucus membranes and is very much a part of our natural environment. There are other Candida varieties such as *tropicalis* and *parapsilosis* that also hang around in our intestines. In fact, just as in the case of our gut bacteria, we are mostly clueless as to identifying the number and characteristics of all of the fungi in our intestines. There may be hundreds or thousands of varieties, and to complicate matters, they can easily change configurations from docile yeast to predatory fungi that can burrow through the intestinal wall and cause systemic infection. Studies of root-canalled teeth and cavitation sites (voids in the jawbone under teeth) show large concentrations of fungi, and a test discussed in the following section can detect them. One reason I do not like to see plastics used as dental restoration materials or even for orthodontics is that they apparently act as ideal surfaces on which Candida can form biofilms that are very hard to eradicate [275].

Mercury is an antifungal, which is one reason why thimerosal is used in vaccines. So at first blush, having a lifetime supply of it in our teeth and cells would sound like a good thing. We know, however, that prolonged use of a single type of antifungal can lead to the development of yeast that has become resistant to that antifungal. Could it be that the constant presence of mercury from amalgams, vaccinations, and fish can spawn mercury and antifungal-resistant yeast? You bet, but it only gets worse. For reasons nobody has yet figured out, yeast loves heavy metals, including mercury, and is happy to form compounds with them. Yeast has actually been used commercially to mop up heavy metal spills, and in mining applications to assist in extraction of metals. The upshot of all this is the creation of yeast that is resistant to most of the natural and pharmaceutical antifungals, as well as yeast that has bonded with mercury in our bodies [276] [277, 278].

There are many theories regarding the implications of the above information. One theory is that the body, in order to protect itself from mercury toxicity, will preferentially support the overgrowth of yeast so that mercury will bond with it, taking it out of circulation [279]. Ironically, one could thus look at yeast as a detox agent, which somehow bonds to heavy metals. However, unlike real detox agents, which escort toxins out of the body, the yeast/metal combination is quite happy to stay put.

Another theory supporting the yeast/mercury relationship is the following. Neutrophils are a form of white blood cell produced by the immune system to fight invading organisms, and they are a first-line defense against fungi such as Candida [280]. Unfortunately, mercury disables neutrophils, severely limiting their ability to control fungal overgrowth [281] [282], and as a result the body is unable to keep Candida in check, permitting a large amount of mercury-bonded Candida to reside in the gut and perhaps elsewhere in the body. Now, let's say you decide you have Candida overgrowth, and start taking antifungals to get rid of it. To the extent the antifungals are successful, you may inadvertently be releasing large amounts of mercury from the damaged yeast cells, and this mercury can now redistribute, potentially causing more damage than the Candida overgrowth.

In light of the above, others and I believe that wholesale antifungal therapy may be counterproductive for those who are mercury toxic, and a more realistic approach is to tolerate, to the extent you are comfortable, Candida overgrowth symptoms while at the same time detoxing the mercury. There are all sorts of tests available that claim to detect fungal overgrowth, including stool and saliva tests. I have found them to be less than reliable, with many false negatives. Another approach that has been proposed is to take an antifungal, such as nystatin, and see what happens. Supposedly, if you get an adverse reaction, you can assume it is the result of a yeast die-off reaction. Conversely, if you do not get a reaction, you supposedly do not have a yeast problem. While it is not a bad idea to try this test, it does not always work, because at most it proves that you no longer have yeast that is sensitive to that antifungal. As stated above, the mercury-Candida connection produces antifungal-resistant strains that do not die when you take some antifungals, so the lack of a reaction may not be a reliable indication of anything other than that the antifungal you are using does not work.

The detox community has found it most puzzling that the symptom list for Candida overgrowth is virtually identical to the symptom list for mercury toxicity. I am going to go out on a limb here, based on years of self-experimentation and research, and make the following statement. If you are mercury toxic, you will have a persistent yeast overgrowth problem, and conversely, if you have a persistent yeast overgrowth problem, you are mercury toxic – period. In fact, the two conditions are intimately related, which is why the symptom list is virtually the same. This really is not rocket science, and what follows is some additional research that has led me to make this conclusion.

Conventional wisdom has concluded that extensive use of antibiotics is a sufficient cause for a Candida overgrowth problem that continues even after the discontinuance of the antibiotic. However, not everyone that takes antibiotics ends up with fungal overgrowth, and many tests have been run on non-immunocompromised rats that show that the gut is quite capable of re-colonizing to normal after antibiotics have been stopped [283]. I believe it is mercury (and/or another heavy metal) overload, which works in combination with antibiotic or hormone use, (either of which itself can become a necessary cause of chronic Candida overgrowth), whereby the combination provides the sufficiency to sustain Candida overgrowth after antibiotics have been stopped. In the autism treatment community, it has become well established that kids with autism respond well to both antifungal therapy as well as mercury chelation therapy, again showing another strong link between the two conditions [284].

Some believe that Candida is limited to the gut and therefore could not cause systemic illness. Candida does not have to leave the gut to produce systemic illness. It produces dozens of toxins that can easily travel throughout the body to do damage. One of these toxins is acetaldehyde, described more fully below. It is also well known that Candida populates virtually all of the mucus membranes of the body, including the vagina and the sinuses. Recent studies have shown that most nasal, sinus and ear infections are really fungal in origin, and using antibiotics or cortisone-based medicines will seriously aggravate the condition [285].

Another parallel between Candida and mercury includes treatments that involve decreasing the amount of copper in the body. Most mercury-detox protocols include attempts to decrease copper, which also happens to be the same protocol for Candida control. It turns out that not only is Candida tolerant of high copper concentrations, copper also increases its virulence [286, 287]. It is also interesting that nystatin, a soil-based antifungal, is known to remove copper, and this may be part of its action against Candida [288]. Molybdenum is another link between mercury and Candida. This metal is often prescribed in mercury-detox protocols, and yet it is also quite important in supporting the enzymes used to render harmless acetaldehyde, a toxic byproduct of Candida. Thiamine (vitamin B-1) is yet another link. It is used as a supplement with some success in treating autistic children, and it is also found to be depleted by acetaldehyde in Candida overgrowth, probably as a result of magnesium deficiency (thiamine requires magnesium to function properly). Lastly, the detrimental and long lasting effect of mercury on neutrophils, a first line body defense against fungal overgrowth [282], seals the deal for me – we are really talking about what probably should be called the "Mercury-Yeast Spectrum Disorder™," so in keeping with "we name it we tame it," I hereby anoint this nasty disorder as MYSD.

Some additional discussion is warranted on the role of acetaldehyde in the Candida overgrowth matrix of symptoms, because I believe it plays such a large role. As you may remember in the diet section above, I described how fruit fallen from a tree can ferment in the presence of yeast, yielding a high alcohol (ethanol) content. When the sugars in carbohydrates are exposed to Candida in the human gut, the same thing happens, and ethanol is produced. It is then broken down into carbon dioxide and water in the same way that alcohol from an alcoholic beverage is processed by the body. During this process, which takes place in the liver and other organs such as the brain and kidneys, a potent neurotoxin is produced called acetaldehyde (AH). From my research, this toxin is the culprit behind many of the symptoms resulting from the mercury-yeast spectrum disorder, which, by the way, also shares many of the symptoms of the autism spectrum disorder, as well as many of the symptoms of chronic alcoholism! Yes, alcoholism. Because of the propensity for yeast to produce alcohol, it occurred to me (and others) that an overgrowth might be akin to having an alcohol still in the gut that is pumping it into our system 24/7. The amounts generated may be too low to be easily measured in the bloodstream, yet its persistence can have a severe impact on health.

I am now going to discuss AH in some depth, based on the combination of a chain of observations that look like the following. There is a mercury-yeast-spectrum-disorder, and it causes chronic alcohol production in the gut, leading to the continuous formation of acetaldehyde (AH), which may well be the cause of or a contributing factor for many of the symptoms related to this disorder. I will also discuss supplements that have been shown to offset the damage caused by AH and ethanol.

Dr. Truss, previously mentioned as a leader in yeast disorder research, came to this conclusion more than 25 years ago: there is a strong relationship between Candida overgrowth (candidiasis) and the symptoms of chronic alcohol poisoning. Much of the following information is derived from his important research paper entitled *Metabolic Abnormalities in Patients with Chronic Candidiasis – The Acetaldehyde Hypothesis* [289]. Dr, Truss, in turn, relied upon experts in the field of alcoholism treatment, including Dr. Charles Lieber, whose study entitled *Alcohol: Its Metabolism and Interaction With Nutrients* also forms a part of my discussion [290].

While most of the research that has been conducted regarding the adverse effects of AH is primarily directed toward the treatment of alcoholism, it turns out that much the same damage takes place in the mercury-yeast disorder. AH causes brain damage by interfering with the oxygen-carrying capability of red blood cells, and causes nerve-cell damage in a manner similar to that in Alzheimer's disease. AH induces magnesium deficiency, thiamine (vitamin B1) deficiency, niacin (vitamin B3) deficiency, coenzyme A (derived in part from vitamin B5) deficiency, and P5P (another reason for vitamin B6 supplementation) deficiency. It also interferes with the body's ability to use delta-6 desaturase to convert essential omega-6 fatty acids to GLA (gamma-linolenic acid), an important fatty acid for mood regulation and to control inflammation.

AH binds to sulfhydryl groups, which are the very groups relied upon by the mercury and lead chelating agents referred to above, hence interfering with their detox action. On the other hand, this sulfhydryl binding also takes AH out of action, reducing its toxicity [291]. AH also bind to amines, the results of which are far reaching, including: abnormalities in porphyrin metabolism (which also happens with mercury toxicity and which lead to the UPPA test, as discussed in the previous section). AH causes glutathione depletion (leading to free-radical damage), interference with liver metabolism of toxins, and derangement of amino acids in the body. AH also interferes with fatty acids, whereby most omega-3 fatty acid levels are depressed. It also uniquely increases the fluidity of membranes lining the gut wall, leading me to speculate that AH is a major cause of the "leaky gut syndrome" where toxins can pass through the intestinal membrane into the bloodstream. AH also produces opiates that cause cravings for things such as sugar and alcohol, which feed the cycle of further AH production [292].

I could go on for many more pages reciting the damage caused by AH and the uncanny similarity to Candida overgrowth and mercury toxicity symptoms, but I will focus on two areas in particular than can have far reaching effects on health, and for which certain supplement therapies has proven successful. The first has to do with the effect of AH on the membranes of the red blood cells. Although as stated above, the fluidity of gut wall membranes is increased, in the case of red blood cells, AH stiffens their membranes. This rigidity interferes with the ability of the blood cells to pass through many of the small capillaries in the body, and disrupts the ability of nutrients to enter the blood cells. The result of these disruptions can range from mineral transport abnormalities (this also happens with mercury toxicity), energy disruption, neurological symptoms, and nutrient and oxygen deprivation. Mitral valve prolapse, carpal tunnel syndrome, non-responsiveness to hormones, and imbalances of the autonomic nervous system are just a few of the problems that may be caused by the membrane stiffness effects of AH.

An unusual supplement has been used to overcome the effects of this membrane stiffness, and it is a particular form of phosphatidylcholine (PC) known as polyenylphosphatidylcholine (PPC). These are long words for fat-soluble molecules that are a natural part of cell membranes in the body, depleted by AH. From my research, there is only one source of PPC in the US. It is made and sold under the name PhosChol by Nutrasal [293], is also sold under the name PPC by Source Naturals, and is sold under the name Hepatopro by Life Extension Foundation [129]. It is derived from soy, not one of my favorite foods, but in this instance, the product appears to be devoid of the proteins and phytosterols that contribute to soy toxicity, so I use it as a detoxification supplement while dealing with MYSD. I take three gelcaps daily (900 mg each), one with each meal.

Liver toxicity is the second major area of health disruption caused by ethanol and AH. It is probably no surprise to anyone that chronic levels of alcohol and its metabolites delivered to the liver for detoxification can result in the classic symptoms of alcoholic liver disease. The supplement of choice in dealing with this issue is S-adenosylmethionine (SAMe), a coenzyme used to support the methylation pathways in the liver. It is sold under a variety of brands such as Source Naturals, and I take 200 to 400 mg twice a day, away from meals. There is also research to show that the amino acid taurine works in conjunction with magnesium, and protects the liver of rats from ethanol damage [294] [295]. It also acts to support neutrophils, the body's defense against Candida [296]. As you recall, one of the suggested oral magnesium supplements is magnesium taurate, which contains a substantial amount of taurine. Note that vitamin B6 also acts to support neutrophils [297].

I mentioned a unique form of vitamin B-5, pantethine, in the stress section above for its ability to support the adrenal glands. It also has been found to lower the blood levels of AH, apparently by increasing the activity of aldehyde dehydrogenase, an enzyme that breaks down AH to acetic acid [298]. Additionally, pantethine appears to have the unique characteristic of not supporting the growth of yeasts, yet it strongly supports the growth of healthy gut bacteria [299]. Add to this the fact that pantethine improves the lipid profile (in ways that are not understood), and you end up with an important supplement for both the fungal and stress detox areas.

There are additional supplement protocols designed to deal with AH by either binding with it or hastening its conversion to acetic acid by the liver. I have experimented at length with many of these and found that they either do not produce any meaningful results, or aggravate the yeast overgrowth. One set of examples is the taking of large doses of vitamins in an attempt to replace those lost due to Candida overgrowth. This can be quite counterproductive because Candida thrives on vitamins, particularly the B vitamins, including biotin, thiamine, B-3 and B-6 [300]. The B vitamin protocols I mentioned earlier, particularly the coenzymated sublingual versions of B-complex and B-6 appear to be a good compromise.

A vitamin-A supplement (unfortunately synthetic) may also be useful because it is depleted by ethanol, and one source is Bio-Ae-Mulsion from Biotics Research. I have used a daily dose of 4000 IU. It is my belief that vitamin A supplements should always be taken with vitamin D3 supplements to prevent toxicity, because they are almost always found together in nature in about a 10:1 ratio (in units of IU), such as in natural cod liver oil. As indicated earlier, I take 4000 IU of vitamin A, and I make sure I take at least 400 IU of synthetic vitamin D3. Additional information regarding the interactions between vitamins A and D can be found on the Weston Price Foundation website [7].

A caution is in order with respect to synthetic vitamin A and beta-carotene supplementation in the presence of ethanol. Lieber has found that ethanol both depletes vitamin A and potentiates its repletion, leaving a rather narrow window for supplementation, since excessive vitamin A can produce liver toxicity. I limit my supplementation to 4000 IU and feel comfortable that adding vitamin D resolves the toxicity issue.

The interaction between ethanol and beta-carotene is quite unusual. As I mentioned earlier, I do not take beta-carotene as an isolated nutrient, but always as part of a carotenoid complex. Well, studies have found that when beta-carotene was taken in combination with ethanol, it increased liver toxicity as compared to ethanol alone. I know of no studies related to the use of the entire carotenoid complex, such as found in red palm oil, but I feel comfortable that sticking with MA's formula will avoid adverse effects.

Yet another compound that is a natural part of the Wellness Diet has been found to protect the liver from the toxic effects of alcohol, and that is the amino acid glycine. As discussed above, gelatin is a major source of glycine, and its inclusion in the Wellness Diet should provide long-term liver recovery and protection [301] [302].

Some in the Candida-supplement world believe that taking additional biotin will prevent the Candida yeast from converting to its invasive form, but that has been shown not to be true [303]. What keeps Candida happy in the gut is glucose. If it is starved of glucose, conversion to an invasive form is likely to take place, where it can burrow through the intestinal wall and become systemic. Now, let's move on to controlling this beast.

As I indicated above, trying to wipe out Candida overgrowth while you still have a significant body-burden of mercury may be counterproductive. Further, the body's defense system remains crippled by mercury, so that it is unable to control Candida regrowth. However, there is a program that I have used to control Candida overgrowth symptoms and some of the damage it causes. My approach is to minimize killing the fungus outright, all while continuing to reduce my mercury body burden using the protocols described above in the heavy metal section. A first approach is not to overfeed it, and I have found the Wellness Diet to be quite helpful in controlling Candida, even though fresh fruit is part of the diet. From my experience, the major Candida culprits related to fruit are dried fruit and fruit juices, both high in sugars and not part of the diet.

Second, I try to support the immune system naturally by taking a supplement designed to do so. The one I use is called ProBoost by Genicel [304], which is a sublingual powder that contains a protein normally provided by the thymus gland, and which supports the entire immune system in a totally natural manner. There is substantial research on their website showing the efficacy of the product in relation to the immune system, as well as having a suppressive effect on Candida overgrowth[305]. I take one packet of the powder daily, but up to three per day can be taken if needed to help suppress infection. I consider this supplement of such importance in this modern world of infectious toxins that I have incorporated it as a part of my regular diet. Finally, a supplement based on the amino acid cysteine, N-Acetyl-cysteine (NAC) has been shown to reduce the damage caused by AH and to stimulate the activity of neutrophils [306] [307] [308, 309] [310]. NAC is a sulfur compound which can weakly bond to mercury and drag it around, so some mercury toxic people do not tolerate it. I have not found any problems using it along with the alkalinity protocol. There are many brands available, and I take one per meal of the 500 mg Jarrow Formulas brand N-A-C during detox [128].

While we are on the topic of sulfur compounds and Candida, there are conflicting data in the research community as to whether sulfur-containing compounds promote or deter Candida overgrowth. Sulfur is the third most abundant mineral in our body and is a component of every cell. In its elemental form, sulfur is a potent antifungal, and has been used as such for millennia. Of course, all of the mercury chelating agents are sulfur-containing compounds, as are SAMe, NAC, and an enormous number of foods. It is unclear from the research as to which sulfur compounds might feed Candida growth in the human intestine, if any. From my point of view, I feel comfortable taking these supplements in conjunction with the overall Candida control protocols outlined in this section. Some people have an adverse reaction to particular sulfur containing foods, and the only one of substance in the Wellness Diet as a possibly acceptable food is egg yolk. These adverse reactions may be due to a Candida issue (either die-off or perhaps an increase in virulence), or some other factor which may involve the ability of the liver to process sulfur compounds.

Bad things happen when you mix Candida (and other yeasts) with cortisone – yeasts really grow out of control. The theory is that cortisone, a hormone, suppresses the immune system, allowing free reign for fungal overgrowth, as demonstrated by several research studies [311] [312] [313]. For those battling with the MYSD, use of cortisone over a period long enough to cause immune suppression is not a very good idea. While it may provide some short-term symptom relief, it is counterproductive in the long haul, leading to a fungal nightmare. This leaves the Jefferies protocol (discussed in the stress section), which theoretically does not involve immune suppressive doses of hydrocortisone (they are typically 5 mg doses four times per day). I have also found the use of cortisone nasal sprays or even excessive use of strong cortisone skin creams can aggravate yeast overgrowth and I avoid them. Other hormones, particularly progesterone, similarly encourage overgrowth, and women on birth control pills are known to be predisposed to yeast infections [15]. I also consider magnesium supplementation a very important part of the Candida protocol, since it is depleted by AH, leading to a further compromise of the immune system, as well as to gut problems [314].

The next part of the Candida control protocol is to make the gut somewhat inhospitable to fungal overgrowth, using the principal of competitive exclusion, discussed above in the dirt section. The objective is to fill many of the gut receptor sites that might be used by Candida with some friendly stuff that can adhere to these sites. At one time I though that conventional probiotics could fill the bill, and it may work for many in controlling overgrowth. However, in the presence of mercury, it seems something stronger is necessary for this task. Enter dirt!

Of the two spore-former species I discussed above, bacillus laterosporus has a history of controlling Candida overgrowth in even the most difficult of cases. I take one per day as part of the Wellness Diet, and when detoxing with the Dirt Detox Protocol I am on a daily dose of two per day to assist in keeping the gut flora under control.

Now that we have added defense system support and competitive exclusion to the fungal protocol, let's move on to a discussion of antifungals themselves (fungicides that actually kill the fungus). Although I said we do not want to do any major Candida destruction to avoid mercury overload, it would be nice to have something available for gentle control. An ideal candidate would be a natural antifungal, which has MA's seal of approval on it for use in the human body, which is only toxic to the bad stuff, and is impervious to the development of resistance. Re-enter iodine!

Not only is iodine an excellent antifungal [315], it is also a detox agent, as we shall see in the halogen section below. To the extent that it liberates mercury by killing yeast, it may assist in pushing it out of the body (it is not a chelator). As a matter of interest, Dr. Truss, one of the first to identify the Candida problem in the 1950s, is said to have successfully used Lugol's solution as an antifungal agent, years before most of the pharmaceutical agents were available. He apparently prescribed 6 to 8 drops four times per day, which is about 150-200 milligrams per day, more than 1000 times the RDA of iodine.

As part of my halogen detox protocol, I routinely take 75 mg of iodine daily (with occasional breaks) which, along with the immune system boosting supplement ProBoost, has kept my Candida overgrowth under control without aggravating the mercury detox side effects. I have found that for Candida control, Lugol's solution is a better choice than iodine tablets. Some iodine tablets have an enteric coating so that they do not dissolve until they have passed the stomach. For Candida control, you may well want the iodine in the mouth, esophagus, and upper intestine, so I swish a diluted amount of it in the mouth, and sip it slowly to get the best effect. Recall that there are now two strengths of Lugol's solution on the market. The Truss formula used the original full-strength version, so adjustments should be made if the new reduced strength product is used. Regarding pre- and probiotics, it remains unclear if one or both of these products actually feed the multitude of fungal strains in the gut, so I would use caution until sufficient fungal and parasite detox has taken place.

To wrap up the Candida discussion, my analysis of the persistent Candida overgrowth problem is that it is intimately involved with mercury toxicity. Further, trying to wipe out Candida in this instance is counterproductive and actually not likely to be successful long term as long as mercury levels remain high. The defense system is sufficiently damaged by mercury that Candida overgrowth would quickly return even if you could temporarily wipe it out. I have outlined a protocol of defense system support (boosting the immune system and magnesium levels), competitive exclusion (using spore-formers), and mild antifungal use (iodine) to keep things under control. I believe this is a good overall approach to a very difficult detoxification problem involving many players. I continue to experiment with the Dirt Detox protocol to evaluate its role in controlling the fungal problem.

Before leaving the fungal area, I would like to mention the problem of mold, which is fungus gone wild. The mold problem, sometimes referred to as the "Sick Building Syndrome," usually originates in a home or building with insufficient ventilation and sunlight, and excess moisture, coupled with building materials that foster fungal growth. If the damage is sufficiently extensive, usually the only solution is total destruction. In this regard, I have some suggestions in the lifestyle section on living environment regarding home construction. Several books on mold toxicity have been written, and they indicate that supplements that bind with bile have been used with success in treating symptoms from mold exposure [316]. The use of apple pectin may be particularly useful in this instance. It is my belief that following The Wellness Project, including the suggestions in this section, will at least free up the defense system to deal with mold to the greatest extent possible.

## The Bacterial Problem

In this section, we are going to visit the issue of toxic bacteria in the body, where it came from, and what to do about it. First, let's look at some of the history related to treatments for bacterial infections. In the dairy discussion of the diet section, I mentioned the Germ Theory, promulgated by Pasteur, which states that microorganisms are the cause of infections. This was in conflict with the Terrain Theory that said a compromised immune system causes infections. Claude Bernard and Antoine Bechamp popularized this theory in the mid 1800's [317]. One of the fundamental precepts of The Wellness Project is to strengthen the internal environment by putting the good stuff in and getting the bad stuff out, and in this regard, The Wellness Project is in alignment with the Terrain Theory. This conflict of theories is yet another example where the medical community has confused necessary causes with sufficient causes. For an infection to occur requires both a pathogenic microorganism *and* a compromised defense system. Each is necessary, but neither in itself is sufficient to result in an infection. Therefore, I will now take the liberty of combining the Germ and Terrain Theories into what I will coin "The Infection Theory™," as follows: An infection requires a potentially pathogenic microorganism and a compromised defense system incapable of controlling the growth and dissemination of that organism.

The parallels between the Germ Theory, the Cholesterol Theory and the Skin Cancer Theory are quite clear. In each case, there are at least two elements necessary to produce the result, and in each case the medical community has chosen to attack what, in hindsight, has proven to be the wrong element. Examples are cholesterol, UV exposure, and germs. In each of these cases, the other element in the equation is a compromised defense system. By ignoring this element, decades have been wasted where defense system research could have been conducted that would now be bearing fruit (pun intended) in preventing these and other maladies. This is why The Wellness Project is all about strengthening the defense system. We now read almost daily that the "Antibiotic Era" is fast coming to an end as bacteria mutate faster than we can create antibiotics, spawning deadly strains that are resistant to everything Big Pharma has to offer. (As you will see, The Wellness Project has a "secret weapon" for these critters, courtesy of MA).

Previously, I mentioned the critical role that intestinal bacteria, sometimes referred to as the microflora or microbiome, plays in keeping us healthy, and it is a very important part of our defense system. Of course, the intent of The Wellness Project is to support the body to establish or reestablish a healthy gut environment, and the suggested soil components play an important role. Enter mercury again.

In spite of all the negative things I have said about mercury, it is a very potent antibiotic and antifungal, and for many years was the preferred medication to treat syphilis. While it sometimes cured the disease, many times it killed the patient. Now, let's think about this: there is finally general consensus, even by the ADA (American Dental Association), that amalgam fillings outgas mercury continuously into the body. If mercury is an antibiotic, theoretically, those with amalgams in place have a built-in lifetime source of antibiotics leaking into their body 24/7. Sounds good, but it is not.

There has been a lot of press lately on how the over-prescription of antibiotics has spawned super-bacteria such as MRSA (methicillin resistant staphylococcus aureus) and other nasty flesh-eating stuff. The problem, of course, is that bacteria are able to become resistant to antibiotics when exposed to them long enough. Further, we know that taking antibiotics, which do not discriminate between good and bad gut bacteria, kills virtually everything, leaving a person vulnerable to regrowth of what could be a very unbalanced mix of flora. Can you image what a lifetime of mercury infusion has done to gut flora? A few bright scientists have undertaken the study of this issue and have found that mercury has not only spawned a host of mercury-resistant bacteria, but that most of these strains have also acquired the traits of resistance to antibiotics in general [318] [319] [320] [321]. If you never had any amalgams, could you still end up with these Frankenbacteria? Well, a group of children was tested who never had amalgam restorations, but who had presumably been vaccinated with thimerosal. They were found to harbor bacteria that were both mercury and general antibiotic resistant [322].

Other than the usual industry denials regarding the above, it is not rocket science to see we have a serious issue here. Considering the number of people that have been exposed to mercury via amalgams or vaccines, I am not sure there are many walking around with what could be called "normal" gut flora. Unless this is accounted for, it would seem that the NIH gut bacteria study might come to the wrong conclusion as to what should be used for a blueprint for healthy gut flora, especially if they do not also account for spore-forming bacteria missing in virtually everyone's gut. From personal experience and other anecdotal reports, I can tell you that mercury can severely influence digestive function by altering gut bacteria, causing what is called intestinal dysbiosis, and making it somewhat impossible to achieve the desired bowel characteristics described in the defecation section above. Symptoms can range from oral thrush (mouth fungus), to GERD, to halitosis, to gut pain, to IBS, to IBD (Irritable Bowel Disease), to constipation, to diarrhea, and to nutrient deficiencies in general. From my point of view, the long-term solution is to follow the Wellness Diet and the detoxification plan to get rid of mercury. Spore-forming bacteria play a critical role in restoring gut function.

Just when you thought we were done with dental issues and bacteria problems, along come root canals, which I refer to as toxic time bombs. A fellow member of the Advisory Board of the Price-Pottenger Nutrition Foundation is Dr. George Meinig, a retired dentist with an extensive career in the field of endodontistry, a sub-specialty dealing with tooth root and pulp issues, including the root canal procedure. Early in his career, Dr. Meinig pioneered in root canal procedures, and was one of the founders of what is now the American Association of Endodontics, who have conferred upon him honorary recognition for his work in the field. When he speaks on the subject of root canals, I listen very carefully. During his career, he became interested in the work of Weston Price, a dentist himself, and by perusing the archives at the Price-Pottenger Nutrition Foundation, discovered reams of research by Price on root canals, documents that had been suppressed by the dental community beginning over 70 years ago. What came out of his research was a book entitled *The Root Canal Cover-up* by George E. Meinig DDS FACD [323] which should be read by everyone who has ever had a root canalled tooth or is contemplating one.

What Price found and Meinig brought to light was that virtually all root-canalled teeth were loaded with bacteria that were producing toxins, and that the toxins were able to travel down the tooth canal to virtually all parts of the body. While a strong defense system is usually able to keep the toxins in check, it just takes some precipitating event that drags down the defense system to enable the toxins to cause major illness. In a fascinating series of experiments, Price was able to take an extracted root-canalled tooth from an ill patient, implant it under the skin of a rabbit, and cause the same illness in the rabbit. Price's studies were conducted over a 25-year period, included a team of 60 scientists, filled 1174 pages, and were conducted under the auspices of the American Dental Association. Unfortunately, some members of that organization decided to bury the results. They also refused to accept the focal theory of infection, where a primary infection can cause systemic illness. We saw this issue resurface in the Candida discussion.

The root canal problem is really not rocket science. There are miles of microtubules that run throughout every tooth. Once a root canal procedure has been performed, the tooth is dead and the blood supply is cut off, so there is no way for the body to control the contents of these tubules, which are filled with bacteria that cannot be reached by antibiotics or anything else. Over time (actually, your lifetime) these bacteria produce virulent toxins that leak down through the tooth canal and, but for the constant vigilance of the defense system, are capable of making the patient ill. Dentists place *gutta percha*, a latex discovered about 150 years ago and derived from the sap of trees grown in Asia, into the opening they made in the tooth when they filed out the pulp, in the hope that it will seal up the opening. Typically, it does not, so more bacteria seeps into the dead tooth.

Recently, new procedures have been tried to fix the problem, but so far there is no proof that they work any better. One is to use a laser to try to sterilize the miles of tubules, and then to use calcium hydroxide (Biocalex® is one brand) as a filler. Approaches that are more recent use ozone and/or oxygen to try to sterilize the tooth. As pointed out in the book *The Roots of Disease* by Robert Kulacz, DDS and Thomas Levy, MD, JD [324], neither the laser nor ozone nor calcium hydroxide do the job. If you are unsure whether your root-canalled teeth are currently toxic, there is a simple and inexpensive test to provide you and your dentist with some answers. It is called the TOPAS test (Toxicity Prescreening Assay), and is available as a research tool to participating dentists [325] while it awaits regulatory approval in the US.

From the perspective of rocket science, root canal procedures are really a technological failure, and would never get you off the launching pad. I share the opinions of Drs. Meinig, Kulacz, Levy and many others that the procedure does not work as intended and has the potential of making someone quite ill. Nevertheless, just like in the diet studies, there is no doubt in my mind that there are folks who can live to 100 in perfect health with a mouth full of root canals. Undoubtedly, they have been endowed with a very strong defense system, and have succeeded in avoiding any catastrophes in life that might impair it. Are you one of them? If not, and if you have root-canalled teeth and wish to keep them, it would be prudent not get sick. The illness list caused by root canal toxins is heavily biased towards heart disease, and the above referenced books have long lists of many other illnesses, which cover virtually everything imaginable.

Root canals are in second place, just behind amalgams, on my list of the major technology errors in the fields of dentistry and medicine. I do applaud the endodontist community for trying hard to find a solution to the problem with new technologies. In the meanwhile, if you have an irreparably damaged tooth, as I did, I believe the safe option is extraction, with a permanent bridge replacement. I have given copies of the above referenced books on root canal issues to friends who have mentioned they are going in for a root canal procedure. Among those who read them, all opted for extraction. Ah, now we get to extractions – and you thought we were finished with the dental industry. Onward to cavitations.

A cavitation is a hole or defect in the jawbone at the site of an old or healed tooth extraction. It may also be present around an infected tooth such as a root canal-treated tooth. The contents of a cavitation typically consist of highly toxic and infected bone and dead tissue, essentially identical in appearance to gangrene as seen in other parts of the body. Studies done with people that have had wisdom tooth extractions show that most have cavitations at these old extraction sites. Many cavitations form when the bone surrounding an extracted tooth is not properly cleansed and treated prior to the closing of the wound.

Procedures for doing this have been developed, and Hal Huggins, mentioned above, has a referral list of oral surgeons trained to perform them. As far as diagnostic tools for detecting cavitations, a trained dentist can use either finger feel, or pin pressure on the bone, or the TOPAS test mentioned above. An even more elegant method is to use ultrasound to view the upper and lower jawbone for cavitation detection. A popular device for accomplishing this is the Cavitat®, and many specially trained oral surgeons use this device [326] because cavitations are sometimes difficult to find, and rarely produce fever or other such signs of infection. In addition to a boatload of illnesses, cavitations are well known for producing facial and other upper body pain, and cleaning them out can remove symptoms almost instantly. I strongly suggest that everyone who has had extractions or root canals be tested at least once for cavitations.

Moving out of the mouth, while there are a plethora of bacteria surrounding us (many of them found in hospitals), one group in particular deserves special attention because of their persistence. These bacteria cause the condition known as Lyme disease, an infectious disease that has stirred up a huge controversy in the medical community, who are busy arguing over the definition. It's clear to me though, and to many doctors, that this is a quite real, serious, and under-diagnosed disease, which can have life-altering consequences, and may be contagious. The disease is believed to be caused by bacteria from the genus *Borrelia* and is transmitted to humans by the bite of infected insects. Symptoms often include fever, headache, fatigue, and sometimes a typical skin rash. The fatigue is bad enough to keep you in bed, and other symptoms, including arthritic-like joint pain, can be disabling.

Officially, the thinking is that most early cases can be treated with large doses of antibiotics for a few weeks. If not caught quickly, some experts advocate massive doses of antibiotics for several years, while others admit that they have not figured out a cure. Dr. Klinghardt has spent many years looking for treatment strategies, and the results of his work can be found in the protocol section of his website [204]. There are interesting parallels between some of the symptoms of Lyme and mercury toxicity, as well as similarities to parasite infestation, and even autism [327]. There is a fascinating protocol in the parasite section below that has given relief to many Lyme sufferers.

To gain control over some of these nasty bacteria as part of a detox program, I have a few natural suggestions. The first is the spore-forming bacteria, for all of the reasons previously mentioned. I have experimented with getting these bacteria into the body by means of nasal sprays, eardrops, skin sprays, and gargles, all with good results. There is no magic formula; I simply put some spore-former powder, say from two capsules, in an ounce or two of mineral water, and put it into a suitable dispenser. I have also added a capsule of humic/fulvic acid to the mix. As far as oral intake, I have experimented with very large spore-former doses (up to 20 capsules per day) for several weeks with no ill effects. An interesting research project would be to treat Lyme suffers with saturation doses of spore-formers to see if they can competitively eliminate or even kill the Borrelia bacteria.

There are many herbal remedies to ward off bacterial infections, and each has a niche. One in particular is somewhat broad-based, and comes from nature's arsenal of plant protectors. It is the seed and pulp of grapefruit, which one would not normally eat on the Wellness Diet because these portions of fruit are naturally toxic. If you are ill or going to be exposed to infections, grapefruit seed extract (GSE), not to be confused with grape seed extract, is a product that has proved helpful, and is widely available as a liquid or tablet. Another herb discussed more fully below is artemesia.

Then there is the latest favorite in non-prescription antibiotics – colloidal silver. As you can tell from some of the earlier discussions in this book, I have done a fair amount of research into silver, which, by the way, can be classified as a heavy metal, is not believed to be an essential mineral, and is known to be toxic at very high exposures. There are many safe colloidal products on the market, and I will tell you about my favorite in a moment. First, some potentially bad news about silver, which, strangely enough, takes us back to amalgam fillings. If you remember, amalgams are about 50% mercury and 50% *silver*. Well, silver does not outgas like mercury, but you can bet that a lifetime of silver in your mouth has caused a certain amount of silver, through abrasion, diffusion, and other processes, to be floating around your body 24/7, and certainly, there would be a very high concentration in the mouth. Could it be that this has spawned silver-resistant bacteria, just as mercury has spawned mercury-resistant bacteria? Apparently so.

A small study conducted on bacteria found on teeth with amalgam fillings identified bacteria strains that were both silver-resistant and also generally resistant to prescription antibiotics [328]. A survey of silver-resistant bacteria shows that several are starting to pop up, which is quite unfortunate. Silver coatings are used widely as microbials in medical procedures, including those involving the insertion of catheters and stents. For the most part, however, silver still has a good track record, and I suggest the brand Sovereign Silver® made by Natural-Immunogenics Corp. [329]. To avoid developing a resistance, I would only use silver sparingly as needed. Alcohol and chlorine are other candidates for antibacterials, but both are toxic. Wouldn't it be great if there was a natural antibiotic, which has MA's seal of approval on it for use in the human body, and (so far) is impervious to the development of resistance? Enter iodine!

I have discussed iodine previously as a detox agent and a potent and natural antibiotic that is also an essential mineral. As far as I am concerned, it is a powerhouse in the category of natural antibiotics. When one studies the literature, there are essentially no reports of any significance showing iodine-resistant bacteria other than an anecdotal report or two. This is good news indeed, since as anyone who has had a hospital medical procedure performed at a hospital is aware, iodine is the antibacterial of choice to clean wounds as well as the surgeon's hands. Speaking of hand cleaning, the many varieties of antibacterial soaps on the market usually contain triclosan as the active ingredient. Reports are starting to surface that widespread use of these products may be creating antibiotic-resistant strains of bacteria, and I avoid their use. My choice for hand cleaners are those containing iodine, including povidone-iodine topical antiseptics such as the line of Betadine products by Purdue Pharma [330], or the many generic products including swabs, sprays and other items listed under povidone or povidone-iodine and sold at most drugstores.

Iodine in the form of Lugol's solution can also be used topically, but it does stain the skin, so one might want to try the Clayodine compound mentioned above. Using iodine topically may well result in systemic absorption, and symptoms of detoxification may arise. For use as a systemic antibiotic, I would take several drops of Lugol's solution in fruit tea and/or gargle with the diluted solution, or take one or more Iodoral tablets. For further discussion, see the halogen section below.

One cannot discuss bacteria without revisiting conventional probiotics. In the discussion in the diet section, I mentioned that probiotics could be helpful or harmful, depending on who benefits more from them, you or the bad guys in your gut. As you can see from the detox discussion so far, there are plenty of bad guys, and there are more to come. My suggestion stands of taking modest doses of only a few strains, at least until a detox program has had a chance to decrease the critter load, which not only includes bacteria, but also fungi and parasites, all of which might indirectly benefit from a large dose of pre- and probiotics. This note of caution arises from my personal experiments, where, based on symptoms, I was able to worsen Candida overgrowth by taking large doses of conventional probiotics. Others have also found that probiotics can feed parasites [331], and prebiotics such as FOS can feed unwelcome bacteria, especially *Klebsiella pneumoniae, hemolytic E. coli, Bacteroides* species, and *Staphylococcus aureus* [332].

This note of caution does not apply to spore-formers, which do not suffer any of the problems associated with conventional probiotics, and that brings me to a discussion of the Dirt Detox Protocol as applied to bacteria. Spore-formers such as bacillus laterosporus have been tested against salmonella and pathogenic strains of E. coli with excellent results, so I would expect the protocol to work well against toxic gut bacteria.

Regarding testing for nasty gut bacteria, there are a number of stool tests that can be performed that may be useful in analyzing gut bacteria, fungi, and parasites. One that I have used is called the CDSA (Comprehensive Digestive Stool Analysis) test by Genova Diagnostics [333].

## The Parasite Problem

Closely allied to the fungal problem is the parasite problem. For purposes of this section, I will define parasites as including worms, amoeba, flukes, and protozoa. Like bacteria and fungi, most parasites reside in our gut, and some are friendly while others are not. Also like bacteria and fungi, we have yet to identify what are probably thousands of different parasites in our gut. Many folks deny they have parasites, but in my opinion, it is virtually impossible to avoid them whenever you open your mouth and put something in it, and they may also enter via the eyes, ears, nose, and skin. I feel comfortable making the statement that virtually everyone who has not been routinely treated for them harbors parasites. At present and for the foreseeable future, it is practically impossible to prove me wrong because there is no foolproof test for parasite infestation, and I have tried many. Obviously, it is hard to test for strains of parasites we have yet to identify, but there is no lack of trying by a multitude of test labs.

We can get many clues about parasites from the animal kingdom (including insects), where this issue is taken very seriously, as it should be. Animals spend a great deal of time managing their parasite infestations and they are highly attuned to know when they are infected. Humans, on the other hand, know virtually nothing about parasites and have lost any instinct regarding whether or not we are infested. Clues from MA such as intestinal discomfort are treated with the usual symptom-suppressing OTC and prescription products, without getting to the source of the problem. For this reason, most of us are walking around with a lifetime load of untreated parasite infestations for which the symptom list goes on for pages. To find clues to infestation, let's look at how animals deal with the problem, as explained in Cindy Engel's book *Wild Health*, a major source of the following information [9].

For parasite control, most animals resort to the toxins in the parts of plants that we avoid as food choices in the Wellness Diet. In their war against parasites, they choose plants that are not part of their normal diet, usually very bitter, and whose levels of toxicity can sometimes approach lethal amounts. They will also eat rough plant parts, mostly folded leaves, in an effort to hook on to and scrape parasites from the intestinal wall, known as the Velcro® effect. Dogs and cats are occasionally known to eat grass, which can have a scouring effect as well as promote vomiting as an additional purge. Actually, tolerance of or a desire for very bitter plants, even in humans, has been directly correlated with the degree of parasite infestation in that person, and as the infestation decreases, so does the tolerance of bitters. The bitters usually include tannins, saponins and other alkaloids toxic to parasites. The plant *vernonia amygdalina* is particularly potent, and studies are underway to investigate its use as a drug.

Another way in which animals control parasites is through the purgative effect of *salt*. Parasite infested camels routinely seek out the very salty plant *Salvadora persica* (commonly known as peelu), as well as salt-rich wells to gain the purging effects of salt. As you will see below, I view this as a major clue from MA regarding parasite control. Yet another animal control method for parasites is our old friend clay. It appears to help in three ways: by adsorbing toxins excreted by the parasites, by physically expelling worm eggs, and by protecting the gut from invasion from migrating worm larvae [334]. Before going into a discussion on parasite control, a caution is warranted on the use of pre- or probiotics when a heavy parasite load may be present, because they may well end up feeding the parasites. Once clearance has occurred, then some higher-dose, broader-strain products might be helpful [331] [335].

So far, from our excursion into the animal world we have discovered that toxic plant parts, clay, and salt are all used as natural remedies. I suggest these same routes for human parasite cleansing. Starting with plant parts, there are many herbal parasite-cleanse products on the market, and here are some of the protocols I have used with good results. The first is an herbal concoction that has been used for many years, and is produced and sold directly by a small company called Humaworm, Inc. [336]. It is a 30-day program of two capsules per day, which can be repeated every 90 days, if necessary. Their website lists the formula, and has some helpful information regarding symptoms and detox reactions. Generally, every six months I repeat the cleanse.

The second suggestion is known as the Clark Para-Cleanse protocol, using green-black walnut hulls, wormwood (artemesia), and common cloves. The ingredients and one-week protocol for using them are widely available in health food stores and on the web. The black walnut hulls and wormwood kill adult and developmental stages of many types of parasites, and the cloves kill the eggs. This protocol is high dose/short time, and can produce some unexpectedly severe die-off reactions such as dizziness and nausea, so you might want to have a partner around during the program. This protocol can also be repeated once every several months. When you have cleaned out everything that these formulas are able to handle, you should notice no symptoms upon redoing the protocol. None of these formulas is perfect, and they are not capable of removing all forms of parasites, so let's move on to clay .

The types of clay and dosages previously mentioned as part of the Dirt Detox Protocol may be incorporated into an herbal parasite cleanse, or even delayed until immediately thereafter. Remember to separate the taking of clay and other soil components from the herbs by about two hours.

At this point, I would like to mention the problem of pollution-linked illnesses involving parasitic organisms, many of which are acquired by eating seafood from polluted waters, another problem totally avoided in the Wellness Diet. Books have been written on this topic [337] and it is my belief that following The Wellness Project, including the suggestions in this section, will at least free up the defense system to deal with this problem to the extent possible.

Now for the real surprise in the human world of parasite cleansing – salt. If we had paid more attention to the animal world in the past, perhaps the role of salt as a parasite cleanser would have surfaced sooner. A few years ago, a group of Lyme disease sufferers tried an experiment of taking large doses of salt (eight grams or more per day) along with vitamin C. What happened next was quite unexpected – parasites of all sorts started to exit their bodies in great numbers from unusual locations such as their eyes, ears, and skin. As a result of this discovery, the Salt/C protocol, as it is called, was launched. Some long-time Lyme sufferers who were getting nowhere with conventional treatment suddenly found major relief using this protocol. A website has been launched showing photos of many types of parasites that have exited bodies, and I caution the reader that some of these photos can be quite unsettling [338]. While the experiments so far have been primarily with Lyme sufferers, there is no reason to suppose this protocol will not work for anyone suffering from parasites for whatever reason. It does raise the question, however, as to whether the insect bite or sting that transfers the Lyme bacteria may also be transferring parasites directly into the bloodstream, which then spread everywhere and rapidly multiply.

From the website, you can find the details of the protocol. There are web support forums for those experimenting with it (look for Yahoo groups with the word *lyme* in the title). For my own experiments, I used ancient seabed unrefined salt, mentioned earlier, and put it into 00 size gelatin capsules. I also used buffered vitamin C capsules and took up to ten grams per day of both for a few weeks. Because I had done extensive parasite cleanses beforehand, I had no surprises. By the way, the objective of these protocols is not necessarily to totally eradicate all parasites from the body. Some studies have shown that having a small amount hanging around may be beneficial for some intestinal illnesses [339].

The dramatic effects of salt as a natural detoxifier (even more on this in the next section) raises the question of whether our low-salt craze, which has been recently escalated to a near hysterical anti-salt movement, has jeopardized the health of millions by essentially eliminating this natural defender. This is not rocket science. I don't think it is a coincidence that MA has provided us with salt taste buds, or that the blood of our prey contains pounds of salt. Here is one more of my predictions. The low-salt craze will eventually make it to the top-ten list of technology blunders in the history of medicine. This brings me to a discussion of bromide.

## The Halogen Problem

I have already acquainted the reader with iodine (a halogen) as a detoxifier, so let's look at what there is left to detoxify (plenty). Iodine's toxic halogen cousins that are of interest to us are the bromides, fluorides and a chlorine compound known as perchlorate. Let's start with bromine, and bromide, which is a reduced form of bromine. Bromine may or may not be an essential micromineral in the body in extremely small doses, but in excess it is very bad news, and we are awash in it. Currently, bromide is found in pesticides (methyl bromide); bread products (potassium bromate); brominated vegetable oil that may be added to citrus-flavored drinks; hot tub disinfectants; certain asthma inhalers and prescription drugs; personal care products like toothpaste and mouthwash; fabric dyes; and as flame retardants (PBDEs) in drapes, coats, pajamas, mattresses, carpeting, and most plastic products in consumer applications such as computers and cell phones.

As reported in Dr. Brownstein's book on iodine, previously cited [240], bromine in sufficient concentrations replaces iodine in the body.

The results: every thyroid condition you can think of, including hypo- and hyperthyroid and autoimmune conditions to thyroid cancer; skin conditions known as bromoderma, which can express as acne-like lesions, cherry angiomas and other strange rashes; mental conditions from depression to schizophrenia; hearing problems; and kidney cancer from bromates such as those used as dough conditioners in bread products. This last application is another technology blunder that should be recognized with some sort of award.

Dough conditioners are used to increase production of bread-making, in other words, to save money. Originally, iodine compounds were used in this application, but because of an erroneous conclusion that consumers would ingest excessive iodine, in the 1980s the industry switched over to potassium bromate, a known carcinogen. This substance is banned in Canada and the UK, but is considered safe in the U.S. Fortunately for Wellness Diet users, we dodge this blunder.

Are there any clues from MA substantiating the bromine debacle? Yes, a very sad one. A recent study was conducted in an attempt to find the causes of an epidemic among cats of feline hyperthyroidism (FH). Brominated flame retardants known as polybrominated diphenyl ethers (PBDEs) came up as a major culprit [340]. Pet cats may be like canaries in coalmines when it comes to evaluating the health impacts of these persistent chemicals, used in carpets, furniture, and electronics. Veterinarians first noticed a dramatic surge in feline hyperthyroidism (FH) in the 1980s, coinciding with the use of PBDEs as flame-retardants in consumer products. FH, the most common endocrine disorder in cats, causes rapid weight loss due to increased concentrations of thyroxine. They found that hyperthyroidal cats had very high body burdens of PBDEs, which are in residential carpeting as well as in cat food, particularly fish-flavored canned brands. Cats swallow PBDEs in food and by licking PBDE-laden house dust from their fur. The bromine atoms in the PBDEs mimic the iodine in thyroxine, displacing it and leading to the FH condition. The potential link between FH and PBDEs suggests that house cats may be sentinels for chronic indoor PBDE exposure in people. As the author of the study speculated, "like cats, toddlers may be inordinately exposed to PBDEs in dust by crawling on floors and placing objects in their mouths."

Wherever you are currently reading this book, the odds are that you are surrounded by this bromine-laden chemical, since it is in most upholstered furniture and in plastic enclosures for electrical and electronic products. Perhaps the human epidemic of subclinical hypothyroidism (bromine can cause hypo- or hyperthyroid conditions) is related to these chemicals, which are also found in high concentrations in lake, river and farmed fish. Even worse, fish also contain PCBs, and a study has shown the combination of the two (PBDEs and PCBs) interact in a manner that enhances their individual neurotoxicity [84].

The cat study mentioned above prompts me to suggest another clue from MA. If you have pets and they are exhibiting illness, perhaps you are at risk, since you share the same environment. As you will see in the lifestyle section, I am not in favor of indoor carpeting, and this is one more reason for my position. While we are on the subject of thyroid glands, there are many studies linking thyroid conditions to deranged cholesterol levels, particularly elevated LDL levels, so the halogen problem may extend its tentacles all the way into the statin drug arena [341].

Under certain conditions, bromide in water may be converted to bromate, a known carcinogen, if ozone is used in the water purification cycle. This has led to some embarrassments for the bottled water industry (a large recall), as well as for the Los Angeles Water Department, who recently announced the dumping of 600 million gallons of bromate-contaminated water, possibly as the result of ozonation of bromide contaminated water. It also seems possible that bromide in the presence of chlorine and sunlight can be converted to bromates. Some forms of charcoal, and RO water filters remove bromates.

Using bromine (or chlorine) for hot tub or swimming pool disinfection is definitely not a good idea, and I suggest ozone instead as the best of the alternatives, notwithstanding the bromate conversion problem I just mentioned. The solution is to start with bromide-free water, and then the bromate conversion problem is moot. Knowledgeable ozone system manufacturers can design pool and spa systems to minimize such conversion. One ozone system manufacturer that I have used is Clearwater Tech LLC, in San Luis Obispo, California [342].

Because bromine interferes with iodine and is so ubiquitous, it may well be a major player in what seems to be an epidemic of thyroid illnesses. Earlier in this book, I discussed my theory regarding autoimmune diseases, pointing to toxins as the ultimate culprit. Two prevalent autoimmune conditions involve the thyroid gland and are named Graves' disease and Hashimoto's disease. Dr. Brownstein has found that proper treatment with iodine can reduce or eliminate the symptoms related to both of these conditions. I believe this occurs because iodine displaces the toxic halogens from occupying iodine receptor sites, and when this occurs, the defense system no longer treats the thyroid cells as foreign. I see no reason why this cannot also apply to the other autoimmune conditions.

In addition to the thyroid gland, recent studies have identified iodine as a critically important element in virtually all of the organs of the body, including the ovaries and mammary glands of women, leading to speculation that bromine may also be a contributor to breast and ovarian diseases, including cancer. Bromine is not the only player in the list of halogen elements that interfere with the body's use of iodine. Enter fluoride.

The health police deliberately put fluoride, a form of fluorine, into our drinking water, supposedly to prevent dental carries. That is almost as irrational as putting mercury in our mouths, and certainly deserves a high place of honor in the technology-blunder hall of fame. Books have been written on this blunder [343], and a recent article in *Scientific American* offers a good summary of the issues [344]. In a nutshell, not only does fluoride not achieve its objective of reducing tooth decay in children (who mostly drink soda!), it poisons the entire community. By now, it should be well known that the dental benefit of fluoride, if any, is only topical, not systemic; the toxic effects of fluoride are sufficiently severe that regulatory agencies caution against making infant formula with fluoridated water, and there is a poison warning on fluoridated toothpaste. Even the FDA will not approve fluoridated water as safe or effective because there is no evidence that it is.

The effects of excess fluoride include weakened bone strength and bone cancer, brain damage, tooth discoloration, decreased thyroid function, and the constellation of illnesses surrounding the interference with iodine. Years ago, fluoride was actually used to treat hyperthyroidism, because of its ability to interfere with iodine. It also interferes with the absorption of magnesium [62], which is already in short supply for most people and is needed to build strong teeth!  As the reader by now knows, and as the studies of Weston Price and PA skeletal evidence have shown, tooth decay is prevented by following the correct diet, one that is in alignment with our heritage.  I have already discussed water filtration for those unfortunate enough to live in a fluoridated community, and I would add to that the avoidance of any product containing fluoride, including toothpaste, most SSRI antidepressants, fluoroquinolone-based antibiotics, dental bonding agents, and some nasal sprays.  More details are available at the Fluoride Action Network [345].

Chlorine and perchlorate round out the toxic halogen family, all of which interfere with iodine.  The elimination of chlorine in drinking and bathing water was discussed above in the water filter section. Perchlorates, which used to be used as a thyroid depressing medication, are used modernly as a rocket fuel, and are also found in car airbags and fireworks.  They also have contaminated many of our wells and rivers. Vegetables such as lettuce contain high amounts from irrigation water (another plus for the Wellness Diet), as does cow and breast milk.

The protocols to offset the halogen problems listed above are not rocket science.  Reduce your exposure to the toxic halogens, and increase your intake of iodine, which acts to displace the other halogens and take their place.  The iodine testing and supplementation procedures have already been covered.  I personally have been taking large doses of iodine daily for some time, so perhaps relating my experiences would be helpful. Shortly after beginning a daily dose of 25 mg of iodine, skin problems characteristic of bromine excretion began to appear on my face.  Others undergoing this protocol have reported redness, rashes, and pustules around the "butterfly" area of the face – over the nose and cheeks.  In my case, the rash was slightly above this area, across my eyebrows and the bridge of my nose, and including the area above my eyelids, forming an exact outline of my sinuses.  It resolved within two weeks.  However, when I increased the dose to 50 mg, the rashes reappeared, only to resolve again a few weeks later.

I have repeated this process several times and as of the writing of this book, I am up to 75 mg, and the bromine (and probably fluoride and perchlorates) continues to be excreted through my skin.  While this process is annoying, I feel good that I am getting rid of a lifetime of this stuff, so I put up with it. Anecdotal reports by clinicians experimenting on themselves and measuring bromine excretion from their bodies indicate that the process may continue for several years, a testament to our lifetime exposure. Because rashes can detract from our appearance, others and I have experimented with cosmetic cover-ups for use during the detox process. Mineral-based powders are a candidate if they do not contain any toxic minerals such as aluminum or titanium, and do not use micronized powders, which increase absorption. If you use a moisturizer (discussed more fully in the lifestyle section), apply the powder over it to minimize the chances of absorption. There is more about safe and natural cosmetics in the lifestyle section.

Through continued experimentation, researchers have found that our old friend salt, in combination with vitamin C, can be used as part of the halogen detox protocol to improve results in some recalcitrant cases [346]. I believe this discovery occurred independently from the salt/C protocol used in connection with parasite cleansing, and I wonder how many more applications we may uncover for this unusual duet. For those readers with a further interest, there are support- and research-oriented groups online that discuss these iodine protocols (look for Yahoo groups with the word *iodine* in their name).

Lastly, the Dirt Detox Protocol may be of benefit in treating the halogen problem. There have been reports of urine alkalization alone having been used successfully to treat fluoride toxicity [215], and I suspect alkalization will speed up the removal of other halogens. Please don't think we are done with the halogen discussion. Wait until we get to the discussion of lighting in the lifestyle section to revisit bromine – think *halogen* lamps.

## The Virus Problem

Viruses are in the news on a regular basis, from AIDS to the constellation of herpes family viruses (oral, genital, shingles), along with the new vaccines for shingles and the human papilloma virus. A relatively new field of scientific investigation known as Paleovirology has undertaken the task of understanding the role of viruses in our genetic heritage, and reports are starting to emerge on the findings from these studies [347]. The researchers have found in our DNA the fragments of long-vanished viruses that probably have been with us for our entire evolutionary history. The supposition is that viruses have been and always will be part of our heritage, and may actually have acted - and will continue to act - to shape our genetic future. My understanding from this is that we are loaded with viruses. Once they have infected us, they are likely to hang around for a lifetime, and our sole defense is our defense system. This is in alignment with my objective in The Wellness Project to do whatever is possible to keep the defense system from being burdened with the wrong foods and other toxins, so that it can deal with important stuff like viruses. Regarding the use of the Dirt Detox Protocol for viral issues, the soil components of fulvic/humic acids and spore-formers have both exhibited antiviral properties. I suggest trying topical as well as oral application of these soil compounds for those with viral outbreaks.

Many years ago, a good friend of mine was plagued with repeated oral herpes outbreaks, and I decided to do some research to see if I could find something to help. What came out of my research were two patents (which I have since donated to the public) for a topical method of exposing the herpes virus to the defense system so that it could more promptly suppress the outbreaks. Please see the separate side box labeled "Viruses and a Topically Applied Food Preservative" for more details.

## Viruses and a Topically Applied Food Preservative

When the book Life Extension [18] came out more than 20 years ago, one of the fascinating topics discussed was the oral use of a widely-used artificial food preservative known as BHT (butylated hydroxytoluene) to suppress herpes simplex eruptions. I read everything I could on the subject and was not comfortable suggesting oral use of BHT to anyone because of the conflicting data on toxicity, ranging from non-toxic and health-promoting to possible toxicity issues [348]. I began experiments with the topical application of BHT bound to various lipids as a way around the potential toxicity issues, and settled on the combination of BHT mixed with Tea Tree Oil. Friends who tried it as a topical preparation achieved good results in suppressing or speeding up the healing of eruptions.  My guess as to how it works is that the BHT dissolves the lipid outer layer of the virus, and the tea tree oil destroys what is left.  I received two patents on the preparation, which I have since donated to the public, so that anyone is free to experiment with the idea.  For those interested, see for example U.S. Patent 5,215,478 for more information [349].

It is well known that many types of viruses, including those in the herpes family, thrive on the amino acid arginine, and one of the simple protocols sufferers have used in the past is either to avoid arginine rich foods, which just happen to be nuts and seeds, or to take large doses of the competing amino acid lysine.  Well, here is yet another plus for the Wellness Diet, which avoids those foods with a high arginine/lysine ratio.  Perhaps this is yet another whisper of wisdom from MA to lay off her nuts and seeds or pay the consequences by feeding the bad guys.

## The EMF Problem

EMF (Electromagnetic Field) radiation toxicity is a hot topic today, involving everything from power lines to cell phones.  I have done some research in the area, and looked for some simple protocols that can be implemented in an effort to reduce the risk of harm.  Because of the long interval of time between cause and effect, it has been difficult to draw firm conclusions as to which type of radiation causes what condition, and to postulate safe levels of exposure.  Therefore, the best approach is to minimize exposure.

Starting with electric field exposure, this issue typically arises in the home (and office), where we are surrounded with miles of wiring, located inside and outside of the walls, which are connected to the 60 Hz AC power system.  The effect of this wiring on the body can be measured easily using a digital meter with an AC millivolt scale.  Such meters are readily available, and one source is *lessemf.com* [350], which is a website that also provides many reference and educational resources that can be useful in this complicated arena.  I am going to give you the short version.

Electric fields cause the buildup of an electrical charge on the human body relative to the earth, and this can be measured in AC volts.

To eliminate this charge is not rocket science. All that needs to be done is electrically to connect your body to the earth, discharging the charge. Of course, PA had no problem with this for several reasons. First, he was not surrounded by electrical wires, and second he/she walked barefoot on native soil, placing him/her in electrical contact with the earth so no charge could have accumulated under any conditions. Well, the goal here is to emulate PA by reproducing the body/native soil connection in our lives as often as possible.

As it turns out, a whole industry was developed about 30 years ago to do just that, and I was a participant in its genesis way back then. At that time, using what is called the CMOS (Complementary Metal Oxide Semiconductor) process, electronic devices were being developed that were acutely sensitive to static charge. One annoying form of this with which we are all familiar is the voltage that accumulates on the body in dry weather and causes "shocks" when we touch a conductor. Well, such discharges also wipe out sensitive electronic parts, so all kinds of products were developed then to connect anyone working around electronics to earth. The industry is called the static control industry and includes wristbands, floor mats, seat pads, table coverings, special shoe and sock bindings, and electrically conductive clothing and packaging materials, all still widely available and in use today. These products employ all sorts of materials such as conductive fibers like silver or carbon that are coated on or woven into fabric. I made great use of these devices in the 1970s, where entire assembly lines of folks were grounded while working on electronic parts. For safety sake, we used resistors in the ground wiring to reduce the potential for shock.

The health benefits of grounding the body are recently being re-investigated, and some believe that it reduces inflammation and has a calming effect. If so, all of those grounded assembly workers have been indirectly getting a health benefit! For those interested in grounding themselves, it is simple to do so using these anti-static devices. The *lessemf.com* website has dozens of such items available, along with special cords to connect you to earth ground through house wiring. One company in particular, called Earth FX [351], is the source of specially designed mattress pads and sheets that can be used to connect you to earth while you sleep, and my wife and I have used one of their pads for some time.  I have also given away several to friends, some of whom claim they sleep better using them.  Their website also lists some of the reported health benefits from using the pads, and they appear to have some patents for their pad designs.

As I mentioned above in connection with the use of FIR saunas, I believe there may be benefit to grounding oneself while inside.  My interest is in the possibility that a charged body may interfere with the excretion of toxins.  I am unaware of any research in this area, but I do feel better when grounded in the sauna.  You can just use one of the many kinds of conductive wrist straps available, and a suitable wire out the door or vent of the sauna to a local AC ground connection.  All commercial wrist straps contain a built-in safety resistor.  A patent application has been filed covering this idea.

Summarizing the electric field discussion, the idea is to emulate PA, who was connected electrically to the earth by walking barefoot on moist soil or grass.  We no longer are grounded because we usually walk with rubber or plastic shoes on cement, all of which are insulators.  We have no path to discharge electrical energy that builds up on our bodies from all the gadgets and lights in our electrical surroundings, with unknown health effects.  Obviously, to the extent possible, we should walk barefoot on earth or a beach.  Barring that, there are many ways to hook yourself up inside the house.

If you remember the discussion above on the flaws of the rat chow experiments, I brought up the question of what effect removing the rats from their native environment and putting them in cages might have on the outcome of the experiment.  Well, that led me to the whole issue of the effects on animals removed from their native habitat, particularly with respect to their disconnection from earth, since most mammals naturally spend their life in direct contact with native soil.

Now, let's move on to magnetic fields, where cell phones are in the spotlight.  Setting aside the usual denials, suppressions, and cover-ups, there is evidence, mostly from European studies, that cell phone radiation may be a predisposing factor in various brain and eye diseases, so let's assume that is the case.  The obvious precautions of using a speakerphone or other hands-free systems seem prudent, but many folks will not implement these measures.  The next best thing is to try to implement some sort of shield for the brain and eye to minimize energy absorption, followed by a warning system to the user whenever certain predetermined parameters have been exceeded, increasing the risk of harm. There are all sorts of devices on the market claiming to channel, divert, filter, and otherwise render the RF (Radio Frequency) energy harmless, and many are by far hoaxes. Out of frustration and concern, I collaborated with some friends, one of whom is an RF genius, to come up with some workable solutions. See the side box entitled "CellFrame" for more information.

For those who live near cell phone towers or other sources of high frequency magnetic fields, an option is to shield yourself from the RF energy. One way to do that is to use electrically conductive paint to paint the room or rooms most used. Once painted, a simple connection between the painted surface and ground will form an RF shield for the entire room. Conductive paints are available that contain copper or carbon particles, and they can be over-painted with suitable sealers and finishes. The website *www.lessemf.com* [350] has information on such paints and methods of making ground connections.

---

### CellFrame™

The objective was to design some inexpensive ways to reduce the absorption of RF energy by the ear, brain and eyes, using shielding, attenuation, and reflection methods. An additional goal was to conceive of a warning system for the user, particularly in view of the adaptive power levels that can be generated by modern cell phones. The way that works is if communications with the cell tower are weak, the phone can increase its transmission power level automatically and significantly without the knowledge of the user. Since radiation damage is clearly dose dependent, it would seem prudent to alert the user to this event so that protective action could be taken. From a few brainstorming sessions, a number of designs were generated, several of which make use of the ubiquitous eyeglass frame, hence the trademark CellFrame. A patent application covering the designs has been filed.

This completes the discussion of physical detoxification protocols, so now let's move on to emotional detoxification.

# Chapter 18 - Emotional Detoxification

You may well ask: what is emotional detoxification? The reason this section is here began with some observations by Dr. Klinghardt several years ago while physically performing heavy metal detoxification protocols on patients that were not responding well. In other words, the usual protocols were not producing any significant toxin excretion in clearly toxic patients. However, when these same patients participated in certain types of emotional therapy techniques and released some deep-rooted emotional issues, lo and behold, the toxic metals began to pour out of their bodies. So, what can be described as a mind-body connection was established where emotional detoxification lead to enhanced physical detoxification, an important finding indeed. Since my wife is a licensed psychotherapist, there was quite a bit of interest generated in our household concerning this phenomenon. So began a journey of exploration, and here are my findings. In each instance, I gravitated toward protocols that have demonstrated that they can produce results very quickly.

## Family Constellations

I want to begin this discussion with a confession. With my science and law backgrounds, I seem to have a built-in skepticism for any protocol for which I cannot find any plausible explanation. In other words, I do not gravitate towards *woo-woo* stuff. This first protocol, Family Constellations, initially fell into that category and I approached it with a great deal of skepticism. However, after participating in the process, personally benefiting from it, and seeing many others who benefited, I can confidently suggest trying it.

While there are many books on the subject, three in particular present cogent explanations of the work and provide examples. The books are *The Healing of Individuals, Families and Nations* by John L. Payne; *The Language of the Soul* by John L. Payne; and *The Healing Power of the Past* by Bertold Ulsamer. John Payne is a facilitator of Family Constellations in South Africa [352], and Bertold Ulsamer is a facilitator in Germany [353]. The Family Constellation concept was developed by Bert Hellinger, a highly controversial German therapist [354], and it is now being practiced worldwide.

Briefly, when an individual wishes to work on a relationship issue, a theme in their life, or an illness, this technique seeks to look at entanglements within a family system that may be at the root of disruptive life patterns. The protocol is event-oriented inasmuch as personality descriptions or any particular bias or "story" that a client may have is not give much attention. In setting up a constellation, the interest is in *who* is a member of the family system and *what* specifically happened. Events of significance that often have impact on a family system include the early death of parents or grandparents; miscarriages, stillbirths and abortions; murders, tragic and accidental deaths; sudden loss of partner/spouse; adoptions; broken engagements and divorce; war experiences; incest; victims and perpetrators of crime and injustice; family secrets; and individuals who have been forced out of a family or disowned.

During a brief pre-constellation interview, the client is asked about who is in the family and if there have been any specific events that have occurred in the family, such as those listed above. Once the information is gathered, the client is then asked to select participants (usually complete strangers) in the workshop to represent members of their family and any other significant individuals, be they grandparents, uncles, aunts, etc., whose lives may have been impacted by events typical of the list above. Once all of the representatives have been chosen, they are placed intuitively in a standing pattern on the workshop floor space and it is at this point that the constellation comes to life.

The great difference between Family Constellation work and psychodrama or "role play" is that the representatives are not acting out roles according to personality descriptions given by the client. With the set-up of a constellation, the representatives move into and become part of *the knowing field* of the family and remarkably take on the actual feelings and impulses of the real family members. This process is a deep experience not only for the representatives, but also for the client as they watch their family come to life in front of them. Once a Family Constellation is set up, the facilitator first views the set-up in silence, observing both the body language and the pattern that has been created. Very often, the facilitator is able to see indications of certain events that have taken place within the family simply from observing how the representatives are standing in relationship to one another and their overall demeanor, even when the client has made no mention of specific events.

Once these preliminary observations have been made, the facilitator then walks to each representative and asks him or her how he or she is feeling. The feelings reported can be physical descriptions or a wide variety of emotional states. When problems and entanglements are identified, the facilitator then uses healing sentences to bring about resolution. An entanglement is identified when an individual is "tied up" in the fate or business of another. Very often, hidden loyalties are revealed to the extent that a client can be literally carrying and living out both the feelings and the fate of another from their extended family system.

The result of this fascinating process is that what might take years of conventional psychotherapy can sometimes be accomplished in an hour. In the US, the facilitators that I have worked with are JoAnna Chartrand and Dyrian Benz in the Santa Barbara, California area [355]. In other parts of the country, see Bert Hellinger's website for a list of facilitators. Both Drs. Klinghardt and Gruenn, referred to above, have used the Family Workshop protocols as part of their heavy metal detoxification practice, and reported good results. Astute readers may see a subtle connection between the premise of Family Constellations and the premise of The Wellness Project. In the case of The Wellness Project, the objective is alignment between heritage and lifestyle by going back in time to reconcile with our ancestry; in Family Constellations, the objective is alignment between our psyche and our family system by going back in time to reconcile with our ancestry. The analogy is so compelling, and the results so gratifying, that it has rooted this work as an important part of The Wellness Project.

## Emotional Freedom Technique (EFT)

This simple technique, known as "tapping," can be learned easily at home at no cost, with results in minutes. This is another instance where

I don't know why or how it works, but it does. The objective is to resolve quickly at least the symptoms associated with emotional and physical illnesses. It involves a specific sequence of tapping on certain acupuncture points on your head and upper body while you orally repeat a basic formula related to your condition. Developed by Gary Craig, an engineer, this method seems to remove subtle energy blockages in the body and lead to all sorts of emotional and physical healing. At the EFT website [356], you can download instructions, watch a video, and get started tapping away on some of your issues. EFT has been proven successful in thousands of clinical cases, and has been endorsed by many medical doctors and therapists, including Dr. Gruenn, who uses it in his practice. One theory I have as to its efficacy has to do with the analogy of tapping to drumming, discussed further in the lifestyle section, which seems to be the most primitive of human-made external sounds and may be one used by PA as a therapeutic form of healing.

## Trauma Healing

Many people traumatized emotionally during episodes of violence or natural disasters often hold on to their experience in a way that takes on a physical life of its own in the form of pain, stiffness, or some distortion in the finely-tuned mechanics of the body. In a real sense, such unresolved traumas add another element of toxicity in the body that needs to be expelled. Peter Levine, a therapist, has developed a theory for dealing with trauma, based on an animal model called the *immobility response*, a survival-enhancing fixed-action pattern that evolved as a protective mode of behavior in prey animals and which is triggered by the perceived imminence of being killed by a predator. As readers know by now, I am a big believer in taking cues from the animal kingdom, and this protocol fits that model. His book *Waking the Tiger* explains the principles and gives examples [357], and his Foundation for Human Experience [358] has a list of practitioners trained in the work.

# Section Four - Lifestyle

*All the sounds of the earth are like music.* - Oscar Hammerstein II

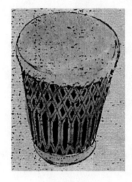 In addition to diet and detoxification, there are many other aspects of PA's lifestyle—to the extent that we know about it or can make educated guesses —that we have abandoned as well. As we grope into our far-distant tropical past for life-style patterns that have relevance to us in today's different world, let's have some fun speculating on what a typical day may have been like for our Paleo Ancestors.

• Awaken by the growing light of dawn.

• Arise from some kind of bedding placed on the ground, maybe outside or in a cave.

• No tooth brushing, mouth washing or flossing, but teeth are naturally perfectly healthy, straight, and free of cavities.

• Begin a day of fruit gathering and animal hunting (while avoiding predators and accidents) barefoot without the use of sunglasses or sunscreen.

• Drinking mineral rich water from streams, ponds, rock and tree depressions, and perhaps taking a dip (no soap).

• The family dress, if any, would probably be limited to primitive loincloths.

• Babies are carried by the mother on gathering trips, and breast-fed on demand, day and night. Pregnant women give birth in a squatting position.

• After eating, individuals squat for bowel movements (no toilet paper needed). If stools are abnormal, remedies are applied to re-establish gut health, including clays and certain anti-parasitic herbs.

• For recreation and relaxation, there would be lovemaking, perhaps primitive drumming and singing, some dancing, and naps.

• After sundown, the clan would retire for at least a nine-hour sleep in a world lit only by moonlight and starlight.

From these general patterns, we can extract ideas that may be useful for us some two million or so years later.

# Chapter 19 - Personal Care

By personal care, I mean dental care and substances we put on our skin and hair for various purposes. Let's start with dental care.

## Dental Care

The ancients did not use toothpaste and yet, remarkably, from the skeletons that have survived, we find perfect dentition—straight teeth evenly spaced, and no cavities. Along with that, we find wide jaws that accommodate all of the teeth, including wisdom teeth, with no problems. I feel confident that following the Wellness Diet and detox protocols will eliminate the tooth decay and gum problems of the modern world, and I do not use any commercial toothpaste, floss or mouthwash.

If we look at animals, such as cats and dogs, we see that they clean their teeth simply by chewing on hides, gristle, and raw bones and some modern indigenous tribes chew on rough bark and twigs as a dental treatment. Taking this as a clue and factoring in the various detox protocols, I arrived at a natural tooth cleaner that is also a detoxifier for the mouth, gums, and the rest of the body – our friend clay.

Ultra-finely-ground clay powder makes a wonderful product for a tooth cleanser, with extremely mild abrasive properties somewhat like baking soda, and no added colorants or sweeteners. Pascalite, the company mentioned earlier as a supplier of an acceptable edible clay, makes such a product called Pasca-Dent which works great [224]. You simply dump some powder in the palm of your hand, wet your toothbrush, stick it in the clay, and use it as toothpaste. There is no significant taste, and besides cleaning your teeth, the clay particles also adsorb bacteria, so after brushing, don't spit it out. Instead, slosh the clay in your mouth for as long as comfortable so it can get between your teeth and around your gums to pick up quantities of oral bacteria. When you are done, you can either spit it out or swallow it.

Mouthwash is also big business, and I have no idea why. It is hardly a solution for bad breath, which is a sign of a gut problem, gum disease, magnesium deficiency, or possibly a sinus or tonsil disorder, all issues that need to be addressed by diet and detoxification. Flossing is a relatively new and somewhat questionable practice. Some dentists feel that flossing can do more harm than good by pushing debris further into gum pockets or hard-to-get areas. I would rather have clay particles between my teeth, on guard 24/7 against a host of nasty stuff. For those who insist on a mouthwash, iodine has been shown to be an excellent choice, particularly for those with root canals or plastic of any kind in their mouth, which fosters fungal overgrowth [359] [360]. Swishing and gargling with a mixture of a few drops of Lugol's solution in mineral water should do the trick. Using the Clayodine concept, I have added a few drops of Lugol's to the clay toothpowder, so I get the effect of an antiseptic toothpaste and mouthwash in one.

## Skin Care

We are a society that slathers our skin with tons of toxic stuff in the hope that we can improve its look. My mantra is that, in general, "if it is on the skin, it is also in (the body)." The skin is a great absorber of both good and bad compounds [361]. The threshold question to ask is: why do we need anything on our skin at all? Heavy metal toxins are well known to mess with the skin, causing chronic dryness and all kinds of rashes. An incorrect diet can also cause skin problems like acne and eczema, and fungal overgrowth is well known to cause many skin ailments from athlete's foot to dandruff to ringworm. For clues from MA on skin care, let's peek into the animal kingdom, once again through the lens of Cindy Engel's book *Wild Health*.

Many animals spend a great deal of time tending to their skin, but not for beauty reasons. They are universally plagued by ectoparasites, better known as mosquitoes, gnats, ticks and everything else that bites and stings. In many instances, animals will groom each other, removing pests. In other cases, they have learned how to use natural substances to protect, soothe, and heal the skin. These include covering themselves with certain plant resins and even covering themselves with insects such as ants! In addition, our old friends fruit, dirt, clay, and salt are widely used for skin care, as is sunlight. Some animals will rub fruit over their bodies, including the pulp and rind, which have antiseptic and repellant characteristics. Other animals will roll in mud or cover themselves with clay for soothing effects and to discourage pests. Still other will rub salt on their skin, which kills mites and is beneficial to healing.

Armed with the above, let's see what might work on human skin from Nature. Regarding using fruit on the skin, modernly, alpha hydroxyl acid (AHA), which is fruit acid, is widely used in skin preparations as an exfoliant and remedy for dry skin. A more natural approach might be to cut up some fruit from the Wellness Diet and smear it over the skin on a regular basis. Regarding dirt and mud, I have found that compounds derived from soil and discussed earlier are very soothing to the skin. Morningstar Minerals makes a soil-based product called Derma Boost™ that contains humic acid and is designed to be sprayed on the skin, with good results [74]. Adding spore-forming bacteria to the spray more closely matches the makeup of soil.

Regarding clay, believe it or not, hydrated clay makes a great substitute for soap, eliminating the concern over toxic ingredients. Hydrated clay is clay already mixed with water, and for this application, a pasty consistency works well. You can easily make your own by mixing clay and water to get the desired consistency. Alternatively, the company Nature's Body Beautiful makes a line of clay/water skin cleansers [362], which take some getting used to, as there is no sudsing action. You can put iodine in the mixture as discussed earlier to add antimicrobial action for skin infections. If you insist on soap, the line of baby soaps (and shampoos) from Weleda, a European manufacturer, seems to have a minimum of potentially toxic ingredients [363]. Another choice is soap made with salt, but I am not aware of any made with unrefined ancient dry seabed salt. Those adventuresome readers who are amateur soap makers might wish to make some. In the bacteria detox section, I have already mentioned using an iodine-based hand soap. Finally, as mentioned above, soap nuts can be used as a body soap and shampoo, and instructions are widely available on the internet.

The subject of antiperspirants and deodorants was covered in the discussion of sweating, but for those that insist on using a deodorant, the miracle mineral magnesium is the natural choice. Taking it orally should do the trick, but if not, try wiping the magnesium chloride lotion directly on areas of concern such as the underarms and feet. Bear in mind that magnesium chloride, like ordinary sea salt, causes a burning sensation if put on cuts or irritated skin. An alternative to magnesium chloride lotion is magnesium hydroxide liquid, well known as Milk of Magnesia! Yes, you can swab some unflavored Milk of Magnesia under your arms and it will dry to a powder form and works great as a deodorant .

I cannot find any substantive research on the skin absorption of magnesium hydroxide, so I do not know if it will aid in replenishing body stores through the skin, as does the chloride form. I will tell you, however, that it can be used as a face and body wash with excellent antifungal and antiseptic properties. It is known to relieve dandruff and acne better than most other products. Original Phillips Milk of Magnesia, widely available, can be left on the skin for five minutes or so, and produce positive results for a host of skin problems. This is yet another feather in the cap of magnesium.

Regarding moisturizers, if you are sufficiently detoxified you should not need any since it is the toxins in our body that mess with the natural fatty acids produced by our skin. For those who do need moisturizers, I have come up with an interesting candidate – our friend red palm oil, which you may remember is from an acceptable fruit. The unfortunate problem with this oil is that it stains clothing and temporarily tints the skin slightly orange. However, there is available a palm oil product where the carotenoids that account for the color, and some other unsaturated fatty acids are removed, leaving a colorless paste known as palm oil shortening (not hydrogenated). It works quite well as a colorless moisturizer, and is available from Tropical Traditions [277].

Yet another natural moisturizer that PA would likely have applied to his/her skin is animal fat. Since soap and towels were not available, one can presume that after eating, hands covered in animal fat would have found their way to the hair and skin. More modernly, a product derived from milk fats has been used as a hair and skin moisturizer. It is called ghee, which is made from butter that has been heated, or clarified, and all of the milk proteins are removed, leaving just animal fats. In modern India, where it appears to have originated, ghee is a popular food but is also used topically with great success. I have experimented with it and it is quite soothing to the skin. A popular brand, derived from grass fed cows, is Purity Farms [364]. Although it is a dairy derived product, because all of the potentially offending sugars and proteins such as lactose, whey and casein, have been removed, I see no problem applying it to the skin. Gelatin, discussed above, is related to collagen, a major component of our skin, and taking it as part of the Wellness Diet is sure to enhance skin tone.

For the most part, cosmetics relate to looking good, reversing the effects of the aging process, and certainly attracting the other sex. Cosmetics are the bottled version of the preening that goes on throughout the animal kingdom—all that peacock strutting and showing off to find a sexual partner to procreate the species. This activity, in one form or another, is obviously built into the genes, humans included. From the study of modern indigenous tribes, we have learned that painting of the body with natural coloring agents is a very old practice, and I recall a particular instance where tribal women used red clay to cover their skin for decorative purposes. This brings me to mineral-based cosmetics.

A recent trend in natural cosmetics is to base them on a variety of naturally colored minerals that have been powdered and combined to match complexions. If you choose to use such a product, you might want some assurance from the manufacturer that no toxic minerals are used, including aluminum and titanium, and that none of the minerals are in nano-particle form, which increases their skin absorption. An example of a manufacturer that provides such products is Earth's Beauty Cosmetics [365].

## Sunscreens

Earlier in this book, I expressed my opinion regarding the precipitating factors contributing to skin cancer, and the folly of using sunscreen. In addition to blocking healthy UV light, the other problem with sunscreens is that most of the active ingredients, which are absorbed through the skin, are themselves toxic and can cause DNA damage, which injures skin cells and in fact may contribute to cancer! They have also been found to be hormone disruptors, including interfering with thyroid hormones [366] [367, 368]. This is yet another reason to take iodine supplementation if you are a sunscreen user.

As discussed above in relation to supplementation, the majority of Americans and Western Europeans are way below minimum levels of vitamin D. For more information on this important issue, I suggest reading *The UV Advantage*, by Michael Holick, M.D., of Boston University, who blatantly challenges mainstream thinking in this area regarding the avoidance of UV light exposure. He shows how lack of proper sun exposure can cause serious health problems, such as osteoporosis, colon, ovarian, breast, and prostate cancer, high blood pressure, multiple sclerosis, and depression [8]. I discuss this further in the next section on how to create a healthy living environment.

From my perspective, following the Wellness Diet and detoxifying will eventually bring you into alignment with your environment, and unless you are an exceptional case where you have moved to a very sunny climate from a heritage country located at a very high or low latitude, your body should be able to handle reasonable amounts of sun without any skin damage. However, if you are very pale-skinned, for example you come from Norway and transplant yourself to Hawaii, you may well have a problem since your naturally low levels of melanin, a trait genetically acquired over generations living in a sun-deprived area, will prevent you from being able to handle a tropical climate without some help.

What should you do in that case or in a situation where you are still detoxing and have not yet reached a healthy equilibrium? Here are my suggestions. First, wear a hat and suitable clothing if you will be getting more than a reasonable amount of UV exposure. Second, be aware of some exciting research using the herb forskolin which, when topically applied, stimulated the formation of additional melanin in rats [369] [370]. This research may produce a new topical treatment to restore melanin in fair-skinned people. Third, be aware of some exciting research into a non-toxic plant- based sunscreen, based on one of my patents (see the box entitled Non-Toxic Plant Based Sunscreen for more information).

Fourth, if you insist on using a sunscreen already on the market while waiting for the advanced products, the only one I can suggest is based on zinc oxide as the active ingredient, and it is called UV Natural [371].

## Non-Toxic Plant-Based Sunscreen

Some time ago, while I was sitting on the lanai of our Hawaii home, my wife came out and said, "grab your hat, and let's go for a walk." At that moment, I looked up at the palm trees and the question popped into my mind: why aren't these trees wearing a hat. Why can they sit 24/7 in the tropical sun for a hundred years and not burn up? The question took me on a quest into botany and the discovery that we really do not fully understand how plants protect themselves from UV light. An early assumption that it was chlorophyll is incorrect, and the speculation has shifted to some natural compounds of a reddish or bluish color called anthocyanins. These substances are what make blueberries blue and raspberries red, and they are found in high concentrations in our friends - fruit. They are very powerful antioxidants, and are the reason why blueberries have become such a celebrated health food recently. Moreover, the blue and red colors effectively filter UV light. So I decided to create a human sunscreen based on anthocyanins as the active ingredient. My hypothesis was that the colors would filter the light and the antioxidant effect would subdue free radical UV-induced skin damage. If this worked, it would be yet another plus for our use of fruit. After my patent issued (U.S. 6,783,754), I funded the Department of Molecular, Cellular, and Developmental Biology at UC Santa Barbara to undertake skin cell studies to determine the efficacy and dose range for topical anthocyanins used to protect against DNA damage. Preliminary results have been extremely positive, indicating the sunscreen preparation actually stops the DNA damage that could lead to skin cancer. Results of the study are slated for publication in 2009, and grant proposals have already been submitted and funded. Eventually, I hope to interest potential licensees in commercial development.

# Chapter 20 - Living Environment

This section will cover some health issues and possible solutions for the unnatural activity of daily living inside a building, be it a house, apartment or office where you spend a significant part of your time. PA did not have these issues, so we are going to have to come up with some innovative solutions to try to align this environment with our heritage, which is to spend a great deal of our time outside. Let's start with the air we breathe.

Ideally, the objective is to simulate indoors the fresh air of a clean outdoor environment. In today's world, this becomes quite a chore because of the many airborne contaminants inside and outside of our living space. My approach to this is to have a continuously circulating supply of indoor air that has been conditioned to remove toxins, similar to the approach used for water filtration. In my house, I have a rather complete conditioning system sold under the Amana® brand, manufactured by Goodman Manufacturing Co. [372]. The system begins with a forced air gas heater and an outside compressor-based air-cooling system. The entire ductwork was vacuumed to ensure a clean starting environment. Filtration begins with a pleated pre-filter such as the Filtrete® brand Ultra Allergen filter to remove particles around 1 micron in size, and it is on a three-month replacement schedule. This is followed by a whole-house HEPA (High Efficiency Particulate Air) filter using dual carbon cartridges rated to remove particles down to 0.3 microns, including lint, dust, mites, pollen, mold spores, fungi, bacteria, viruses, pet dander, smoke, and grease.

Next in line is a whole-house electronic air cleaner using electrostatic charge to remove these same types of particles down to 0.01 microns in size. Also placed throughout the system are UV air purifiers designed to destroy bacteria, viruses, mold, and volatile organic compounds (VOCs) that either have slipped through the other filters or have collected in the system. The system circulating air fan is kept running continuously, day and night, so the air is continuously filtered. If this sounds like overkill, it is a reflection of the importance I assign to clean air. After all, our interface with the environment is dominated by air, water, and food, so it seems foolish not to pay equal attention to all three.

For those whose indoor environment is not conducive to whole house filtration, room-sized units would be appropriate. I would look for those with a combination of HEPA, electrostatic, and UV filters, and a fan large enough to circulate the room air several times per day. Ceiling fans are also a good idea to keep the air circulating, and in very humid environments, a dehumidifier can aid in reducing mold formation. Air ozonation, which can be used to control mold, is a controversial subject, because large concentrations of ozone can be quite toxic to humans and pets. If mold is a serious and continuous problem, my suggestion is to use ozonators, but only when the area is unoccupied, and then turn them off during occupancy. In our Hawaii home, when we were off-island, we had an ozone generator running continuously along with ceiling fans for circulation, and mold was never a problem.

While it is fine to establish an air filter system, it is equally important to take measures to reduce the amount of contaminants either brought into the home or resulting from the construction of the home itself. Regarding home construction, there are many books regarding the use of home construction materials that have low VOC (Volatile Organic Compound) levels. In addition, I avoid the use of wall-to-wall carpeting, as it usually is manufactured with toxins such as brominated fire retardants (PBDEs) as discussed in the halogen section above, and also acts to accumulate additional toxins by trapping and holding contaminants brought into the home. In my house, I used wood, tile and stone floors partially covered with thin area rugs that are easy to remove and clean. As far as bringing in contaminants, the Japanese custom of removing shoes at the door is a very good one. In addition, for anyone who has been in a toxic environment, such as public parks, golf courses, medical and dental offices, hospitals, factories, etc., it would be prudent to have a place to change clothing and shoes before entering the home. Grass shades are becoming popular for window covering instead of heavy drapes that also tend to accumulate toxins. Of, course, whenever possible, it is a wise idea to open windows to let in sunlight and fresh air, assuming it is not polluted.

I realize that there is a Catch-22 in several of the proposals mentioned above, which increase electricity consumption, raising the issue of increased environmental air pollution from coal- and gas-fired generating stations. Fortunately, fan motors of the type used in air handling systems are now quite efficient and do not consume anywhere near the power used for indoor lighting, our next topic.

Indoor lighting is also filled with a plethora of Catch-22 choices, as we shall see. The ideal objective is to recreate indoors full-spectrum sunlight ranging from infrared to ultraviolet. The classic incandescent bulb produces a yellowish light, is wasteful of energy, and may contain lead in the base. Next, we have the halogen lamp, filled at high pressure with a halogen gas. Remember our halogen detox problem? Well, here it is again. From what little information I can gather of the lighting industry, the gas originally used was our friend iodine, but now they have switched over to *bromine*, one of the dreaded toxic halogens. Halogen lamps are slightly more energy-efficient that plain filament lamps and they are capable of creating light covering most of the visible spectrum. Fortunately, they are produced with thick quartz walls, so that breakage, and possible bromine contamination, is extremely rare. However, their commercial proliferation does contribute to the continued production of bromine, which is already in excess in our environment.

Next, we have fluorescents, which have been around for many years in long-tube form for commercial lighting applications, and are more energy efficient than filament bulbs. More recently, we have compact fluorescent lights (CFLs) that will shortly be mandated for use in new homes, and incandescents will be phased out. Well, in each CFL sits about 5 mg of *mercury*, the most toxic substance of all those discussed in this book. Complicate this with the fact that CFLs are made with a very thin and fragile glass enclosure that is easily broken, spilling mercury. If that happens in your home, you may have a serious problem on your hands. If you do an online search, you will find several horror stories of homeowners who broke these bulbs and were faced with enormous cleanup costs, or ended up contaminating portions of their home. New guidelines are being considered for a warning on the bulbs regarding cleanup procedures.

So here is the environmental Catch-22 for CFLs. Whether or not shifting from incandescent lighting to more energy-efficient fluorescent light will result in a net reduction of mercury emissions due to the displacement of coal-fired electricity generation is questionable at this time. More highly polluting production plants using mercury will need to be established to make fluorescent bulbs to replace incandescent bulbs. In addition, the lack of recycling will put this mercury into landfills where it will contaminate them and leach into drinking water sources. Readers already know my feelings regarding mercury, so I have minimized the use of these bulbs in my home. In the mean time, I have installed low-voltage halogens in readiness for the next wave in interior lighting technology – LEDs.

Full-spectrum LED bulbs are already in production, but the price for total home replacement is still prohibitive. These bulbs are quite energy efficient and at first look, seem to be the preferred choice. However, the fabrication of LED chips is not without environmental issues. Having been involved in semiconductor design and fabrication during the time I was designing and manufacturing solid state relays, I am familiar with the toxic waste disposal issues in that industry, which uses such toxins as arsenic, antimony and hydrofluoric acid (a fluoride compound). Since life is full of informed trade-offs, considering all of the above, my lighting choice at the moment is LEDs, and I intend to start replacement of my halogens in the near future, using full-spectrum whenever possible in an effort to duplicate sunlight. Which brings up the issue of UV light.

It turns out that most residential full-spectrum bulbs on the market are not really full spectrum at all. They deliberately block the ultraviolet portion of the spectrum in the mistaken belief that UV is harmful. From all of the previous discussions in this book regarding UV, vitamin D, and skin cancer, you know that my position is to expose one's body to at least modest amounts of sunlight daily, or else take vitamin D supplements. One way to get UV exposure is by use of a UVB sunlamp, recreating the portion of the solar spectrum responsible for generating vitamin D in the skin. I realize some dermatologist readers out there are cringing at the thought, but mild, non-burning exposure, not designed to give you a deep tan, but to replenish vitamin D, is natural and healthy. This subject is discussed by dermatologist Michael Holick in his book *The UV Advantage*, previously mentioned above [8]. In my home, I have mounted a simple fixture, containing a UVB fluorescent bulb (which I treat with great respect!), on the inside roof of my FIR sauna, and use it for a few minutes several times a week. There are many sources for sunlamps, and one should take care not to go beyond the point that causes a slight pinkness of the skin, and to use eye protection because of the concentrated energy radiated by the lamp. A caveat to those who are, or should be, undergoing detox protocols, your skin may not be able to tolerate any substantial UV exposure until toxins are eliminated, your diet is cleaned up, and normal fatty acid synthesis is restored. In such instance, vitamin D3 supplements are the way to proceed. This brings me to a discussion of sunglasses.

PA obviously did not wear shades, so why do we? Actually, other than the marketing hype and making a fashion statement, I cannot find any good reason for wearing them, sort of like sunscreen. Some in the health field believe that excessive UV light can cause eye diseases such as cataracts. If that is the case, I suggest that UV light may be a necessary, but certainly not sufficient cause, since millions of people who do not wear sunglasses do not get eye disease. My guess is that faulty diet and a body loaded with toxins are the real culprits. The downside to wearing sunglasses is that it interferes with a portion of the endocrine system involving the pineal gland, which is light responsive. We do not fully understand the operation of the pineal gland, but from what we do know, you do not want to mess with it. Some animal tests show that it prolongs lifespan, and it is known to produce melatonin and possibly other hormones that affect the entire endocrine system. I was somewhat shocked to find research that points to the accumulation of *fluoride* in high concentrations in the pineal gland [373], yet another reason to consider the halogen-detox protocol. Another reason to avoid wearing sunglasses is that they can become addictive, because the eyes get used to the reduced light and then become at least temporarily oversensitive to normal sunlight. While there are certainly applications where, for safety reasons, glare-reducing polarized sunglasses should be used, it might be a good idea from a health point of view to forgo sunglasses when they are unnecessary.

Because we rarely base our sleep patterns on sunlight, as PA did, there are a few things that can be done to help keep the body synchronized to natural light. In particular, the release of the hormone melatonin by the pineal gland is stimulated by darkness, and melatonin can contribute to normal sleep patterns. Many of us stay awake in a bright environment until bedtime, not giving the gland much time to adjust to darkness and begin melatonin production. Recent studies have shown that it is the blue portion of the visible light spectrum that shuts off melatonin production [374]. Enterprising companies have developed blue-light blocking eyeglasses and light bulbs that can be used indoors for, say, three hours prior to bedtime to acclimate the pineal gland to darkness. The other portions of the light spectrum do not appear to suppress this hormone production. A company called Photonic Developments [375] makes glasses and light bulbs for this purpose.

Imagine a lifestyle habit that increases alertness, boosts creativity, reduces stress, improves perception, stamina, motor skills, and accuracy, helps you make better decisions, keeps you looking younger, reduces the risk of heart attack, elevates your mood, and strengthens memory. The answer is a daily nap. Research studies continue to show physiological benefits from naps, and I try to nod off for 15 to 30 minutes in the early afternoon. Dr. Sara Mednick has researched and written extensively on the subject, and her website provides the details [376].

## Exercise and Relaxation

No book on health seems to be complete without a discussion of exercise. I do not believe exercise can restore an unhealthy person to health, but it certainly can improve their fitness. There has been a lot of research on the life-extending effects of exercise at the cellular level, but if your diet is wrong and you are loaded with toxins, it seems to me that exercise will have a hard time correcting these problems.

What we do know from a study of the animal kingdom and indigenous tribes is that physical exertion in the adult is reserved for obtaining food, dealing with predators including other humans, and reproduction. In fact, energy conservation is an important survival strategy because if you are too fatigued to obtain food, you are history. Since we are privileged not to have to hunt, gather, or evade predators, it takes a conscious effort to get moving, because our immediate survival is not on the line. No wonder exercise is a struggle for many. In search of an answer for this dilemma, I invented and patented a device called the Officizer™, which is described in the side box with that title. In addition to using the Officizer (which I have used daily while writing this book), my personal preferences are walking and resistance training, neither to excess.

The use of a pedometer to monitor walking progress can be a helpful motivator.

It is well known that above a certain level of exertion, carbohydrate loading becomes important to avoid severe fatigue. Although PA might have been able to accomplish this on the Wellness Diet by pigging-out on fruit, I truly have a hard time imagining such a scenario on a regular basis. So, for me this is another whisper of wisdom from MA not to overexert. In particular, excessive exercise rapidly depletes the body of magnesium, which may persist for months [135].

## The Officizer™

When I was working in an office environment, like many others, I had a room full of exercise equipment at home, which I bought and used for a while. Then one day, sitting at my desk at work, I realized that *now* was when I was ready for some exercise. I wondered, why can't I exercise while I do my work? So I came up with a chair-based exerciser product that straps onto any swivel chair. An adjustable, stretchable band is attached to the center chair post, and at the other end is a bar that resembles a footrest with wheels at either end. You put your feet on it and push, which makes it a combination of a leg press and a leg extension. I designed it to be force balanced so I could push on it without swiveling, which allowed me to read or type at my computer and still be working out. Since it is designed specifically for use in an office environment the Officizer represents a new category of fitness equipment that allows you to be pumping away underneath your desk without anybody knowing what you're doing! The four patents that cover the technology include using the computer you are working on at your desk to monitor your exercise progress. A special mouse design monitors your pulse rate via your fingertip, and a small software program is designed to pop up on the screen every so often to let you know your pulse rate and to spur you on toward meeting pre-established goals. Eventually, I hope to get around to either mass-producing the device or licensing others to do so.

The ideal exercises for us would be based on hunter/gatherer physical behavior, including bending, lunging, squatting, pushing, pulling, and twisting. For those who do tend to overexert when exercising and end up pulling muscles, over-stretching, or otherwise doing some physical injury to their body, I suggest a particular form of chiropractic therapy based on the use of a low-force, spring-driven hammer known as an Activator Adjusting Instrument. The website for this type of therapy lists practitioners proficient in this method and explains how it works [377].

The photos taken by Weston Price of the women in the various indigenous tribes around the world have impressed me because of their round faces and bodies, hardly the model look of today. A recent study points to the observation that women with relatively small waists and relatively large hips and thighs store higher body levels of omega-3s, and their children enjoy an edge when it comes to brain development [378]. This might account for the observation that "real women do have curves," in keeping with the movie of a similar name. Perhaps sometime in the future Rubenesque figures will become popular again.

I am not sure whether to characterize making love as exercise, as recreation, or both. However, there is a fascinating book on the subject as it pertains to our genetic heritage written by Jared Diamond, entitled *Why is Sex Fun?,* and it is a great read [379].

Another form of relaxation that seems to be universally portrayed as a pastime of native cultures is drumming. I have no idea if PA drummed, but it is easy to imagine people making drumming sounds as a natural part of living around items such as branches and animal bones that can be knocked together to make noise. There is something primal about drumming that, for me, may be related to the sound of a heartbeat as heard in the womb. Others in the healthcare field have found drumming and other forms of percussion to be particularly healing to those with a variety of health-related problems.

One organization in particular, known as The Rhythmic Arts Project (TRAP), has had great success in working with people with disabilities. Employing drums and percussion, the program teaches and enhances basic life skills such as maintaining focus, using memory, taking turns, developing leadership, using numbers, and following instructions. Issues of spatial awareness, fine and gross motor skills, and speech are also addressed [380]. Once you have music available, dancing is the next logical step, and it is a superb form of exercise that also stretches muscles.

Relating exercise to the air we breathe, there is speculation that the atmospheric oxygen content has been decreasing since the Paleo era, and we do know that the carbon dioxide concentration has more than doubled. This fuels further speculation that increasing the availability of oxygen to the body today might be another way in which to align our environment with our heritage. A few methods of doing so have been suggested. One of them is called EWOT (Exercise With Oxygen Therapy), proposed by Dr. William C. Douglass, who has written a book on the subject [381].

Basically, you hook yourself up to a source of oxygen such as an oxygen tank or an oxygen concentrator using conventional tubing and a nasal cannula, and breathe this oxygen, along with room air, while performing light exercise for 15 minutes. It actually feels quite good to do so, and certainly floods the body's tissues with oxygen, which is normally depleted by exercise. Since you generally need a prescription for oxygen, I presume your MD will want to review this protocol. For details on its use and some case studies, consult the Douglass book.

# Section Five - The Future

*The significant problems we have cannot be solved at the
same level of thinking with which we created them.* –

Albert Einstein

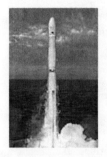 The purpose of this section is to summarize a few areas of future research that I believe will be most beneficial to the health of our population (and humans in general). The first area is that of nutritional research. I'm referring to studies such as those that purportedly show saturated fat contributes to heart disease; that salt is a cause of high blood pressure; that eating according to the FDA pyramid will make you healthy; or that following any of the dietary guidelines put out by diabetes, heart, or cancer societies will in any way provide a health benefit.

My suggestion is that in the future, for the sake of accuracy, peer-reviewed journals should, for all nutrition study participants, publish a list of all of the foods they were and are eating. This should include the source of those foods (e.g. was the meat grain-fed, and were all foods organic or GMO) along with an inventory of all known toxins in the body of study participants, such as a count of each person's amalgams and root canals, and a list of all medications taken and being taken during the study. Because of its unique importance, magnesium levels should also be tested and reported in any study having to do with cardiovascular issues. In other words, the objective is to establish a baseline control for these studies, just as we have established a baseline diet in The Wellness Project. To do otherwise is just inadequate science. Of course, what I would ideally like to see are existing studies repeated with participants that have followed The Wellness Project for some time, to see what the difference would be in outcome. It is unlikely that any commercial enterprise would fund such studies because, not only is there no money in it, the results could very well dramatically curtail existing sales of drugs and supplements. So private funding is the only alternative.

In the fruit arena, efforts should be made to halt any genetic modifications to fruit-bearing plants, since the effects on humans are unknown, and the potential for harm is enormous.

In the dirt arena, I believe that research into the missing components of our diet from soil, including humic and fulvic acids and soil bacteria such as the spore-formers, could produce dramatic health benefits for virtually all categories of illness. In a broader sense, such a study should also encompass the study of gut bacteria as it applies to health.

The next area is in the field of detoxification. Research is sorely needed to develop new non-toxic agents that bind strongly to toxins such as heavy metals, pesticides, certain halogens, fungi, etc. and to escort them out of the body without depositing them elsewhere along the way. Perhaps the alkalinity theory is one answer, but controlled experiments should be conducted as part of a research program. Magnesium's role in the field of detoxification should be researched in great depth, just based on the limited studies that have already been conducted. The treatment of autoimmune conditions should be broadened to include the possibility that they stem from toxins in cells, as opposed to a defective immune system.

In the vaccination arena, rules should be made that anyone dispensing vaccinations must have on hand preservative-free single-dose vials for those who ask for them. Also, alternate vaccination schedules should be provided where inoculations are spread out over time to enable a child's defense system to better deal with them. Lastly, methods for parents to opt out of the programs should be made universal.

In the halogen arena, water fluoridation needs to be banned immediately, and I suggest replacing the fluoride in our water supplies with magnesium! I believe this could have a profound effect on reducing the rates of cardiovascular disease, bone fractures, dental caries, viral infections, and psychological disturbances in our population, and may well be the most important and cost-effective public health measure to be implemented in our lifetime. Of course, whole house water softeners should be banned because they remove magnesium and calcium from the drinking water. Substantial funding should be devoted to high-dose iodine research, covering everything from breast, thyroid, and ovarian cancer to ovarian and breast cysts. Iodine should also be investigated as an alternative to prescription antibiotics and antifungals. The use of bromine should be banned in foods such as bread and soda, as well as in clothing and plastics as a flame retardant. This is another area where private funding will be required, as it has a very negative impact on many commercial enterprises.

I realize that several of the protocols disclosed in this book are not easy to implement, due to a variety of factors such as availability of products, space limitations, and a general reluctance to make radical lifestyle modifications. Therefore, I propose the establishment of neighborhood detoxification centers where many of the diet and detox protocols of The Wellness Project would be made available to the public. A patent application has been filed covering this concept.

It is my intention to devote a portion of the profits from the sale of this book and the licensing of my inventions in the health field to research efforts such as those described above, and I hope there are some readers who will share my passion.

Lastly, I would like to propose a new paradigm for the relationship between a prospective patient and an internist or family doctor. I believe that such a relationship should always begin with the following queries by the doctor:

➢ Provide a one-week diary of everything you put into or on your body, where the entries are made in real time (record the information when you are ingesting or applying the item). Include how food is cooked, what kind of containers are used, and brand names of products. Be sure to include all medications, supplements, cleansers, and cosmetics.

➢ Provide a one-week diary of everything that comes out of your body, including frequency of urinations and their color and odor; stool frequency and description, using the Bristol test; and sweat odor.

➢ Describe your environment – whether mostly indoor or outdoor, age and construction of house, use of carpeting, water supply and filtration, air filtration, use of spas and pools, and use of pesticides.

➢ Provide complete dental records, including the placement of restorations, materials used, and dates of placement. List all root-canalled teeth, and the age of them.

In addition, I believe the prospective patient is entitled to request from the doctor a list of all of the medications the doctor is taking. The objective is to enable the patient to determine if the side-effect profile of any of these medications might impair the doctor's ability to perform.

As a final note, it is my intention to continue my research into The Wellness Project and generate periodic updates to the information in this book. A website is under construction to facilitate communication with readers, and it will appear at *www.projectforwellness.com.*

# Appendix A

## Publications

➢ NASA Tech Brief Document ID: 19660000034 Valve Driver Circuits

➢ NASA Tech Brief – Triple Redundant Spacecraft Attitude Control System

➢ NASA Tech Report #JPL-TR-32-1011. DIANA – A Digital-Analog Simulation Program

➢ NASA Tech Report Document ID: 19680052463 Attitude Control of an Electrically Propelled Spacecraft Utilizing the Primary Thrust System

➢ NASA Tech Report #JPL-TR-32-1104. The Analysis and Configuration of a Control System for a Mars Propulsive Lander

➢ NASA Tech Report Document ID: 19670060448. Computer Analysis and Simulation of Mars Soft Landing Descent Control System Combining Inertial and Radar Sensing Techniques

➢ NASA Tech Report Document ID: 19670006377. Propulsive Planetary Landing Capsule Control System

➢ NASA Tech Report Document ID: 19670005459 Sterilization of Guidance and Control Systems and Components

➢ The Analysis and Configuration of a Control System for a Mars Propulsive Lander (Computer analysis and simulation of Mars soft landing descent control system combining inertial and radar sensing techniques) Mankovitz, R J, International Federation Of Automatic Control, Symposium On Automatic Control In Space, 2nd, Vienna, Austria; 4-8 Sept. 1967. P. 21.

➢ MIL-R-28750 Solid State Relay Military Specification

➢ EIA RS-433 Solid State Relay Standards

➢ Author of "THE LAW," a monthly column in Electronic Engineering Times discussing intellectual property law.

AFFILIATIONS    Intellectual Property Section- CA State Bar

AND HONORS:    Eta Kappa Nu- Engineering Honor Society

                    Who's Who in California – 1983

# Patents

(Health related patents are in **bold**):

| PAT. # | Title |
|--------|-------|
| 6,987,842 | Electronic television program guide delivery system using telephone network idle time |
| RE38,600 | Apparatus and methods for accessing information relating to radio television programs |
| **6,783,754** | **Plant-based non-toxic sunscreen products** |
| 6,760,537 | Apparatus and method for television program scheduling |
| 6,701,060 | Enhancing operations of video tape cassette players |
| 6,687,906 | EPG with advertising inserts |
| 6,606,747 | System and method for grazing television channels from an electronic program guide |
| 6,549,719 | Television program record scheduling and satellite receiver control using compressed codes |
| 6,487,362 | Enhancing operations of video tape cassette recorders |
| 6,477,705 | Method and apparatus for transmitting, storing, and processing electronic program guide data for on-screen display |
| 6,441,862 | Combination of VCR index and EPG |
| **6,361,397** | **Garments which facilitate the drainage of lymphatic fluid from the breast area of the human female** |
| 6,341,195 | Apparatus and methods for a television on-screen guide |
| 6,321,381 | Apparatus and method for improved parental control of television use |
| 6,253,069 | Methods and apparatus for providing information in response to telephonic requests |
| 6,239,794 | Method and system for simultaneously displaying a television program and information about the program |

RE37,131    Apparatus and methods for music and lyrics broadcasting

6,154,203    System and method for grazing television channels from an electronic
program guide

6,147,715    Combination of VCR index and EPG

6,125,231    Method of adding titles to a directory of television programs recorded on a
video tape

6,122,011    Apparatus and method for creating or editing a channel map

**6,117,050    Exercise apparatus for use with conventional chairs**

6,115,057    Apparatus and method for allowing rating level control of the viewing of a
program

6,091,884    Enhancing operations of video tape cassette players

**6,086,450    Brassieres which facilitate the drainage of lymphatic fluid from the breast
area of the human female**

6,072,520    System for improved parental control of television use

6,028,599    Database for use in method and apparatus for displaying television
programs and related text

**6,010,430    Exercise apparatus for use with conventional chairs**

5,995,092    Television system and method for subscription of information services

5,987,213    System and method for automatically recording television programs in
television systems with tuners external to video recorders

5,949,492    Apparatus and methods for accessing information relating to radio
television programs

5,949,471    Apparatus and method for improved parental control of television use

**5,921,900    Exercise apparatus for use with conventional chairs**

5,915,026    System and method for programming electronic devices from a remote site

5,734,786    Apparatus and methods for deriving a television guide from audio signals

5,703,795   Apparatus and methods for accessing information relating to radio and television programs

**5,690,594   Exercise apparatus for use with conventional chairs**

5,677,895   Apparatus and methods for setting timepieces

5,640,484   Switch for automatic selection of television signal sources for delivery of television guide data

5,633,918   Information distribution system

5,581,614   Method for encrypting and embedding information in a video program

5,577,108   Information distribution system with self-contained programmable automatic interface unit

5,561,849   Apparatus and method for music and lyrics broadcasting

5,559,550   Apparatus and methods for synchronizing a clock to a network clock

5,552,837   Remote controller for scanning data and controlling a video system

5,543,929   Television for controlling a video cassette recorder to access programs on a video cassette tape

5,541,738   Electronic program guide

5,526,284   Apparatus and methods for music and lyrics broadcasting

5,523,794   Method and apparatus for portable storage and use of data transmitted by television signal

5,515,173   System and method for automatically recording television programs in television systems with tuners external to video recorders

5,512,963   Apparatus and methods for providing combining multiple video sources

5,499,103   Apparatus for an electronic guide with video clips

5,465,240   Apparatus and methods for displaying text in conjunction with recorded audio programs

5,408,686   Apparatus and methods for music and lyrics broadcasting

5,385,733   **Topical preparation and method for suppression of skin eruptions caused by herpes simplex virus**

5,382,983   Apparatus and method for total parental control of television use

5,215,748   **Topical preparation and method for suppression of skin eruptions caused herpes simplex virus**

5,161,251   Apparatus and methods for providing text information identifying audio program selections

5,159,191   Apparatus and method for using ambient light to control electronic apparatus

5,134,719   Apparatus and methods for identifying broadcast audio program selections in an FM stereo broadcast system

5,119,507   Receiver apparatus and methods for identifying broadcast audio program selections in a radio broadcast system

5,119,503   Apparatus and methods for broadcasting auxiliary data in an FM stereo broadcast system

3,691,426   Current Limiter Responsive to Current Flow and Temperature Rise

3,648,075   Zero Voltage Switching AC Relay Circuit

## Some health related pending patent applications

Food Compositions and Methods

A Method Of Providing An Eating Plan Having A Very Low Concentration Of Natural Toxins

Silver/Plastic Combination that Binds Hazardous Agents and Provides Anti-Microbial Protection

Iodine Containing Compositions

Systems and Methods for Electrically Grounding Humans to Enhance Detoxification

Apparatus and Methods for Reducing Exposure to RF Energy Produced by Portable Transmitters

Soil Based Composition and Method for Removal of Toxins from Mammals

Methods of Providing to the Public Healthy Diet, Detoxification and Lifestyle Protocols in the Form of Neighborhood Centers

# Appendix B - Food and Supplement Schedule

| TIME | DIET | DETOX |
|---|---|---|
| Awakening<br><br>&<br><br>Bedtime | Mineral Water – 10 oz<br>Dolomite – 1 tablet<br>  Optional: HCl Plus – 1 tab<br>Optional per magnesium test:<br>  Magnesium taurate -<br>    1 cap or tab<br><br>Fulvic/Humic acid – 1 capsule/AM<br>Spore-formers – 1 capsule/AM<br>ProBoost – 1 packet/PM<br>Sublingual P5P – 2 tablets | Magnesium and Zinc on skin<br>Magnesium Crystals -<br>  Bath/Footbath (PM)<br>Sauna (once or twice daily)<br>Grounding Whenever Possible<br>SAMe – 200 to 400 mg<br><br>For Three Days per 2 Weeks<br>(MYSD):<br>  DMPS (every 8hrs<br>or DMSA (every 3-4 hrs);<br>  ALA (every 3-4 hrs)<br><br>For Five Other Days Every 2<br>Weeks (MYSD):<br>  Clay – 2 capsules<br>  Fulvic/Humic acid –<br>      1 capsule/PM<br>  Spore-formers –<br>      1 capsule/PM |
| Breakfast<br><br>&<br><br>Lunch<br><br>&<br><br>Dinner | Animal Foods<br>Fruit<br>Salt<br>Hot Water or Fruit Tea – 8 oz<br>Red Palm Oil – 1 tsp<br>  (or: vit. E, K, carotenoids/AM)<br>Eggs (optional)<br>Vitamin C – 500 mg<br>Desiccated Liver – 5 tablets/1 tsp<br>Vitamin D3 – per test results<br>    (or UV light)<br>Multimineral – 1 capsule<br>Gelatin – 1 Tsp./Bone Broth<br>Probiotic – 1 capsule<br>Glandular – 2 tablets<br>Optional:<br>  Digestive Enzymes<br>  Betaine HCl<br>  Bile Salts<br>  Pantethine – 300 mg<br>  Vitamin B-5 - 500 mg | Apple Pectin – 2 + capsules<br>Vitamin A – 4,000 IU/AM<br>PhosChol (PPC) – 1 gelcap<br>Coenzymated B-Complex/AM<br>  (all optional with MYSD<br>detox)<br><br>Zinc per taste test<br><br>During the eight days of<br>MYSD detox:<br>  Potassium/sodium Citrates –<br>    for alkaline urine<br>  NAC – 500 mg<br><br>For three weeks every month<br>(halogen detox):<br>  Iodine – per test results<br>  Salt/C protocol  (optional) |
| Between<br>Breakfast<br>and Lunch<br>&<br>Between<br>Lunch and<br>Dinner | Mineral Water – 16 oz<br>  Dolomite 1 tablet<br>  Vitamin C  500 mg<br>    Optional:  HCl Plus – 1 tab<br>Optional per magnesium test:<br>  Magnesium taurate –<br>    1 cap or tab<br>Gut Repair as necessary | Charcoal as needed to<br>minimize detox symptoms<br><br>Every three to six months:<br>  Parasite Cleanse –<br>    Humaworm |

# Appendix C - Food and Supplement Resources

(see www.montecitowellness.com for a list of website links)

| Food or Supplement | Resource | Website |
|---|---|---|
| Animal Foods | Local health food stores or farmers' markets;  US Wellness Meats; North Star Bison; Blackwing Ostrich | www.uswellnessmeats.com<br>www.northstarbison.com<br>www.blackwing.com |
| Fruits | Local health food stores or farmers' markets;  Brownwood Acres fruit supplements | www.brownwoodacres.com |
| Eggs | Local health food stores or farmers' markets – look for high omega-3 feed;<br>    Example: Christopher Eggs | www.christophereggs.com |
| Salt | RealSalt | www.realsalt.com |
| Glandulars;<br>Vitamin A;<br>Vitamin D;<br>HCl Plus | Neonatal Glandular;<br>Bio-Ae-Mulsion;<br>Bio-D-Mulsion;<br>HCl Plus<br>    by Biotics Research | www.bioticsresearch.com |
| Apple Pectin;<br>Betaine HCL;<br>Potassium citrate | Apple Pectin USP;<br>Betaine HCL with pepsin;<br>Potassium Citrate<br>    by Twinlab | www.twinlab.com |
| Water filters | Doulton Water Filters;<br>Wellness Filters | www.doulton.ca<br>www.wellnessfilter.com |
| Dolomite;<br>Vitamin C | Dolomite 44 grain;<br>Vitamin C 500 mg<br>    by Nature's Plus | www.naturesplus.com |
| Probiotic | Kyo-Dophilus by Wakunaga | www.kyolic.com |
| Humic/Fulvic Acids | Immune Boost 77 (capsules) and Vitality Boost HA  by MorningStar Minerals;<br>Metal Magnet by PhytoPharmica | www.msminerals.com<br>www.phytopharmica.com |
| Spore-formers | Flora Balance by O'Donnell Formulas;<br>Lactobacillus Sporongenes by Thorne and Pure Encapsulations | www.flora-balance.com<br>www.thorne.com<br>www.purecaps.com |
| Edible Clay | Pascalite;<br>Terramin;<br>Redmond Clay | www.pascalite.com<br>www.terrapond.com<br>www.redmondclay.com |
| Multimineral | Citramin II<br>    by Thorne Research | www.thorne.com |
| Vit K complex;<br>Vit E complex | Super K;<br>Gamma E Tocopherol/Tocotrienols;<br>    by Life Extension Foundation | www.lef.org |

| | | |
|---|---|---|
| Liver tablets and powder; Slippery Elm Bromelain | Liver; Slippery Elm Bark Powder; Bromelain     by NOW Foods | www.nowfoods.com |
| Red Palm Oil | Tropical Traditions Organic | www.tropicaltraditions.com |
| Gelatin | Beef Gelatin     By Great Lakes Gelatin | www.greatlakesgelatin.com |
| Magnesium taurate | Magnesium Taurate caps by Cardiovascular Research; Magnesium Taurate 400 tabs     by Douglas Labs | www.douglaslabs.com |
| Magnesium Lotion and bath crystals | Dr. Shealy's Biogenics Magnesium Lotion; Magnesium Chloride Crystals | www.selfhealthsystems.com |
| Zinc Lotion | Zinc Sulphate Lotion     by Kirkman Labs | www.kirkmanlabs.com |
| Sublingual B-6; Sublingual B Complex; Zinc; SAMe; Mastic Gum | Coenzymated B-6, sublingual; Coenzymated B Complex; OptiZinc; SAMe; Mastic Gum capsules     By Source Naturals | www.sourcenaturals.com |
| Toilet Squatting Stool | HealthStep by Ginacor | www.healthstep.com |
| Bile Salts | Cholacol by Standard Process; or Beta Plus by Biotics Research | www.standardprocess.com www.bioticsresearch.com |
| FIR Sauna | High Tech Health | www.hightechhealth.com |
| FIR heating pads | Thermotex | www.thermotex.com |
| pH Paper | Micro Essential Lab | www.microessentiallab.com |
| Clay for baths | Microfine Volclay HPM-20     by American Colloid Company.     Distributed by Laguna Clay | www.colloid.com www.lagunaclay.com |
| Charcoal | Activated Charcoal | www.buyactivatedcharcoal.com |
| Iodine | Iodoral tablets from Vitamin Research; Lugol's Solution from J. Crow | www.vrp.com www.jcrowsmarketplace.com |
| Heavy Metal hypersensitivity test | Melisa test | www.melisa.org |
| Hair Mineral Analysis | Doctor's Data;     Ordered from Direct Labs | www.directlabs.com |
| Iodine skin cleansers | Betadine by Purdue Pharma;     widely available from drugstores | www.pharma.com |
| Stool Tests | Comprehensive Stool Analysis     by Genova Diagnostics | www.gdx.net |
| Parasite cleansers | Humaworm | www.humaworm.com |
| Grounding equipment | Wrist straps, meters, paint, cords; Bedpads | www.lessemf.com www.earthfx.net |
| Clay cleansers | Nature's Body Beautiful | www.naturesbodybeautiful.com |

| Mineral Cosmetics | Earth's Beauty | www.earthsbeauty.com |
|---|---|---|
| DMPS | Prescription – supplied by compounding pharmacies | www.amalgam.org |
| Alpha Lipoic Acid | Lipoic Acid – 25 mg capsules by Kirkman Labs | www.kirkmanlabs.com |
| DMSA | DMSA – 25 mg capsules by Vitamin Research Products | www.vrp.com |
| Water Bottles | Glass bottles by ebottle.com | www.ebottle.com |
| ProBoost | ProBoost Immune System Booster | www.proboostmed.com |
| NAC, Pantethine, Carotenoids | N-A-C; Pantethine 300; CarotenALL by Jarrow Formulas | www.jarrow.com |
| PPC | PhosChol by Nutrasal   or PPC by Source Naturals  or Hepatopro by Life Extension Foundation | www.phoschol.com www.sourcenaturals.com www.lef.org |
| TOPAS Test | TOPAS test by ALT Bioscience | www.altbioscience.com |
| EXATEST | EXATEST by IntraCellular Diagnostics | www.exatest.com |
| Iodine Test | Flechas Family Practice or Vitamin Research Products or Hakala Research Laboratory | www.helpmythyroid.com www.vrp.com www.hakalalabs.com |
| Cavitat Test | Cavitat by Cavitat Medical Technologies | www.cavitat.com |
| Soap Nuts soap | Maggie's Pure Land Cleanut  by AlmaWin | www.maggiespureland.com www.almawin-usa.com |
| Magnesium hydroxide | Original Phillips Milk of Magnesia by Bayer Drugs | Widely available |

# Bibliography

1.     www.ppnf.org, *Price-Pottenger Nutrition Foundation*

2.     Price, W.A., *Nutrition and Physical Degeneration: A Comparison of Primitive and Modern Diets and Their Effects*. 1970: Price-Pottenger Foundation.

3.     Hawks, J., et al., *Recent acceleration of human adaptive evolution*. Proceedings of the National Academy of Sciences, 2007. **104**(52): p. 20753-20758.

4.     Gershon, M.D., *The Second Brain: A Groundbreaking New Understanding of Nervous Disorders of the Stomach and Intestine*. 1999: HarperPerennial.

5.     Cohen, M.N. and G.J. Armelagos, *Paleopathology at the Origins of Agriculture*. 1984: New York: Academic Press.

6.     Diamond, J., *The Worst Mistake in the History of the Human Race*. Discover, 1987. **8**(5): p. 64-66.

7.     www.westonaprice.org, *Weston A. Price Foundation*

8.     Holick, M.F. and M. Jenkins, *The UV Advantage*. 2004: Simon & Schuster.

9.     Engel, C., *Wild Health: How Animals Keep Themselves Well and What We Can Learn from Them*. 2002: Houghton Mifflin.

10.    Cordain, L., *The Paleo diet*. 2002: Wiley.

11.    Pottenger, E., *Pottenger's Cats: A Study in Nutrition (edited writings of Francis Pottenger)*. La Mesa, California: The Price-Pottenger Nutrition Foundation, 1983.

12.    Barger, J.L., et al., *A Low Dose of Dietary Resveratrol Partially Mimics Caloric Restriction and Retards Aging Parameters in Mice*. PLoS ONE, 2008. **3**(6): p. e2264.

13.    www.informedchoice.info, *Glossary of Vaccines*

14.    Randal Bollinger, R., et al., *Biofilms in the large bowel suggest an apparent function of the human vermiform appendix*. J Theor Biol, 2007.

15.    Truss, C.O., *The Missing Diagnosis*. 1986.

16.    Crook, W., *The Yeast Connection: A Medical Breakthrough*. 1983, Jackson, Tenn.: Professional Books,.

17.    Trowbridge, J.P., *The Yeast Syndrome*. Bantam Books.

18.    Pearson, D. and S. Shaw, *Life Extension: A Practical Scientific Approach*. 1982: Warner Books.

19.     Dantzig, P.I., *Age-related macular degeneration and cutaneous signs of mercury toxicity.* Journal of Toxicology: Cutaneous and Ocular Toxicology, 2005. **24**(1): p. 3-9.

20.     www.paleodiet.com, *Paleolithic Diet Page*

21.     Diamond, J., *The Third Chimpanzee.* 1993, New York: HarperCollins.

22.     www.northstarbison.com, *Grassfed American Bison*

23.     www.blackwing.com, *Blackwing Ostrich Meat*

24.     Lame Deer, J. and R. Erdoes, *Lame Deer, Seeker of Visions.* 1972: Simon and Schuster.

25.     Fallon, S., P. Connolly, and M.G. Enig, *Nourishing Traditions: The Cookbook that Challenges Politically Correct Nutrition and the Diet Dictocrats.* 1999: NewTrends Pub.

26.     Anderson, A.K., H.E. Gayley, and A.D. Pratt, *Studies on the Chemical Composition of Bovine Blood.* Journal of Dairy Science, 1930. **13**(4): p. 336.

27.     www.uswellnessmeats.com, *U.S. Wellness Meats*

28.     www.lifelinescreening.com, *Life Line Screening*

29.     www.thincs.org, *The International Network of Cholesterol Skeptics*

30.     Kauffman, J.M., *Misleading Recent Papers on Statin Drugs in Peer-Reviewed Medical Journals.* Journal of American Physicians and Surgeons Volume, 2007. **12**(1): p. 7.

31.     Kauffman, J.M., *Malignant Medical Myths.* 2006: Infinity Publishing.

32.     Graveline, D., *Thief of Memory: Statin Drugs and the Misguided War on Cholesterol.* 2004: Infinity Publishing, Havenford, PA.

33.     Seelig, M.S. and A. Rosanoff, *The Magnesium Factor.* 2003: Avery.

34.     Dean, C., *The Miracle of Magnesium.* 2003: Ballantine Books.

35.     Purvis, J.R. and A. Movahed, *Magnesium disorders and cardiovascular diseases.* Clin Cardiol, 1992. **15**(8): p. 556-68.

36.     Rosanoff, A. and M.S. Seelig, *Comparison of Mechanism and Functional Effects of Magnesium and Statin Pharmaceuticals.* Journal of the American College of Nutrition, 2004. **23**(5): p. 501-505.

37.     Menzel, P. and F. D'Aluisio, *Man Eating Bugs: The Art and Science of Eating Insects.* 1998: Ten Speed Press.

38.     Leopold, A.C. and R. Ardrey, *Toxic Substances in Plants and the Food Habits of Early Man.* Science, 1972. **176**(4034): p. 512-514.

39.     Whittaker, R.H. and P.P. Feeny, *Allelochemics: Chemical Interactions between Species.* Science, 1971. **171**(3973): p. 757-770.

40.     Liener, I., *Toxic constituents of plant foodstuffs.* 1980, New York: Academic Press.

41.     NRC, *Lost Crops of Africa: Volume III: Fruits.* 2008, Washington DC: National Academies Press.

42.     Peters, C.R., E.M. O'Brien, and R.B. Drummond, *Edible Wild Plants of Sub-Saharan Africa.* Royal Botanical Gardens, Kew, 1992.

43.     www.maggiespureland.com, *Maggie's Pure Land Soap Nuts*

44.     Baker, L.C., L.H. Lampitt, and O.B. Meredith, *Solanine glycoside of the potato III. An improved method of extraction and determination.* J. Sci. Food and Agric, 1955. **6**: p. 197-202.

45.     Sizer, C.E., J.A. Maga, and C.J. Craven, *Total glycoalkaloids in potatoes and potato chips.* Journal of Agricultural and Food Chemistry, 1980. **28**(3): p. 578-579.

46.     Rayburn, J.R., J.A. Bantle, and M. Friedman, *Role of Carbohydrate Side Chains of Potato Glycoalkaloids in Developmental Toxicity.* Journal of Agricultural and Food Chemistry, 1994. **42**(7): p. 1511-1515.

47.     Lachman, J., et al., *Potato Glycoalkaloids and their significance in plant protection and human nutrition–Review.* Czechoslovkia, Series Rostlinna Vyroba, 2001. **47**(4): p. 181-191.

48.     Johns, T., *Detoxification function of geophagy and domestication of the potato.* Journal of Chemical Ecology, 1986. **12**(3): p. 635-646.

49.     Dashwood, R.H., *Indole-3-carbinol: Anticarcinogen or tumor promoter in brassica vegetables?* Chemico-Biological Interactions, 1998. **110**(1-2): p. 1-5.

50.     Park, J., M. Shigenaga, and B. Ames, *Induction of cytochrome P4501A1 by 2, 3, 7, 8-tetrachlorodibenzo-p-dioxin or indolo (3, 2-b) carbazole is associated with oxidative DNA damage.* Proc Natl Acad Sci US A, 1996. **93**(6): p. 2322-2327.

51.     Altmann, S.A., S.L. Garrigues, and A.B. Stahl, *More on Hominid Diet Before Fire.* Current Anthropology, 1985. **26**(5): p. 661-663.

52.     Blumenschine, R.J., A. Whiten, and K. Hawkes, *Hominid Carnivory and Foraging Strategies, and the Socio-Economic Function of Early Archaeological Sites [and Discussion].* Philosophical Transactions: Biological Sciences, 1991. **334**(1270): p. 211-221.

53.     Luchterhand, K., *On Early Hominid Plant-Food Niches.* Current Anthropology, 1982. **23**(2): p. 211-218.

54.     Peters, C.R., et al., *The Early Hominid Plant-Food Niche: Insights From an Analysis of Plant Exploitation by Homo, Pan, and Papio in Eastern and Southern Africa [and Comments and Reply].* Current Anthropology, 1981. **22**(2): p. 127-140.

55.     Stahl, A.B., et al., *Hominid Dietary Selection Before Fire [and Comments and Reply].* Current Anthropology, 1984. **25**(2): p. 151-168.

56.     Milton, K., *Nutritional characteristics of wild primate foods: do the diets of our closest living relatives have lessons for us?* Nutrition, 1999. **15**(6): p. 488-498.

57.     Seelig, M.S., *Epidemiology of water magnesium; evidence of contributions to health.* The Magnesium Web Site.

58.     Durlach, J., M. Bara, and A. Guiet-Bara, *Magnesium level in drinking water: its importance in cardiovascular risk.* Magnesium in Health and Disease, 1989: p. 173-182.

59.     www.mgwater.com, *The Magnesium Web Site*

60.     www.ntllabs.com, *Water Testing: National Testing Labs*

61.     www.naturesplus.com, *.: Nature's Plus*

62.     Rodale, J.I. and H.J. Taub, *Magnesium, the Nutrient that Could Change Your Life.* 1968: Pyramid Books.

63.     Kok, F.J., et al., *SERUM COPPER AND ZINC AND THE RISK OF DEATH FROM CANCER AND CARDIOVASCULAR DISEASE.* American Journal of Epidemiology, 2002. **128**(2): p. 352-359.

64.     www.doulton.ca, *Doulton Water Filters*

65.     www.wellnessfilter.com, *Wellness Filters*

66.     Shotyk, W., M. Krachler, and B. Chen, *Contamination of Canadian and European bottled waters with antimony from PET containers.* Journal of Environmental Monitoring, 2006. **8**(2): p. 288-292.

67.     Robbins, W.J. and A. Hervey, *Toxicity of Water Stored in Polyethylene Bottles.* Bulletin of the Torrey Botanical Club, 1974. **101**(5): p. 287-291.

68.    Le, H.H., et al., *Bisphenol A is released from polycarbonate drinking bottles and mimics the neurotoxic actions of estrogen in developing cerebellar neurons.* Toxicology Letters, 2008. **176**(2): p. 149-156.

69.    www.ebottle.com, *Glass Bottles*

70.    www.humichealth.info, *HumicHealth.info*

71.    Fung-Jou Lu, H.-P.H.H.Y.Y.Y., *Fluorescent humic substances-arsenic complex in well water in areas where blackfoot disease is endemic in Taiwan.* APPLIED ORGANOMETALLIC CHEMISTRY, 1991. **5**(6): p. 507-512.

72.    www.humates.com, *Mesa Verde Resources - Humate Supplier*

73.    www.hagroup.neu.edu, *NEU Humic Acid Research Group*

74.    www.msminerals.com, *Morningstar Minerals*

75.    Huynh A Hong , L.H.D., Simon M Cutting *The use of bacterial spore formers as probiotics.* FEMS Microbiol Rev, 2005. **29**(4): p. 813-35.

76.    Ricca, E., A.O. Henriques, and S.M. Cutting, *Bacterial spore formers: probiotics and emerging applications.* 2004: Horizon Bioscience Wymondham, UK.

77.    De Oliveira, E.J., et al., *Molecular Characterization of Brevibacillus laterosporus and Its Potential Use in Biological Control.* Applied and Environmental Microbiology, 2004. **70**(11): p. 6657-6664.

78.    www.thorne.com, *Thorne Research, Inc.*

79.    www.purecaps.com, *Pure Encapsulations*

80.    Corsello, S., MD, *Bacillus Laterosporus BOD.* 1996, New York: Healing Wisdom.

81.    www.flora-balance.com, *Flora Balance: Bacillus Laterosporus*

82.    Stefansson, V., *The Fat of the Land.* 1956: Macmillan.

83.    www.celestialpets.com, *Celestial Pets*

84.    Eriksson, P., C. Fischer, and A. Fredriksson, *Polybrominated Diphenyl Ethers, A Group of Brominated Flame Retardants, Can Interact with Polychlorinated Biphenyls in Enhancing Developmental Neurobehavioral Defects.* Toxicological Sciences, 2006. **94**(2): p. 302.

85.    Enser, M., et al., *The polyunsaturated fatty acid composition of beef and lamb liver.* Meat Science, 1998. **49**(3): p. 321-327.

86.    www.vitalchoice.com, *Vital Choice Wild Seafood*

87.    Nakajima, Y., et al., *Ingestion of Hijiki seaweed and risk of arsenic poisoning.* APPLIED ORGANOMETALLIC CHEMISTRY, 2006. **20**(9): p. 557.

88.    www.diagnostechs.com, *Diagnostechs, Inc.*

89.    www.realmilk.com, *A CAMPAIGN FOR RAW) MILK*

90.    Mandavgane, S.A., V.V. Pattalwar, and A.R. Kalambe, *Development of cow dung based herbal mosquito repellent.* Natural Product Radiance, 2005. **4**(4): p. 270-272.

91.    Campbell, T.C., *The China Study.* 2005: BenBella Books, Dallas.

92.    Bohn, T., et al., *Phytic acid added to white-wheat bread inhibits fractional apparent magnesium absorption in humans.* American Journal of Clinical Nutrition, 2004. **79**(3): p. 418-423.

93.    Duncan, C.W., C.C. Lightfoot, and C.F. Huffman, *Studies on the Composition of Bovine Blood: I. The Magnesium Content of the Blood Plasma of the Normal Dairy Calf.* J. Dairy Sci., 1938. **21**(11): p. 689-696.

94.    Odvina, C.V., et al., *Severely Suppressed Bone Turnover: A Potential Complication of Alendronate Therapy.* 2005, Endocrine Soc. p. 1294-1301.

95.    Ruggiero, S.L., et al., *Osteonecrosis of the jaws associated with the use of bisphosphonates: a review of 63 cases.* Journal of Oral and Maxillofacial Surgery, 2004. **62**(5): p. 527-534.

96.    Sabrina C. Agarwal, M.D.G., *Bone quantity and quality in past populations.* The Anatomical Record, 1996. **246**(4): p. 423-432.

97.    Bischoff-Ferrari, H.A., et al., *Calcium intake and hip fracture risk in men and women: a meta-analysis of prospective cohort studies and randomized controlled trials.* American Journal of Clinical Nutrition, 2007. **86**(6): p. 1780.

98.    www.breastpumpsdirect.com, *Electric Breast Pumps*

99.    www.llli.org, *La Leche League International*

100.   Alvarez, H.P., *Grandmother hypothesis and primate life histories.* AMERICAN JOURNAL OF PHYSICAL ANTHROPOLOGY, 2000. **113**(3): p. 435-450.

101.   Martin, M.C., et al., *Menopause without symptoms: the endocrinology of menopause among rural Mayan Indians.* Am J Obstet Gynecol, 1993. **168**(6 Pt 1): p. 1839-45.

102.   Stewart, D.E., *Menopause in highland Guatemala Mayan women.* Maturitas, 2003. **44**(4): p. 293-7.

103.    Lock, M., *Menopause: lessons from anthropology*. 1998, Am
        Psychosomatic Soc. p. 410-419.
104.    www.bioticsresearch.com, *Biotics Research*
105.    Cronin, C.C. and F. Shanahan, *Why is celiac disease so common
        in Ireland*. Perspect Biol Med, 2001. **44**(3): p. 342-52.
106.    Gotthoffer, N.R., *Gelatin in nutrition and medicine*. 1945.
107.    Daniel, K.T., *The Whole Soy Story: The Dark Side of America's
        Favorite Health Food*. 2005: New Trends Publishing.
108.    Finley, J.W., et al., *Bioavailability of selenium from meat and
        broccoli as determined by retention and distribution of 75 Se*.
        Biological Trace Element Research, 2004. **99**(1): p. 191-209.
109.    Zheng, J.J., et al., *Measurement of zinc bioavailability from beef
        and a ready-to-eat high-fiber breakfast cereal in humans:
        application of a whole-gut lavage technique*. Am J Clin Nutr,
        1993. **58**(6): p. 902-7.
110.    Schuiling, M. and H.C. Harries, *The coconut palm in East Africa*.
        East African Tall. Principes, 1994. **38**(1): p. 4-11.
111.    Petroianu, G.A., *Green coconut water for intravenous use: Trace
        and minor element content*. The Journal of Trace Elements in
        Experimental Medicine, 2004. **17**(4): p. 273-282.
112.    Mercola, J., *Sweet Deception: Why Splenda, NutraSweet, and the
        FDA May Be Hazardous to Your Health*. 2006: Nelson Books.
113.    Ming, D. and G. Hellekant, *Brazzein, a new high-potency
        thermostable sweet protein from Pentadiplandra brazzeana B.*
        FEBS Lett, 1994. **355**(1): p. 106-8.
114.    Parke, D.V. and A.L. Parke, *Rapeseed oil: An autoxidative food
        lipid*. Journal of clinical biochemistry and nutrition, 1999. **26**(2):
        p. 51-61.
115.    www.brownwoodacres.com, *Brownwood Acres Fruit Supplements*
116.    Hirsch, J., et al., *Indicators of Erythrocyte Damage after
        Microwave Warming of Packed Red Blood Cells*. Clin Chem, 2003.
        **49**(5): p. 792-799.
117.    Lubec, G., C. Wolf, and B. Bartosch, *Aminoacid isomerisation
        and microwave exposure*. Lancet, 1989. **2**(8676): p. 1392-3.
118.    Arvanitoyannis, I. and L. Bosnea, *Migration of Substances from
        Food Packaging Materials to Foods*. Critical Reviews in Food
        Science and Nutrition, 2004. **44**(2): p. 63-76.

119.    Said, Z.M., et al., *Pyridoxine uptake by colonocytes: A specific and regulated carrier-mediated process.* Am J Physiol Cell Physiol, 2008: p. 00015.2008.

120.    Ershoff, B.H., *Protective Effects of Liver in Immature Rats Fed Toxic Doses of Thiouracil.* Journal of Nutrition, 1954. **52**(3): p. 437.

121.    Ershoff, B.H., *Increased Survival of Liver-Fed Rats Administered Multiple Sublethal Doses of X-Irradiation.* Journal of Nutrition, 1952. **47**(2): p. 289.

122.    www.nowfoods.com, *NOW Foods*

123.    Leklem, J.E. and C.B. Hollenbeck, *Acute ingestion of glucose decreases plasma pyridoxal 5'-phosphate and total vitamin B-6 concentration.* Am J Clin Nutr, 1990. **51**(5): p. 832-6.

124.    Wei, I.L., Y.H. Huang, and G.S. Wang, *Vitamin B6 deficiency decreases the glucose utilization in cognitive brain structures of rats.* The Journal of Nutritional Biochemistry, 1999. **10**(9): p. 525-531.

125.    www.sourcenaturals.com, *Source Naturals*

126.    www.tropicaltraditions.com, *Tropical Traditions - Palm Oil*

127.    www.palmoilworld.org, *Palm Oil World*

128.    www.jarrow.com, *Jarrow Formulas*

129.    www.lef.org, *Life Extension Foundation*

130.    www.vitamindcouncil.com, *Vitamin D Council*

131.    Binkley, N., et al., *Low Vitamin D Status despite Abundant Sun Exposure.* Journal of Clinical Endocrinology & Metabolism, 2007. **92**(6): p. 2130.

132.    Bastuji-Garin, S. and T.L. Diepgen, *Cutaneous malignant melanoma, sun exposure, and sunscreen use: epidemiological evidence.* British Journal of Dermatology, 2002. **146**(s61): p. 24-30.

133.    Elwood, J.M., *Melanoma and sun exposure: An overview of published studies.* International Journal of Cancer, 1997. **73**(2): p. 198-203.

134.    Whang, R., D.D. Whang, and M.P. Ryan, *Refractory potassium repletion. A consequence of magnesium deficiency.* Archives of Internal Medicine, 1992. **152**(1): p. 40-45.

135.    Seelig, M.S., *Consequences of magnesium deficiency on the enhancement of stress reactions; preventive and therapeutic implications (a review).* 1994, Am Coll Nutrition. p. 429-446.

136.    Gontijo-Amaral, C., et al., *Oral magnesium supplementation in asthmatic children: a double-blind randomized placebo-controlled trial.* Eur J Clin Nutr, 2006. **61**: p. 54–60.

137.    www.magnesiumresearchlab.com, *Magnesium Research Lab*

138.    Arnold, A., et al., *Magnesium deficiency in critically ill patients.* Anaesthesia, 1995. **50**(3): p. 203-205.

139.    www.exatest.com, *Magnesium Deficiency - IntraCellular Diagnostics' EXAtest for Minerals Electrolytes*

140.    www.bodybio.com, *BodyBio Company*

141.    Durlach, J., et al., *Taurine and magnesium homeostasis: new data and recent advances.* Magnesium in cellular processes and medicine. Basel: S Karger publ, 1987: p. 219-38.

142.    www.douglaslabs.com, *Douglas Labs*

143.    www.selfhealthsystems.com, *Self-Health Systems - Magnesium Lotion*

144.    Shealy, C.N., *Holy Water, Sacred Oil.* 2000, Fair Grove, MO: Biogenics.

145.    Gaby, A.R., *Intravenous nutrient therapy: the "Myers' cocktail.".* Altern Med Rev, 2002. **7**(5): p. 389-403.

146.    Turnlund, J.R., et al., *Vitamin B-6 depletion followed by repletion with animal-or plant-source diets and calcium and magnesium metabolism in young women.* Am J Clin Nutr, 1992. **56**(5): p. 905-10.

147.    Holman, P., *Pyridoxine–vitamin B-6.* Journal of the Australasian College of Nutritional and Environmental Medicine (ACNEM), 1995. **14**: p. 5-16.

148.    Schauss, A. and C. Costin, *Zinc as a nutrient in the treatment of eating disorders.* Am J Nat Med, 1997. **4**: p. 8-13.

149.    www.kirkmanlabs.com, *Kirkman Labs*

150.    www.realsalt.com, *RealSalt*

151.    Brownstein, D., *Salt Your Way to Health.* 2007: Medical Alternatives Press.

152.    www.thyroid.about.com, *Thyroid Disease Information*

153.    www.stopthethyroidmadness.com, *Stop The Thyroid Madness*

154.    Resnick, D. and G. Niwayama, *Diagnosis of Bone and Joint Disorders.* 1988: Philadelphia.

155.    Wald, A. and S.A. Adibi, *Stimulation of gastric acid secreted by glycine and related oligopeptides in humans.* American Journal of

Physiology- Gastrointestinal and Liver Physiology, 1982. **242**(2): p. 85-88.

156.    Grobben, A.H., et al., *Inactivation of the bovine-spongiform-encephalopathy (BSE) agent by the acid and alkaline processes used in the manufacture of bone gelatine.* Biotechnology and Applied Biochemistry, 2004. **39**(3): p. 329-338.

157.    Prudden, J.F. and L.L. Balassa, *The biological activity of bovine cartilage preparations. Clinical demonstration of their potent anti-inflammatory capacity with supplementary notes on certain relevant fundamental supportive studies.* Semin Arthritis Rheum, 1974. **3**(4): p. 287-321.

158.    Samonina, G., et al., *Protection of gastric mucosal integrity by gelatin and simple proline-containing peptides.* Pathophysiology, 2000. **7**(1): p. 69-73.

159.    Moskowitz, R.W., *Role of collagen hydrolysate in bone and joint disease.* Seminars in Arthritis and Rheumatism, 2000. **30**(2): p. 87-99.

160.    www.greatlakesgelatin.com, *Great Lakes Gelatin, Grayslake, Illinois*

161.    Yehuda, S. and R. Carasso, *Modulation of learning, pain thresholds, and thermoregulation in the rat by preparations of free purified alpha-linolenic and linoleic acids: determination of the optimal omega 3-to-omega 6 ratio.* Proc Natl Acad Sci US A, 1993. **90**(21): p. 10345-10349.

162.    Erasmus, U., *Fats that heal, fats that kill.* 1993: Alive Books.

163.    Hansen, A.E., et al., *ROLE OF LINOLEIC ACID IN INFANT NUTRITION: Clinical and Chemical Study of 428 Infants Fed on Milk Mixtures Varying in Kind and Amount of Fat.* Pediatrics, 1963. **31**(1): p. 171-192.

164.    Daley, C.A., et al., *A Literature Review of the Value-Added Nutrients found in Grass-fed Beef Products*, College of Agriculture, California State University, Chico.

165.    www.christophereggs.com, *Christopher Eggs*

166.    Milinsk, M.C., et al., *Fatty acid profile of egg yolk lipids from hens fed diets rich in n-3 fatty acids.* Food Chemistry, 2003. **83**(2): p. 287-292.

167.    Gower, J.D., *A role for dietary lipids and antioxidants in the activation of carcinogens.* Free Radical Biology & Medicine, 1988. **5**(2): p. 95-111.

168.    Mozaffarian, D., E.B. Rimm, and D.M. Herrington, *Dietary fats, carbohydrate, and progression of coronary atherosclerosis in postmenopausal women.* American Journal of Clinical Nutrition, 2004. **80**(5): p. 1175-1184.

169.    Fujiyama-Fujiwara, Y., et al., *Effects of sesamin on the fatty acid composition of the liver of rats fed N-6 and N-3 fatty acid-rich diet.* J Nutr Sci Vitaminol (Tokyo), 1995. **41**(2): p. 217-25.

170.    Shimizu, S., et al., *Sesamin is a potent and specific inhibitor of delta-5 desaturase in polyunsaturated fatty acid biosynthesis.* Lipids, 1991. **26**(7): p. 512-516.

171.    Wagner, S. and H. Breiteneder, *The latex-fruit syndrome.* Biochem Soc Trans, 2002. **30**(pt 6): p. 935-940.

172.    Fernandez-Rivas, M., R. van Ree, and M. Cuevas, *Allergy to Rosaceae fruits without related pollinosis.* J Allergy Clin Immunol, 1997. **100**(6 Pt 1): p. 728-33.

173.    Wright, J. and L. Lenard, *Why Stomach Acid Is Good for You.* 2001, M. Evans and Company.

174.    www.twinlab.com, *Twinlab Supplements*

175.    www.standardprocess.com, *Standard Process*

176.    Alverdy, J.C., *The re-emerging role of the intestinal microflora in critical illness and inflammation.* J Leukoc Biol, 2007: p. 1-6.

177.    Mitsou, E.K., et al., *Fecal microflora of Greek healthy neonates.* Anaerobe, 2007.

178.    Gibson, G.R. and R.A. Rastall, *When we eat, which bacteria should we be feeding.* ASM News, 2004. **70**: p. 224-231.

179.    Vogel, G., *CLINICAL TRIALS: Deaths Prompt a Review of Experimental Probiotic Therapy.* Science, 2008. **319**(5863): p. 557a-.

180.    Rodenburg, W., et al., *Impaired barrier function by dietary fructo-oligosaccharides (FOS) in rats is accompanied by increased colonic mitochondrial gene expression.* BMC Genomics, 2008. **9**(1): p. 144.

181.    Kirsch, M., *Bacterial overgrowth.* American Journal of Gastroenterology, 1990. **85**(3): p. 231-237.

182.    Bouhnik, Y., et al., *Bacterial populations contaminating the upper gut in patients with small intestinal bacterial overgrowth syndrome.* The American Journal of Gastroenterology, 1999. **94**(5): p. 1327-1331.

183.   www.kyolic.com, *Wakunaga -Kyolic Brand*

184.   Majamaa, H. and E. Isolauri, *Probiotics: a novel approach in the management of food allergy.* J Allergy Clin Immunol, 1997. **99**(2): p. 179-85.

185.   Lewis, W.H. and M.P.F. Elvin-Lewis, *Medical Botany: Plants Affecting Human Health.* 2003: Wiley.

186.   Odenyo, A.A. and P.O. Osuji, *Tannin-tolerant ruminal bacteria from East African ruminants.* Canadian Journal of Microbiology, 1998. **44**: p. 905-909.

187.   Jones, R.J. and R.G. Megarrity, *Successful transfer of DHP-degrading bacteria from Hawaiian goats to Australian ruminants to overcome the toxicity of Leucaena.* Aust Vet J, 1986. **63**(8): p. 259-62.

188.   www.terrapond.com, *Terramin Clay*

189.   Hibberd, A.R., M.A. Howard, and A.G. Hunnisett, *Mercury from Dental Amalgam Fillings: Studies on Oral Chelating Agents for Assessing and Reducing Mercury Burdens in Humans.* Journal of Nutritional & Environmental Medicine, 1998. **8**(3): p. 219-231.

190.   O'Donnell, L., J. Virjee, and K. Heaton, *Detection of pseudodiarrhoea by simple clinical assessment of intestinal transit rate.* BMJ, 1990. **300**(6722): p. 439-440.

191.   www.healthstep.com, *HealthStep*

192.   Singer, S. and S. Grismaijer, *Dressed to Kill: The Link Between Breast Cancer and Bras.* 1995: Avery Pub. Group.

193.   www.intimatehealth.net, *Intimate Health - Brassage*

194.   Exley, C., *Does antiperspirant use increase the risk of aluminium-related disease, including Alzheimer's disease?* Molecular Medicine Today, 1998. **4**(3): p. 107-109.

195.   Wilson, L., *Sauna Therapy for Detoxification and Healing* 2006, Prescott: L.D. Wilson Consultants.

196.   Sylver, N., *The Holistic Handbook of Sauna Therapy.* 2003: Center for Frequency Education.

197.   Dantzig, P., *The role of mercury in pustulosis palmaris et plantaris.* Journal of Occupational and Environmental Medicine, 2003. **45**(5): p. 468-469.

198.   Dantzig, P.I., *A new cutaneous sign of mercury poisoning?* Journal of the American Academy of Dermatology, 2003. **49**(6): p. 1109-1111.

199. Dantzig, P.I., *Persistent Palmar Plaques—Another Possible Cutaneous Sign of Mercury Poisoning.* Cutaneous and Ocular Toxicology, 2005. **23**(2): p. 77-81.

200. Dantzig, P.I., *Parkinson's Disease, Macular Degeneration and Cutaneous Signs of Mercury Toxicity.* Journal of Occupational and Environmental Medicine, 2006. **48**(7): p. 656.

201. Boyd, A.S., et al., *Mercury exposure and cutaneous disease.* J Am Acad Dermatol, 2000. **43**(1 Pt 1): p. 81-90.

202. www.hightechhealth.com, *High Tech Health Saunas*

203. www.drlwilson.com, *Dr. Larry Wilson*

204. www.neuraltherapy.com, *Dr. Dietrich Klinghardt, AANT, KMT, American Association of Neuraltherapy*

205. www.drgruenn.com, *Hans Gruenn MD*

206. www.soapnut.com, *Soapnut Powder*

207. www.almawin-usa.com, *AlmaWin Cleanut*

208. www.thermotex.com, *FIR Heating Pads*

209. Christl, I., et al., *Relating ion binding by fulvic and humic acids to chemical composition and molecular size. 2. Metal binding.* Environ. Sci. Technol, 2001. **35**(12): p. 2512-2517.

210. Liu, A. and R.D. Gonzalez, *Adsorption/Desorption in a System Consisting of Humic Acid, Heavy Metals, and Clay Minerals.* Journal of Colloid And Interface Science, 1999. **218**(1): p. 225-232.

211. Mullen, M.D., et al., *Bacterial sorption of heavy metals.* Appl Environ Microbiol, 1989. **55**(12): p. 3143-3149.

212. Beveridge, T.J. and R.G.E. Murray, *Uptake and retention of metals by cell walls of Bacillus subtilis.* J. Bacteriol, 1976. **127**(3): p. 1502-1518.

213. Fowle, D.A. and J.B. Fein, *Experimental measurements of the reversibility of metal–bacteria adsorption reactions.* Chemical Geology, 2000. **168**(1-2): p. 27-36.

214. www.microessentiallab.com, *Mircroessential Lab- pH paper*

215. Proudfoot, A.T., E.P. Krenzelok, and J.A. Vale, *Position Paper on Urine Alkalinization.* Clinical Toxicology, 2005. **42**(1): p. 1-26.

216. Minich, D.M. and J.S. Bland, *ACID-ALKALINE BALANCE: ROLE IN CHRONIC DISEASE AND DETOXIFICATION.* PHYSIOLOGY. **6**(11): p. 12.

217. Diamond, J., *Eat Dirt*, in *Discover Magazine*. 1998. p. pp70-76.

218.    Dextreit, R., *Our Earth, Our Cure*. 1974: Swan House.

219.    A~, P., *Living Clay*. 2006: Perry Productions.

220.    Abehsera, M., *The Healing Power Of Clay*. 2001: Citadel.

221.    Callahan, G.N., *Eating dirt*. Emerg Infect Dis, 2003. **9**(8): p. 1016-
        1021.

222.    Graham , C., *The Clay Disciples*. 2006.

223.    www.eytonsearth.org, *Healing With Clay, Earth and Mud*

224.    www.pascalite.com, *Pascalite Clay*

225.    www.redmondclay.com, *Redmond Clay*

226.    www.colloid.com, *Amercian Colloid Company - Volclay HPM-20*

227.    www.lagunaclay.com, *LagunaClay2007*

228.    Heintze, U.L.F., et al., *Methylation of mercury from dental
        amalgam and mercuric chloride by oral streptococci in vitro*.
        European Journal of Oral Sciences, 1983. **91**(2): p. 150-152.

229.    Rowland, I.R., P. Grasso, and M.J. Davies, *The methylation of
        mercuric chloride by human intestinal bacteria*. Cellular and
        Molecular Life Sciences (CMLS), 1975. **31**(9): p. 1064-1065.

230.    Trevors, J.T., *Mercury methylation by bacteria*. Journal of Basic
        Microbiology, 1986. **26**(8): p. 499-504.

231.    www.humet.hu, *HUMIFULVATE*

232.    www.phytopharmica.com, *PhytoPharmica*

233.    Noyes, R., *Handbook of Pollution Control Processes*. 1991: Noyes
        Publications.

234.    Shastri, Y. and U. Diwekar, *Optimal Control of Lake pH for
        Mercury Bioaccumulation Control*. 2006.

235.    www.buyactivatedcharcoal.com, *BUY ACTIVATED CHARCOAL*

236.    www.optimox.com, *The Optimox Corporation - Iodoral*

237.    www.drbrownstein.com, *Dr. David Brownstein, MD*

238.    www.helpmythyroid.com, *Flechas Family Practice2005*

239.    Abraham, G.E., *The historical background of the iodine project*.
        The Original Internist, 2005. **12**(2): p. 57-66.

240.    Brownstein, D., *Iodine: Why You Need It, why You Can't Live
        Without it*. 3rd edition ed. 2007: Medical Alternatives Press.

241.    www.helpmythyroid.com, *Flechas Family Practice*

242.    www.vrp.com, *Vitamin Research Products*

243.    www.jcrowsmarketplace.com, *J.Crow's® Marketplace - Lugol's
        Solution*

244.    Trevorrow, V., *STUDIES ON THE NATURE OF THE IODINE IN BLOOD*. Journal of Biological Chemistry, 1939. **127**(3): p. 737-750.

245.    Seidell, A. and F. Fenger, *SEASONAL VARIATION IN THE IODINE CONTENT OF THE THYROID GLAND*. Journal of Biological Chemistry, 1913. **13**(4): p. 517-526.

246.    FDA, *April 25, 2000. Total Diet Study Statistics on Element Results. Revision 1, 1991–1998. Washington, DC: Food and Drug Administration.*

247.    Guiet-Bara, A., M. Bara, and J. Durlach, *Magnesium: a competitive inhibitor of lead and cadmium. Ultrastructural studies of the human amniotic epithelial cell.* Magnes Res, 1990. **3**(1): p. 31-6.

248.    Soldatovic, D., et al., *Compared effects of high oral Mg supplements and of EDTA chelating agent on chronic lead intoxication in rabbits.* Magnes Res, 1997. **10**(2): p. 127-33.

249.    Soldatovic, D., V. Matovic, and D. Vujanovic, *Prophylactic effect of high magnesium intake in rabbits exposed to prolonged lead intoxication.* Magnes Res, 1993. **6**(2): p. 145-8.

250.    Djukic-Cosic, D., et al., *Effect of supplemental magnesium on the kidney levels of cadmium, zinc, and copper of mice exposed to toxic levels of cadmium.* Biological Trace Element Research, 2006. **114**(1): p. 281-291.

251.    Rooney, J.P.K., *The role of thiols, dithiols, nutritional factors and interacting ligands in the toxicology of mercury.* Toxicology, 2007. **234**(3): p. 145-156.

252.    Baldewicz, T., *Plasma pyridoxine deficiency is related to increased psychological distress in recently bereaved homosexual men.* 1998, Am Psychosomatic Soc. p. 297-308.

253.    Jefferies, W.M.K., *Safe Uses of Cortisol.* 2004: Charles C. Thomas, Publisher Ltd.

254.    Cutler, A.H., *Amalgam Illness.* 1999: Andrew Hall Cutler.

255.    Imura, N., et al., *Chemical Methylation of Inorganic Mercury with Methylcobalaiin, a Vitamin B12 Analog.* Science, 1971. **172**(3989): p. 1248-1249.

256.    www.iaomt.org, *IAOMT International Academy of Oral Medicine and Toxicology*

257.    www.toxicteeth.org, *Consumers for Dental Choice*

258.    www.melisa.org, *MELISA® Medica Foundation*

259. Woods, J.S., *Altered porphyrin metabolism as a biomarker of mercury exposure and toxicity*. Can J Physiol Pharmacol, 1996. **74**(2): p. 210-215.

260. Geier, D.A., *A Prospective Study of Mercury Toxicity Biomarkers in Autistic Spectrum Disorders*. Journal of Toxicology and Environmental Health, Part A, 2007. **70**(20): p. 1723-1730.

261. www.directlabs.com, *Direct Labs*

262. www.doctorsdata.com, *Doctor's Data Lab*

263. Cutler, A.H., *Hair Test Interpretation: Finding Hidden Toxicities*. 2004: Andrew Hall Cutler.

264. Ibrahim, D., et al., *Heavy Metal Poisoning: Clinical Presentations and Pathophysiology*. Clinics in Laboratory Medicine, 2006. **26**(1): p. 67-97.

265. www.ccrlab.com, *Clifford Reactivity Test*

266. www.hugnet.com, *Huggins Applied Healing*

267. www.amalgam.org, *DAMS Intl. Dental Amalgam Mercury Solutions*

268. Segermann, J., et al., *Effect of alpha-lipoic acid on the peripheral conversion of thyroxine to triiodothyronine and on serum lipid, protein and glucose levels*. Arzneimittelforschung, 1991. **41**(12): p. 1294-8.

269. Khamaisi, M., et al., *Lipoic acid acutely induces hypoglycemia in fasting nondiabetic and diabetic rats*. Metabolism, 1999. **48**(4): p. 504-10.

270. Barnes, B., *Hope for Hypoglycemia*. 1989, Robinson Press, Incorporated.

271. Waters, R.S., et al., *EDTA chelation effects on urinary losses of cadmium, calcium, chromium, cobalt, copper, lead, magnesium, and zinc*. Biological Trace Element Research, 2001. **83**(3): p. 207-221.

272. De Lucca, A., *In Vitro Inhibitory and Fungicidal Properties of Edta for Aspergillus and Fusarium*. Interscience Conference on Antimicrobial Agents & Chemotherapy Proceedings, 2006: p. 27-30.

273. Duhr, E.F., et al., *HgEDTA complex inhibits GTP interactions with the E-site of brain beta-tubulin*. Toxicol Appl Pharmacol, 1993. **122**(2): p. 273-80.

274.    Omura, Y., *Radiation Injury and Mercury Deposits in Internal Organs.* Acupuncture and Electro- Therapeutics Res., Int. J., 1995. **Vol.20**: p. pp. 133-148.

275.    Chandra, J., et al., *Modification of Surface Properties of Biomaterials Influences the Ability of Candida albicans To Form Biofilms.* Applied and Environmental Microbiology, 2005. **71**(12): p. 8795.

276.    Harrison, J.J., et al., *Metal resistance in Candida biofilms.* FEMS Microbiol Ecol, 2006. **55**(3): p. 479-91.

277.    Harrison, J.J., et al., *Metal Ions May Suppress or Enhance Cellular Differentiation in Candida albicans and Candida tropicalis Biofilms?†.* Applied and Environmental Microbiology, 2007. **73**(15): p. 4940-4949.

278.    Baklayan, A., *Parasites: The Hidden Cause of Many Diseases.* 2005: Dr. Clark Research Association.

279.    Klinghardt, D., *Amalgam/mercury detox as a treatment for chronic viral, bacterial, and fungal illnesses.* Annual Meeting of the International and American Academy of Clinical Nutrition.

280.    Djeu, J.Y., et al., *Function associated with IL-2 receptor-beta on human neutrophils. Mechanism of activation of antifungal activity against Candida albicans by IL-2.* J Immunol, 1993. **150**(3): p. 960-970.

281.    Worth, R.G., et al., *Mercury Inhibition of Neutrophil Activity: Evidence of Aberrant Cellular Signalling and Incoherent Cellular Metabolism.* Scandinavian Journal of Immunology, 2001. **53**(1): p. 49-55.

282.    Perlingeiro, R.C. and M.L. Queiroz, *Measurement of the respiratory burst and chemotaxis in polymorphonuclear leukocytes from mercury-exposed workers.* Hum Exp Toxicol, 1995. **14**(3): p. 281-6.

283.    Savage, D.C., *Microbial interference between indigenous yeast and lactobacilli in the rodent stomach.* J Bacteriol, 1969. **98**(3): p. 1278-1283.

284.    www.autism.asu.edu, *ASU's Autism/Asperger's Research Program*2007

285.    Corey, J.P., C.F. Romberger, and G.Y. Shaw, *Fungal diseases of the sinuses.* Otolaryngol Head Neck Surg, 1990. **103**(6): p. 1012-5.

286.    Vaughn, V.J. and E.D. Weinberg, *Candida albicans dimorphism and virulence: Role of copper.* Mycopathologia, 1978. **64**(1): p. 39-42.

287.    Weissman, Z., et al., *The high copper tolerance of Candida albicans is mediated by a P-type ATPase.* Proceedings of the National Academy of Sciences of the United States of America, 2000. **97**(7): p. 3520.

288.    Kujan, P., et al., *Removal of copper ions from dilute solutions by Streptomyces noursei mycelium. Comparison with yeast biomass.* Folia Microbiol (Praha), 2005. **50**(4): p. 309-13.

289.    Truss, C.O., *Metabolic abnormalities in patients with chronic candidiasis. The acetaldehyde hypothesis.* Journal of orthomolecular psychiatry, 1984. **13**(2): p. 66-93.

290.    Lieber, C.S., *A LCOHOL: Its Metabolism and Interaction With Nutrients.* Annual Review of Nutrition, 2000. **20**: p. 395-430.

291.    Agarwal, D.P. and H.K. Seitz, *Alcohol in Health and Disease.* 2001: Marcel Dekker.

292.    South, J.A., *Acetaldehyde: a common and potent neurotoxin.* VRP's Nutritional News, July. Internet, 1997.

293.    www.phoschol.com, *PhosChol*

294.    Xie, Y., et al., *Ethanol-induced gastric mucosal injury and the protection of taurine against the injury in rats.* Sheng Li Xue Bao, 1999. **51**(3): p. 310-4.

295.    Guiet-Bara, A. and M. Bara, *Ethanol effect on the ionic transfer through isolated human amnion. II. Cellular targets of the in vitro acute ethanol action and of the antagonism between magnesium, taurine and ethanol.* Cell Mol Biol (Noisy-le-grand), 1993. **39**(7): p. 715-22.

296.    Masuda, M., K. Horisaka, and T. Koeda, *Role of taurine in neutrophil function.* Folia Pharmacologica Japonica, 1984. **84**(3): p. 283-292.

297.    Stern, F., et al., *Effect of vitamin B6 supplementation on degradation rates of short-lived proteins in human neutrophils.* The Journal of Nutritional Biochemistry, 1999. **10**(8): p. 467-476.

298.    Watanabe, A., et al., *Lowering of blood acetaldehyde but not ethanol concentrations by pantethine following alcohol ingestion: different effects in flushing and nonflushing subjects.* Alcohol Clin Exp Res, 1985. **9**(3): p. 272-6.

299.     Craig, J.A. and E.E. Snell, *THE COMPARATIVE ACTIVITIES OF PANTETHINE, PANTOTHENIC ACID, AND COENZYME A FOR VARIOUS MICROORGANISMS.* J. Bacteriol, 1951. **61**: p. 238-291.

300.     Firestone, B.Y. and S.A. Koser, *GROWTH PROMOTING EFFECT OF SOME BIOTIN ANALOGUES FOR CANDIDA ALBICANS.* Journal of Bacteriology, 1960. **79**(5): p. 674.

301.     Iimuro, Y., et al., *Glycine prevents alcohol-induced liver injury by decreasing alcohol in the rat stomach.* Gastroenterology, 1996. **110**(5): p. 1536-1542.

302.     Yin, M., et al., *Glycine Accelerates Recovery from Alcohol-Induced Liver Injury.* Journal of Pharmacology and Experimental Therapeutics, 1998. **286**(2): p. 1014.

303.     Vidotto, V., et al., *Importance of some factors on the dimorphism of Candida albicans.* Mycopathologia, 1988. **104**(3): p. 129-135.

304.     www.proboostmed.com, *ProBoost*

305.     Mankowski, Z.T., *Influence of cell-free thymus extracts on the course of experimental Candida albicans infection in mice.* Mycopathologia, 1968. **36**(3): p. 247-256.

306.     Rajakrishnan, V., P. Viswanathan, and V.P. Menon, *Adaptation of siblings of female rats given ethanol effect of N-acetyl-L-cysteine.* Amino Acids, 1997. **12**(3): p. 323-341.

307.     ÖHman, L., et al., *N-acetylcysteine enhances receptor-mediated phagocytosis by human neutrophils.* Collection sécurité, 1992. **36**(3-4): p. 271-277.

308.     Urban, T., et al., *Neutrophil function and glutathione-peroxidase (GSH-px) activity in healthy individuals after treatment with N-acetyl-L-cysteine.* Biomedicine & Pharmacotherapy, 1997. **51**(9): p. 388-390.

309.     Vasdev, S., et al., *N-acetyl cysteine attenuates ethanol induced hypertension in rats.* Artery, 1995. **21**(6): p. 312-6.

310.     Sprince, H., et al., *Protection against Acetaldehyde Toxicity in the rat by l-cysteine, thiamin and l-2-Methylthiazolidine-4-carboxylic acid.* Inflammation Research, 1974. **4**(2): p. 125-130.

311.     Blyth, W. and G.E. Stewart, *Systemic candidiasis in mice treated with prednisolone and amphotericin B. 1. Morbidity, mortality and inflammatory reaction.* Mycopathologia, 1978. **66**(1): p. 41-50.

312. DeMaria, A., H. Buckley, and F. von Lichtenberg, *Gastrointestinal candidiasis in rats treated with antibiotics, cortisone, and azathioprine.* Infection and Immunity, 1976. **13**(6): p. 1761.

313. Larsen, B., et al., *Key physiological differences in Candida albicans CDR1 induction by steroid hormones and antifungal drugs.* Yeast, 1911. **2006**: p. 795-802.

314. Eaton, K.K., et al., *Abnormal Gut Fermentation: Laboratory Studies reveal Deficiency of B vitamins, Zinc, and Magnesium.* Journal of Nutritional & Environmental Medicine, 2004. **14**(2): p. 115-120.

315. Kariuki, E., R. Ngugi, and J. Muthotho, *Povidone iodine therapy for recurrent oral Candidiasis to prevent emerging Antifungal resistant Candida Strains.* Int Conf AIDS, 2000: p. 13.

316. Shoemaker, R.C., *Mold Warriors.* 2005: Gateway Press.

317. Hume, E.D., *Bechamp or Pasteur?* 2006: DLM.

318. Summers, A.O., et al., *Mercury released from dental" silver" fillings provokes an increase in mercury- and antibiotic-resistant bacteria in oral and intestinal floras of primates.* Antimicrobial Agents & Chemotherapy, 1993. **37**(4): p. 825-834.

319. Lorscheider, F.L., et al., *The dental amalgam mercury controversy—inorganic mercury and the CNS; genetic linkage of mercury and antibiotic resistances in intestinal bacteria.* Toxicology, 1995. **97**(1-3): p. 19-22.

320. Ready, D., et al., *The effect of amalgam exposure on mercury-and antibiotic-resistant bacteria.* International Journal of Antimicrobial Agents, 2007. **30**(1): p. 34-39.

321. Wireman, J., et al., *Association of mercury resistance with antibiotic resistance in the gram-negative fecal bacteria of primates.* Appl Environ Microbiol, 1997. **63**(11): p. 4494-4503.

322. Ready, D., et al., *Oral bacteria resistant to mercury and to antibiotics are present in children with no previous exposure to amalgam restorative materials.* FEMS Microbiology Letters, 2003. **223**(1): p. 107-111.

323. Meinig, G., *Root canal cover-up.* 1994: Bion Pub.

324. Kulacz, R. and T.E. Levy, *The Roots of Disease: Connecting Dentistry and Medicine.* 2002: Xlibris Corp.

325. www.altbioscience.com, *ALT BioScience - TOPAS Test*

326. www.cavitat.com, *Cavitat Medical Technologies*

327.    www.lymeinducedautism.com, *L.I.A. Foundation*

328.    Davis, I.J., H. Richards, and P. Mullany, *Short Communication Isolation of silver-and antibiotic-resistant Enterobacter cloacae from teeth.* Oral Microbiology and Immunology, 2005. **20**(3): p. 191.

329.    www.natural-immunogenics.com, *Natural-Immunogenics - Silver*

330.    www.pharma.com, *Purdue Pharma - Betadine*

331.    Galland, L., M.D., *Dysbiotic Relationships in the Bowel*, in *American College of Advancement in Medicine Conference.* Spring 1992.

332.    Mitsuoka, T., *Intestinal flora and aging.* Nutr Rev, 1992. **50**(12): p. 438-46.

333.    www.gdx.net, *Genova Diagnostics*

334.    Hunter, J.M., *Geophagy in Africa and in the United States: A Culture-Nutrition Hypothesis.* Geographical Review, 1973. **63**(2): p. 170-195.

335.    Shanahan, F., *Probiotics: Promise, Problems, and Progress.* Science. **1**(3): p. 6-8.

336.    www.humaworm.com, *HUMAWORM*

337.    Shoemaker, R.C., *Desperation Medicine.* 2001: Gateway Press.

338.    www.lymephotos.com, *lymephotos*

339.    Elliott, D.E., *Does the failure to acquire helminthic parasites predispose to Crohn's disease?* The FASEB Journal, 2000. **14**(12): p. 1848-1855.

340.    Potera, C., *Chemical Exposures: Cats as Sentinel Species.* Environmental Health Perspectives, 2007. **115**(12): p. A580.

341.    Berkenstam, A., et al., *The thyroid hormone mimetic compound KB2115 lowers plasma LDL cholesterol and stimulates bile acid synthesis without cardiac effects in humans.* Proceedings of the National Academy of Sciences, 2008. **105**(2): p. 663-667.

342.    www.cwtozone.com, *ClearWater Tech, LLC*

343.    Bryson, C., *The Fluoride Deception.* 2004: Seven Stories Press.

344.    Fagin, D., *Second Thoughts about Fluoride*, in *Scientific American.* 2008. p. 74-81.

345.    www.fluoridealert.org, *Fluoride Action Network*

346.    Abraham, G.E. and D. Brownstein, *Evidence that the administration of Vitamin C improves a defective cellular transport mechanism for iodine: A case report.* The Original Internist, 2005. **12**(3): p. 125-130.

347.    Specter, M., *Darwin's Surprise*, in *New Yorker*. January 3, 2008. p. 64-73.

348.    Mann, J., *Wipe Out Herpes With BHT*. 1983: MegaHealth Society.

349.    www.google.com/patents, *Google Patents*

350.    www.lessemf.com, *EMF Safety Superstore*

351.    www.earthfx.net, *Earth FX Bed Pads*

352.    www.familyconstellations.net, *John Payne - Family Constellations International*

353.    www.ulsamer.com, *Bertold Ulsamer*

354.    www.hellinger.com, *Bert Hellinger*

355.    www.essentialsolutions.info, *Family Constellations - Santa Barbara*

356.    www.emofree.com, *EFT Emotional Freedom Technique*

357.    Levine, P.A., *Waking the Tiger: Healing Trauma*. 1997: North Atlantic Books.

358.    www.traumahealing.com, *Trauma Healing*

359.    Bhatt, B.M., et al., *Suppression of Mixed Candida Biofilms with an Iodine Oral Rinse*. 2007.

360.    Waltimo, T.M., et al., *In vitro susceptibility of Candida albicans to four disinfectants and their combinations*. Int Endod J, 1999. **32**(6): p. 421-9.

361.    Janjua, N.R., et al., *Sunscreens in human plasma and urine after repeated whole-body topical application*. J Eur Acad Dermatol Venereol, 2008.

362.    www.naturesbodybeautiful.com, *Nature's Body Beautiful - Clay Cosmeceuticals*

363.    www.usa.weleda.com, *Weleda North America*

364.    www.purityfarms.com, *Purity Farms - Ghee*

365.    www.earthsbeauty.com, *Earth's Beauty Mineral Cosmetics*

366.    Hanson, K.M., E. Gratton, and C.J. Bardeen, *Sunscreen enhancement of UV-induced reactive oxygen species in the skin*. Free Radical Biology and Medicine, 2006. **41**(8): p. 1205-1212.

367.    Schlumpf, M., et al., *In Vitro and in Vivo Estrogenicity of UV Screens*. Environmental Health Perspectives, 2001. **109**(3): p. 239-244.

368.    Schmutzler, C., et al., *The Ultraviolet Filter Benzophenone 2 Interferes with the Thyroid Hormone Axis in Rats and Is a Potent in Vitro Inhibitor of Human Recombinant Thyroid Peroxidase*. Endocrinology, 2007. **148**(6): p. 2835.

369.		D'Orazio, J.A., et al., *Topical drug rescue strategy and skin protection based on the role of Mc1r in UV-induced tanning.* Nature, 2006. **443**(7109): p. 340-4.

370.		Wickelgren, I., *SKIN BIOLOGY: A Healthy Tan?* Science, 2007. **315**(5816): p. 1214.

371.		www.uvnaturalusa.com, *UV Natural Sunscreen*

372.		www.goodmanmfg.com, *Goodman Manufacturing Co. - Amana*

373.		Luke, J., *Fluoride Deposition in the Aged Human Pineal Gland.* Caries Research, 2001. **35**: p. 125-128.

374.		Sasseville, A., et al., *Blue blocker glasses impede the capacity of bright light to suppress melatonin production.* Journal of Pineal Research, 2006. **41**(1): p. 73-78.

375.		www.lowbluelights.com, *Photonic Developments - Low Blue Lights*

376.		www.saramednick.com, *Take a nap!*

377.		www.activator.com, *Chiropractic Activator Methods*

378.		Lassek, W., Gaulin, SJ., *Waist-hip ratio and cognitive ability: is gluteofemoral fat a privileged store of neurodevelopmental resources?* . Evol Hum Behav., 2008. **Vol. 29**(Issue 1): p. 26-34.

379.		Diamond, J., *Why is sex fun?* 1997: Basic Books.

380.		www.traponline.com, *The Rhythmic Arts Project*

381.		Douglass, W., *Stop Aging or Slow the Process: How Exercise with Oxygen Therapy (EWOT) Can Help.* 2003, Rhino Publishing.

# INDEX

LaVergne, TN USA
13 January 2010
169823LV00001B/15/P